Building Bridges: A European Perspective on Interprofessional Education, Practice, Policy and Research

Andreas Xyrichis • Maria Kvarnström
Marion Huber • Cornelia Mahler
Editors

Building Bridges: A European Perspective on Interprofessional Education, Practice, Policy and Research

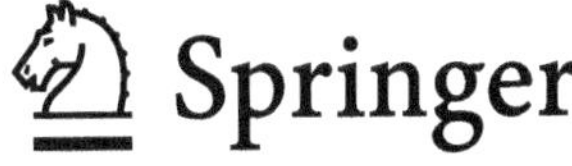

Editors
Andreas Xyrichis
Faculty Nursing, Midwifery,
and Palliative Care
King's College London
London, UK

Marion Huber
Center of Interprofessional Learning
and Practice, Institute of Public Health
at the Department of Health Sciences,
Zurich University of Applied Sciences
Zurich, Switzerland

Maria Kvarnström
Health, Medicine and Caring Sciences
Linköping University
Linköping, Sweden

Cornelia Mahler
Nursing Science
University of Tübingen
Tübingen, Germany

ISBN 978-3-032-23221-2 ISBN 978-3-032-23222-9 (eBook)
https://doi.org/10.1007/978-3-032-23222-9

This Springer imprint is published by the registered company Springer Nature Switzerland AG
The registered company address is: Gewerbestrasse 11, 6330 Cham, Switzerland

Foreword

Health workforce pressures across Europe are now widely recognised as structural and persistent. The October 2025 report of the European Parliament's Committee on Employment and Social Affairs calling for a European Union (EU) Health Workforce Crisis Plan reflects this recognition [1]. The Plan brings renewed parliamentary and political attention to shortages, retention failures, uneven distribution, evolving skill requirements, and an anticipated reliance on productivity gains through service redesign and digital/AI transformation.

While the Plan addresses education, training, workforce optimisation, and new models of care—rooted in a *productivist* economic framing—it also reveals a critical underlying assumption: that health professionals can work together effectively across occupational boundaries. This assumption has significant implications. Interprofessional collaboration is no longer framed as an aspirational ideal but as a prerequisite for health systems resilience, workforce efficiencies, and sustainability. Yet the Draft Plan, like many contemporary policy instruments, tends to treat collaboration as an outcome of structural reform rather than as a *human capability* and *human economy* outcome that must be deliberately cultivated, embedded, and sustained to allow interdisciplinary teams to *be*, *do*, and *flourish*.

It is against this backdrop that this most timely compilation of evidence, insights, and policy options should be read. While the academic research and analysis is distinct from the parliamentary discourse in Brussels and other European capitals, the editors and authors address the foundational question on which European policy ambitions will increasingly depend, namely, how health professionals are prepared, incentivised, and supported for interprofessional collaborative practice.

Despite decades of research and advocacy on *interprofessional education and collaborative practice*—including my personal championing for it as the World Health Organization's (WHO) Director for Health Workforce—the global implementation remains uneven. Many of the strongest examples we read in the literature, or which are showcased at international conferences, can be traced to the commitment of individual Deans, Professors, or clinical champions who believe deeply in the value of collaboration. To all those individuals let me extend my professional appreciation. However, while these initiatives demonstrate what is possible, they also expose an underlying structural fragility: interprofessional practice is too often reliant on personal leadership rather than embedded as institutional and system-level expectations.

The most striking contribution of this volume lies in moving beyond individual exemplars towards a more coherent and durable understanding of interprofessional education and practice. Chapter "Bridging Interprofessional Education, Practice, Research, and Policy: Towards an Interprofessional Science" situates this work within the European context and introduces the concept of *interprofessional science* as a unifying framework linking education, practice, research, and policy. The subsequent chapters extend this analysis through practice-based perspectives drawn from across much, though not all, of Europe.

Read in the context of the motion for a European Parliament [1] Resolution on an EU Health Workforce Crisis Plan, this book offers scholarly evidence and conclusions to support the transition to the systemic implementation of interprofessional education and collaborative practice. In doing so, it offers options to build the bridge between emerging workforce policy assumptions and the educational and professional infrastructures required to make collaboration routine, safe, and sustainable.

King's College London; Former Director,
Health Workforce, World Health Organization
London, UK

Jim Campbell

Reference

1. European Parliament. An EU health workforce crisis plan: sustainability of healthcare systems and employment and working conditions in the healthcare sector. (Procedure 2025/2062(INI)). European Parliament. 2025. Retrieved from https://oeil.europarl.europa.eu/oeil/en/procedure-file?reference=2025/2062(INI)

Contents

Bridging Interprofessional Education, Practice, Research, and Policy: Towards an Interprofessional Science

Andreas Xyrichis, Cornelia Mahler, Maria Kvarnström, and Marion Huber

Introduction

With this chapter, we, the Editors, seek to situate the book within the existing scholarship on interprofessional education and collaborative practice (IPECP), with a particular focus on the European context. In doing so, we aim to draw the conceptual linkages that will guide the analyses in the chapters that follow.

It is widely acknowledged that the complexity of modern healthcare systems poses significant challenges to the delivery of safe, high-quality, patient- and family-centred care [8, 9, 14, 16] . Health service users often present with multifaceted needs that require the coordinated expertise of diverse health and social care professionals. However, the traditional siloed organisation of healthcare and educational systems can hinder effective interprofessional collaboration, putting patient outcomes at risk [7, 17]. This underscores the critical importance of

A. Xyrichis (✉)
Faculty of Nursing, Midwifery, and Palliative Care, King's College London, London, UK
e-mail: andreas.xyrichis@kcl.ac.uk

C. Mahler
Department of Nursing Science, Institute of Health Sciences, University of Tübingen, Tübingen, Baden-Württemberg, Germany
e-mail: cornelia.mahler@med.uni-tuebingen.de

M. Kvarnström
Department of Health, Medicine and Caring Sciences, Division of Society and Health, Linköping University, Östergötland, Sweden
e-mail: maria.kvarnstrom@liu.se

M. Huber
Center of Interprofessional Learning and Practice, Institute of Public Health at the Department of Health Sciences, Zurich University of Applied Sciences, Zurich, Switzerland
e-mail: marion.huber@zhaw.ch

A. Xyrichis et al. (eds.), *Building Bridges: A European Perspective on Interprofessional Education, Practice, Policy and Research*,
https://doi.org/10.1007/978-3-032-23222-9_1

cultivating a culture of collaboration and communication across professional boundaries. Fostering such a culture is essential for enabling health and social care professionals to work together effectively, share knowledge and expertise, and provide integrated, comprehensive care centred on the needs of patients and families [10, 14]. By breaking down professional silos and facilitating cross-professional dialogue and collaboration, organisations can empower their workforce to deliver the highest standards of integrated, person-centred care.

While the necessity of interprofessional collaboration is well-established, the pathways to achieving it are not always clear. Interprofessional education (IPE) is our most powerful intervention to socially engineer the future health workforce necessary for collaborative practice. IPE offers learners opportunities to develop the knowledge, skills, and attitudes required for effective interprofessional working [11]. Yet all too often, IPE has been implemented as a peripheral add-on, rather than being fully integrated into core health professions curricula [12]. This structural marginalisation reflects the broader gaps that exist between the realms of research, practice, education, and policy in the field of IPECP.

These disconnected silos highlight the pressing need for conceptual linkages that can bridge divides and foster a more cohesive, systems-level approach. It is in this context that we adopt the concept of "interprofessional science" as a unifying framework [18]. Interprofessional science encompasses the scholarly inquiry, evidence-base, and theoretical foundations required to advance IPECP, while also attending to the complex system-level factors that shape its implementation and impact. It is defined as the "scientific field of study devoted to advancing pedagogies, applied processes and research methods to promote uptake and evaluation of interprofessional collaborative approaches in health and social care education, practice and research; contributing to patient-centred, quality, safe, sustainable and resilient health systems" [18: 1].

By bringing together teachers, researchers, and clinical practitioners from across Europe, this book aims to collaboratively explore the state of IPECP in the European setting. Through this collaborative endeavour, the Editors wish to situate the book as a significant contribution to the scholarly discourse and to chart a path forward for advancing IPECP in the European region. Recognising the diversity of healthcare systems, educational models, and professional traditions within the European context, the book examines both the common challenges and unique considerations that shape the IPECP landscape across the continent. Ultimately, we aspire for this book to catalyse the establishment of enduring networks and collaborations that extend far beyond its pages, galvanising the European IPECP community towards a more integrated, evidence-informed, and impactful future.

The European Context

Mapping the context is, as always, crucial for discussing issues related to higher education and healthcare. We aim to view Europe as a whole, recognising that while there are certain similarities, there are also distinct differences within Europe. The current European landscape reflects a complex interplay of supranational directives, national implementations, and institutional innovations that collectively shape the advancement of IPECP across the continent.

Foundational Frameworks Driving European IPECP Development

The World Health Organization's "Framework for Action on Interprofessional Education and Collaborative Practice" [14] as well as the Lancet Report on "Health professionals for a new century: transforming education to strengthen health systems in an interdependent world" [7], while having a global focus, helped establish the definitional foundation for European initiatives, identifying IPE as occurring "when students from two or more professions learn about, from and with each other to enable effective collaboration and improve health outcomes" [14]. This framework has been substantially reinforced by WHO Europe's Framework for Action on the Health and Care Workforce 2023–2030, which explicitly identifies interprofessional collaboration competencies as essential for future healthcare workers [15].

The Bucharest Declaration on Health and Care Workforce (2023), unanimously adopted by representatives from 50 of 53 WHO European Region member states, operationalises these principles through five strategic pillars emphasising workforce retention, supply building, performance optimisation, strategic planning, and investment [15]. This European-specific adaptation demonstrates the region's commitment to systematic IPECP integration whilst acknowledging diverse national healthcare contexts.

The Winterthur-Doha Declaration (2023) has further advanced European IPECP discourse by explicitly calling for "task shifting" towards interprofessional collaborative practice as the norm rather than the exception. Developed through Swiss leadership at the Winterthur Interprofessional.Global Symposium, this declaration emphasises and exemplifies COVID-19 pandemic experiences as demonstrating the critical importance of interprofessional collaboration-ready teams, whilst specifically addressing European regulatory frameworks requiring IPE as part of accreditation standards [1].

European Regulatory Architecture Shaping IPECP Implementation

European Union regulatory frameworks create both facilitators and barriers for IPECP advancement. For example, the Bologna Process, encompassing 49 countries of the European Higher Education Area, provides foundational mechanisms through its three-cycle degree structure, the European Credit Transfer and Accumulation System, and quality assurance mechanisms [2]. Enhanced student mobility facilitated by ECTS credits could be leveraged to enable health profession student exposure to diverse healthcare systems, and collaborative practices. Moreover, the development of a common, standardised competency framework for

IPE could support interprofessional competency development across healthcare programmes in Europe [4].

However, systematic review evidence from 32 studies across 14 EHEA countries reveals significant implementation challenges [3]. Most IPE interventions in Europe appear to lack robust theoretical frameworks, with 25 of 32 studies included in that review reporting no theoretical background, and many programmes involving only two professions. This suggests substantial implementation gaps, despite the opportunities for interprofessional integration presented by the Bologna Process.

Fundamentally, Directive 2005/36/EC on recognition of professional qualifications, as amended by Directive 2013/55/EU, establishes the legal basis for automatic recognition mechanisms for seven professions, including doctors, nurses, dentists, pharmacists, and midwives. Whilst this framework facilitates professional mobility through harmonised minimum training requirements and the European Professional Card system, it primarily focuses on individual professional qualifications rather than interprofessional competencies. Although aspects of collaborative working, such as communication and teamwork, are included in the minimum training requirements and curricula, specific mention of IPE is absent, representing a missed opportunity for IPECP integration [5].

Task Shifting as a European Policy Driver

Task shifting has emerged as a key policy instrument within the broader policy discourse aimed at optimising, rather than simply ensuring, the sustainability of the health workforce in Europe. It serves both as a policy discussion tool and as a mechanism to foster dialogue on IPECP.

The European Commission's Expert Panel on Effective Ways of Investing in Health report on task shifting (2019) provides a crucial policy foundation for IPECP advancement by defining task shifting as "the rational assignment of tasks currently undertaken by the health workforce" [5]. The report emphasises that traditional role divisions in European health systems are based on "custom and practice rather than evidence," highlighting opportunities for evidence-based redistribution of tasks across health professions.

This policy framework identifies three types of task shifting relevant to IPECP: enhancement of existing professional roles, substitution or delegation of tasks between professional groups, and innovation through entirely new care delivery approaches. The report explicitly recognises the need to challenge outdated legislative and regulatory barriers across European countries whilst emphasising robust evidence requirements for role changes.

In that vein, IPE is discussed as essential—not optional—to equip health professionals for new roles and ways of working. The report states that changes in traditional professional boundaries "must be supported in implementing it," which entails embedding structured, interprofessional learning opportunities during training to build shared competencies and mutual understanding. It argues that task shifting, where deemed necessary, must be "evidence-based," with professionals' "participation ... supported by appropriate training," affirming that IPE underpins safe, effective, and sustainable transformations in workforce roles.

Not only is task shifting a policy driver, but it is also a driver for the dynamic changes within the health professions themselves, leading to new professions and qualifications emerging within health care systems. These changes underline the need to equip all health professionals with the necessary interprofessional competencies to work together collaboratively to ensure safe and person-centred care. At the same time, this shift also offers a wide field for research activities to answer questions addressing health care provision [13].

Workforce Demographics and Mobility Patterns Informing IPECP Development in Europe

Eurostat data reveals significant workforce composition and mobility patterns affecting IPECP implementation across Europe. The European health workforce comprises over 8 million professionals, including approximately 1.8 million physicians and 4.1 million nursing professionals in the EU-27 countries [6]. Foreign-trained healthcare professionals—that is, those trained in a different European country from where they currently practise—make up between 5% and 25% of the workforce, demonstrating significant intra-European professional mobility [6].

Migration patterns within the EU predominantly demonstrate an East-West and South-North movement, with emigration countries including Romania, Slovakia, Spain, Lithuania, Latvia, Portugal, Bulgaria, Greece, Croatia, Hungary, Italy, and Slovenia. In contrast, Luxembourg, Ireland, Malta, and Sweden serve as primary destination countries. This mobility pattern creates both opportunities for interprofessional experience diversity and challenges for maintaining collaborative practice continuity.

Eurostat [6] figures highlight marked disparities in physician availability across Europe. Greece reports the highest density, with approximately 632 physicians per 100,000 inhabitants, whereas Poland registers one of the lowest at around 233 per 100,000. Nursing workforce densities also vary significantly. In 2018, countries like Germany, Denmark, the Netherlands, and Slovenia had more than 1000 nurses per 100,000 inhabitants, while Bulgaria, Greece, Spain, Italy, Cyprus, and Latvia fell below 500 per 100,000. Eurostat further reports that nine EU Member States—many from southern and eastern Europe—experienced net reductions in practising nurses between 2012 and 2017, which are expected to worsen.

These disparities suggest substantially different contexts for IPECP implementation capacity across European healthcare systems and highlight the importance of locally adapted and targeted policy interventions.

Future Skills and Digital Transformation

The OECD Future of Education and Skills 2030 framework provides interesting implications for IPECP evolution through its Learning Framework 2030 and transformative competencies model. The framework identifies three core transformative competencies particularly relevant to healthcare, to which IPECP can contribute: creating new value through innovation and entrepreneurial thinking, reconciling tensions and dilemmas through ethical decision-making, and taking responsibility through agency and sustainability mindset.

The OECD framework's emphasis on student agency, co-agency between learners and educators, and anticipation-action-reflection cycles aligns closely with interprofessional practice requirements for collaborative decision-making and continuous learning adaptation. The integration of cognitive skills (critical thinking, problem-solving), social-emotional skills (empathy, collaboration, communication), technical skills (digital literacy, AI awareness), and values (ethics, responsibility, global citizenship) can provide a comprehensive foundation for twenty-first-century healthcare professional development grounded in IPECP.

Moving forward, digital competencies become critical elements for future IPECP implementation, with WHO Europe's 2023 Framework specifically identifying "*the ability to use digital health tools, including artificial intelligence, to work in interprofessional teams*" as essential future competencies.

European IPECP Networks

In Europe, there are several regional networks which in different ways promote the concept of interprofessional learning and collaborative practice, and there are connections between the networks to collaborate in spreading the word and promoting each other´s conferences, etc. In addition to these regional networks, there are a number of national networks which are not presented here. Often, the national networks are part of a regional network. Examples of regional networks are presented in Table 1.

Table 1 Examples of regional interprofessional education networks

Network	Website	Countries	Established	Membership	Description	Conferences
CAIPE (Centre for the Advancement of Interprofessional Education)	www.caipe.org	United Kingdom	1987	Open to individuals and organisations	United Kingdom-based organisation, with international activity and profile, promoting interprofessional education through research, policy, and practice development	Annual conferences and events
EIPEN (European Interprofessional Practice & Education Network)	www.eipen.eu	8 European countries	2010	Institutional members from European countries	Network promoting interprofessional education and collaborative practice across some European institutions	Biannual conferences
IP-Health (Interprofessional Health Network of German-Speaking Countries)	www.ip-health.org	Germany, Austria, Switzerland	2015	Open to organisations from German-speaking countries	Platform for sharing research, experiences, and projects in interprofessional education and collaborative practice	Annual conferences and workshops
IPINN (Interprofessional Network of Dutch-Speaking Countries)	www.ipinn.org	Netherlands, Belgium, Aruba, Curaçao, Sint Maarten, Suriname	2012	Open to organisations from Dutch-speaking regions	Collaborative network promoting interprofessional education and collaborative practice across Dutch-speaking countries and territories	Biannual conferences
NIPNET (Nordic Interprofessional Network)	nipnet.org	Denmark, Finland, Iceland, Norway, Sweden	2001	No formal membership; open platform	Platform for sharing research, experiences, and projects to promote interprofessional education and collaborative practice across Nordic countries	Biannual conferences rotating between countries

Discussion

While the value of IPECP appears well-established in Europe, at least within academia and to some extent policy, a comprehensive understanding of the state of adoption and implementation across Europe remains elusive. Gaps persist in mapping the European landscape, leaving policymakers, educators, and researchers without a clear shared baseline. A Europe-wide assessment of the progress and challenges in embedding IPE within health and social care curricula is sorely needed. The chapters that follow offer a path forward in this direction.

The convergence of workforce mobility data, future skills frameworks, and policy imperatives suggests that European IPECP development is approaching a critical juncture. The COVID-19 pandemic experience, reflected in the Bucharest Declaration and recent WHO Europe frameworks, has demonstrated both the necessity and feasibility of interprofessional collaboration at scale. Success in advancing European IPECP will require coordinated action to align regulatory frameworks, integrate interprofessional competencies into professional qualification standards, and develop systematic approaches to implementation and evaluation that acknowledge the diversity of European healthcare systems whilst promoting collaborative practice as the norm rather than the exception.

It is evident that the field lacks a cohesive European perspective on the core interprofessional competencies required for collaborative practice. Diverse national and regional approaches to defining and assessing these competencies hinder the development of a shared framework. Examining how such competencies are currently integrated, or not, into educational programs across the continent would shed valuable light on the state of IPE implementation.

Beyond curricular considerations, the unique contextual factors shaping IPECP in Europe also warrant closer examination. Differences in healthcare systems, professional training traditions, workforce mobility, and higher education structures pose distinct challenges that are not always captured in the broader international literature. Mapping these European-specific barriers and enablers is crucial for developing tailored, contextually relevant strategies for advancing IPECP.

Parallel to these educational and practice-focused gaps, the landscape of interprofessional research across Europe remains fragmented. A coordinated effort to synthesise the existing European evidence base, identify research priorities, and foster cross-border collaborations could significantly strengthen the scholarly foundations of this field. Similarly, a comprehensive mapping of policies and regulations pertaining to interprofessional working would provide valuable insights to guide policy development and implementation.

Underlying all of these gaps, we posit, is a pervasive issue of siloed thinking and fragmented action. While IPECP is widely espoused as a necessity, the reality on the ground reflects persistent divides between the realms of education, practice, research, and policy. Bridging these divides and cultivating a more cohesive, systems-level approach to advancing IPECP in Europe emerges as a critical priority.

Critical Gaps

Our analysis reveals several interconnected gaps that hinder progress in European IPECP development. The absence of coherent conceptual frameworks represents perhaps the most significant challenge, as it prevents the establishment of common ground between education, practice, research, and policy domains. Without overarching frameworks that can bridge these divides, efforts remain fragmented and potentially contradictory, limiting the cumulative impact of individual initiatives.

The limited Europe-wide understanding of IPECP implementation and interprofessional practice creates additional barriers to progress. Whilst some countries may have developed sophisticated approaches to IPECP, the absence of comprehensive, continent-wide assessments prevents the identification of common challenges and the development of tailored solutions that could benefit the broader European community. This gap is compounded by insufficient local-level insights, which limit our understanding of what is needed to improve interprofessional practice within the diverse national and regional contexts that characterise European healthcare systems.

The challenges in overcoming these gaps are multifaceted and deeply rooted in structural limitations. The absence of coordinating mechanisms at the European level means that valuable experiences, innovations, and lessons learned often remain confined within national boundaries. Without a dedicated mechanism to facilitate cross-border dialogue and collaboration, the European IPECP community cannot leverage its collective expertise effectively.

Furthermore, the lack of focused academic work specifically examining IPECP within the European context represents a significant scholarly gap. Whilst global literature on interprofessionalism continues to expand, the unique characteristics, challenges, and opportunities within European healthcare systems require dedicated academic attention. This scholarly deficit limits our ability to develop contextually appropriate solutions and evidence-based recommendations for European IPECP advancement.

Policy direction remains another critical challenge, with clearer frameworks and initiatives needed to enhance workforce mobility, cross-border healthcare delivery, and formal interprofessional collaborations. The complexity of European healthcare systems, combined with varying regulatory frameworks and professional standards, creates barriers that require coordinated policy responses.

Interprofessional science, through the concerted efforts of health professions, educational institutions, and research communities, offers a pathway to bridge these identified gaps. The development of closer collaboration among European health profession representatives, educators, researchers, and policymakers will be crucial in creating a shared vision and implementing a practical roadmap for advancing IPECP across the continent. This collaborative approach must be sustained, systematic, and sensitive to the diverse contexts that characterise European healthcare whilst maintaining focus on the common goals that unite the interprofessional community.

Conclusion

This chapter sought to explore the persistent gaps between education, practice, research, and policy on IPECP across Europe. Through the earlier discussion of similarities, differences, and developments within the European context, we have identified some critical blind spots that impede the advancement of IPECP. These insights form the foundation for our recommendations, which centre on fostering coordinated action and developing shared frameworks to strengthen IPECP throughout the European continent.

First, the European IPECP landscape requires a fundamental shift towards coordinated work at the European level. Progress in IPECP cannot be achieved through isolated national efforts or fragmented professional initiatives. Instead, a collaborative approach that transcends borders, professional boundaries, and sectoral divisions is essential. This coordinated effort could manifest through the establishment of a European mechanism or platform designed to bring together diverse stakeholders from education, practice, research, and policy domains. Such a platform would provide the necessary infrastructure for joint problem-solving, resource sharing, and strategic alignment across the complex IPECP ecosystem.

Second, a systematic charting of IPECP initiatives, frameworks, and evidence across Europe would help address the lack of continent-wide understanding. This inventory could inform the development of tailored solutions, facilitate knowledge exchange, and enable the identification of best practices adaptable to diverse national and regional contexts.

Third, we propose the development of a comprehensive European roadmap for advancing interprofessional science. This roadmap would serve as a strategic guide for the European IPECP community, outlining shared priorities whilst respecting national and regional variations in healthcare systems and educational approaches. The roadmap should align strategies across countries and sectors, foster meaningful cross-border collaborations, and strengthen the conceptual foundations that underpin IPECP implementation. Through this coordinated approach, the European community can develop a more robust evidence base and create sustainable pathways for interprofessional advancement.

Realising the vision of an integrated, evidence-informed, and impactful IPECP landscape across Europe will require dedicated funding and policy directives at the European level. Such support would help catalyse the advancement of IPECP, enabling the creation of joint educational programmes, research initiatives, and interprofessional practice models that transcend geographical boundaries. By providing the necessary resources and institutional backing, the European community can empower IPECP stakeholders to bridge divides, develop shared frameworks, and implement tailored, context-sensitive strategies for cultivating a culture of collaborative practice. Through this coordinated, systems-level approach, the European IPECP community can unlock the full potential of interprofessional science, positioning it as a transformative force for delivering high-quality, patient-centred care throughout the continent.

Reflective Questions

- What does IPECP mean for you and your context?
- How do you experience IPECP where you live and work?
- What do you see as the IPECP gaps in your country?
- In what way are the issues raised in this chapter relevant/specific to your setting/country?

References

1. Babiker A, El Husseini M, Al Nemri A, Al Frayh A, Al Juryyan N, Faki MO, Assiri A, Al Saadi M, Shaikh F, Al Zamil F. Interprofessional collaboration in complex patient care transition: a qualitative multi-perspective analysis. Healthcare. 2023;11(3):359. https://doi.org/10.3390/healthcare11030359.
2. Bologna Declaration. The European Higher Education Area: joint declaration of the European ministers of education. Bologna, Italy; 1999.
3. Colonnello V, Kinoshita Y, Yoshida N, Bustos Villalobos I. Undergraduate interprofessional education in the European Higher Education Area: A systematic review. International Medical Education, 2023;2(2):100–112. https://doi.org/10.3390/ime2020010.
4. European Commission/EACEA/Eurydice. The European Higher Education Area in 2020: Bologna Process Implementation Report. Publications Office of the European Union. 2020.
5. European Commission. Digital health and care in the EU: building a healthier future for all. Publications Office of the European Union; 2021.
6. Eurostat. Healthcare personnel statistics. European Commission 2022. https://ec.europa.eu/eurostat/databrowser/view/hlth_rs_prs2/default/table?lang=en.
7. Frenk J, Chen L, Bhutta ZA, Cohen J, Crisp N, Evans T, Fineberg H, Garcia P, Ke Y, Kelley P, Kistnasamy B, Meleis A, Naylor D, Pablos-Mendez A, Reddy S, Scrimshaw S, Sepulveda J, Serwadda D, Zurayk H. Health professionals for a new century: transforming education to strengthen health systems in an interdependent world. The Lancet. 2010;376(9756):1923–58. https://doi.org/10.1016/S0140-6736(10)61854-5.
8. Institute of Medicine. To err is human: building a safer health system. National Academies Press; 2000.
9. Institute of Medicine. Crossing the quality chasm: A new health system for the 21st century. National Academies Press 2001. https://doi.org/10.17226/10027.
10. Institute of Medicine. Health professions education: a bridge to quality. National Academies Press; 2003.
11. Interprofessional Education Collaborative. IPEC core competencies for interprofessional collaborative practice: Version 3. Interprofessional Education Collaborative; 2023.
12. Thistlethwaite J, Forman D, Matthews LR, Rogers GD, Steketee C, Yassine T. Competencies and frameworks in interprofessional education: a comparative analysis. Acad Med. 2014;89(6):869–75. https://doi.org/10.1097/ACM.0000000000000249.
13. Ullrich C, Mahler C, Stengel S, Wensing M. Dynamic landscapes of health professions. In: Wensing M, Ullrich C, editors. Foundations of health services research: principles, methods, and topics. Springer; 2023. p. 235–47. https://doi.org/10.1007/978-3-031-29998-8.
14. World Health Organization. Framework for action on interprofessional education and collaborative practice. World Health Organization; 2010.
15. World Health Organization Regional Office for Europe. Framework for action on the health and care workforce in the WHO European Region 2023–2030. WHO Regional Office for Europe 2023. https://iris.who.int/handle/10665/372563.

16. World Health Organization. WHO global report on patient safety. World Health Organization; 2024.
17. World Health Professions Alliance. WHPA statement on interprofessional collaborative practice. World Health Professions Alliance; 2025.
18. Xyrichis A. Interprofessional science: an international field of study reaching maturity. J Interprof Care. 2020;34(1):1–3. https://doi.org/10.1080/13561820.2020.1707954.

Dr. Andreas Xyrichis is a Reader in Interprofessional Science at the Florence Nightingale Faculty of Nursing, Midwifery and Palliative Care, King's College London. An intensive care nurse by background, he researches interprofessional practice-based interventions for quality, safety, and equity, working with collaborators across and beyond Europe. Andreas is a Trustee of the UK Centre for the Advancement of Interprofessional Education (CAIPE), co-founder of the European Academy for Interprofessional Science, and Editor-in-Chief of the Journal of Interprofessional Care, the leading international journal in interprofessional science.

Prof. Dr. Cornelia Mahler is the director of the Department of Nursing Science at the Medical Faculty, Eberhard Karls University, Tuebingen, Germany, and dean of studies of the bachelor nursing programme. In 2011, she developed and implemented a bachelor degree in Interprofessional Health Care at the Medical Faculty, University of Heidelberg, Germany, and led the development of interprofessional education and research there. She co-founded and co-led the interprofessional working group within the German Association for Medical Education and has extensive experience in the translation and validation of instruments for research and evaluation in IPE and IPC. She is a nurse by background, co-founder of the European Academy for Interprofessional Science, and serves as an Associate Editor for the Journal of Interprofessional Care.

Dr. Maria Kvarnström is an Associate Professor in Medical Education at the Department of Health, Medicine and Caring Sciences at Linköping University which has the longest European tradition of interprofessional education at a faculty of medicine. She is a member of the strategic area for interprofessional learning and collaboration at the medical faculty at Linköping University, a member of the board of the Nordic Interprofessional network, and co-founder of the Swedish network for IPE. She is a biomedical laboratory scientist by profession, an Associate Editor for the Journal of Interprofessional Care, and a co-founder of the European Academy for Interprofessional Science.

Prof. Dr. Marion Huber is the Head of the Center of Interprofessional Learning and Practice at the Zurich University of Applied Sciences, Department Health Sciences, and leads the research group of interprofessionalism. She is a qualified physiotherapist, psychologis, and neuroscientist and is responsible for the evaluation of the Zurich interprofessional clinical training wards—ZIPAS. She is a co-founder of the European Academy for Interprofessional Science, the Chair of Interprofessional.Global (IP.G)—the Global Confederation for Interprofessional Education and Collaborative Practice—and the Chair of the International Society of Interprofessional Health Care (IP-Health).

Exploring European IPECP Frameworks: A Comprehensive Overview and Analysis

Matthias J. Witti, Bettina Heinzelmann, Claudia De Weerdt, Ingrid Aerts, Hugh Barr, Marion Huber, and Doreen Herinek

Matthias J. Witti and Bettina Heinzelmann contributed equally to this work.

M. J. Witti (✉)
Institute of Medical Education, LMU University Hospital, LMU Munich, Munich, Germany
e-mail: Matthias.Witti@med.uni-muenchen.de

B. Heinzelmann
Institut für Gesundheitsforschung und Bildung (IGB), Universität Osnabrück, Osnabrück, Germany
e-mail: bheinzelmann@uni-osnabrueck.de

C. De Weerdt · I. Aerts
Department of Health and Sciences, Nutrition and Dietetics Program, AP University of Applied Sciences and Arts, Antwerp, Belgium
e-mail: claudia.deweerdt@ap.be; ingrid.aerts@ap.be

H. Barr (Deceased)
University of Westminster, Westminster, UK

M. Huber
Center of Interprofessional Learning and Practice, Institute of Public Health at the Department of Health Sciences, Zurich University of Applied Sciences, Zurich, Switzerland
e-mail: marion.huber@zhaw.ch

D. Herinek
Charité – Universitätsmedizin, Corporate member of Freie Universität Berlin and Humboldt-Universität zu Berlin, Institute of Health and Nursing Science, Berlin, Germany
e-mail: doreen.herinek@charite.de

A. Xyrichis et al. (eds.), *Building Bridges: A European Perspective on Interprofessional Education, Practice, Policy and Research*,
https://doi.org/10.1007/978-3-032-23222-9_2

Introduction

> Prior exposure to interprofessional education is essential for anyone aspiring to work collaboratively across professions (cf. Ewers and Schaeffer [17] p. 55).

This quote highlights the significance of interprofessional education (IPE) as a prerequisite for successful interprofessional collaborative practice (IPCP). Research suggests that IPCP leads to enhanced patient outcomes (e.g. [10, 32]) and increased job satisfaction among healthcare professionals (e.g. [28, 30]). Merely sharing educational experiences is insufficient. Instead, similarities and disparities among professions must inform curricula, learning methods, and assessment criteria. In doing so, students and their teachers will be able to relate interprofessional outcomes to the professional programmes in which they are embedded. Only then can the professions foster a genuine value for both shared commonalities and unique contributions that each brings to practice. This chapter focuses on European frameworks developed to facilitate interprofessional education and collaborative practice (IPECP), considering and comparing their practicality, applicability, intended audiences, objectives, and methodological foundations.

Several frameworks have been developed worldwide to facilitate IPECP by providing different sets of defined competencies to be acquired. These competencies cover, for example, (1) role clarity and responsibilities, (2) interprofessional communication, (3) skills in terms of ethics and values, and (4) teamwork, leadership, and conflict resolution [42].

The WHO "Framework for Action on Interprofessional Education & Collaborative Practice" [49], published in 2010, can also be seen as an important cornerstone for the promotion of IPECP in the European scientific discourse. Based on the assumption that individual interprofessional competencies lead to optimised collaboration and thus to improved healthcare practice, many European institutions have since introduced competency frameworks. In the last 20 years, organisations from the Anglo-Saxon world (USA, Canada, Australia, New Zealand, UK) have become increasingly committed to promoting IPECP. Nevertheless, the movements have also arrived in Europe nowadays and are leading to the IPECP receiving more attention.

In the meantime, various frameworks have been developed in the European region that deal with the question of acquiring interprofessional competencies in education and practice, and which are used as the basis for the respective implementation of IPECP. In this chapter, we describe these frameworks in detail by identifying their similarities and differences. We start by highlighting their historical "origins", impact, and effects. Then, we present seven frameworks and subject them to a comparative analysis, e.g. in terms of content, structure, addressed domains, as well as teaching and learning outcomes. We aim to elaborate on the relevant and trend-setting aspects of the identified frameworks, specifically for the European region. In conclusion, we examine the potential for implementing and adapting these frameworks within the context of curricular and formal requirements.

Background

> Theories are nets cast to catch what we call 'the world': to rationalize, to explain, and to master it. We endeavour to make the mesh ever finer and finer. (Popper [36], p. 59)

We will first differentiate between theories, models, and frameworks to clarify the terminology. While these terms are occasionally used interchangeably, each holds a distinct meaning. To help the reader discern between the different terms within the context of frameworks and to elucidate the conceptual foundation upon which this discussion rests, we will first provide a brief overview of the significance of each term.

Theories are generally understood to be empirically or theoretically derived systematic statements about certain relationships that aim to describe, explain, predict, and—under certain circumstances—control a phenomenon or group of phenomena [4]. Theories are based on empirical evidence and are filled, developed, and tested through research. The product of theories are constructs that are causally related. They therefore serve as a basis for understanding interrelationships in a field of study. In this way, a theoretical reference helps explain the complex and extensive differences between the different cultures and organisations in the healthcare system. Regarding IPECP, organisational structures and cultures, as well as human interactions in an interprofessional context, are the scientific-theoretical starting points. Theories help explain the multifaceted dimensions of IPECP and can thereby generate a framework for understanding [38].

A *model*, on the other hand, can be useful for theorising. In this process, illuminated objects are placed in relation to each other against the background of theoretical references and analysed or modified/adapted within the framework of research activities [13]. It is important to note that a model represents a situation, and as such, it inherently does not encompass all facets of reality. It is also characterised by a function aiming at fulfilling a purpose [40]. Accordingly, it is a simplified representation of complex processes or systems. Whether conceptual, physical, mathematical, or visual in nature [8], a model can be an invaluable asset for both the practical application of theory and the empirical testing of hypotheses. For example, the "Leicester Model of Interprofessional Education" [3] was developed to train health and social care professionals to work together. Central to this model is the assumption that effective interprofessional collaboration is essential for delivering high-quality patient care. The model encourages learning from, with and about other professions to improve communication, teamwork and understanding of different roles within a health and social care team. Its overarching goal is to break down barriers between professional groups, strengthen collaboration amongst them, and improve the overall quality of care. The Leicester Model focuses on practical experience, reflection, and exchange between participants to promote a deep understanding of the values and skills required for effective interprofessional practice [3].

Frameworks are often based on different foundations such as theories, concepts, and/or empirical data. They thus provide a theoretical base of varying quality, integrating ontological, epistemological, and methodological assumptions [25]. In this context, they provide the content and methodological basis for IPE and interprofessional training.

They legitimise decisions by describing competency profiles for different domains, including knowledge, skills, values/attitudes, and—in some cases—provide indications of intended learning outcomes to be achieved [2]. Frameworks, therefore, provide an overview and structure for analysing and understanding IPECP. Existing frameworks ultimately serve as the conceptual basis for the design of IPE on the one hand, delineating the essential competencies for IPCP on the other.

Notwithstanding a steady increase in research activities investigating the effectiveness of IPCP across stakeholders, a consensus on the theoretical basis for IPECP has yet to be reached [11, 38].

In pursuit of synthesising and standardising competency-oriented educational programmes, numerous frameworks on interprofessional competency dimensions have emerged globally. These frameworks have also found their way into curricula and research efforts in Europe [9, 24, 49]. The overarching aim of these IPECP frameworks is to provide learners from different healthcare professions, their educators, and interprofessional practitioners with a content-related basis and thus a common perspective. On the one hand, this enables the selection and adaptation of intended learning outcomes to the requirements of practice. On the other hand, the content of the frameworks points the way forward with regard to the existing theoretical foundation, the goals of IPCP, and the competencies required for this [42].

The IPECP frameworks published beyond Europe address both IPE as well as interprofessional healthcare practice. These frameworks articulate overarching competencies and, when applicable, delineate processes for their attainment, alongside establishing goals for fostering successful IPCP. The central idea is that by acquiring competencies specific to the interprofessional domain, learners will be able to contribute to effective and patient-centred healthcare in (existing) teams [42]. In particular, these frameworks address competency development in the following areas as common ground: (1) values and ethics for interprofessional practice, (2) interprofessional teamwork, (3) roles and responsibilities in the interprofessional team, (4) interprofessional communication, (5) interprofessional conflict resolution [39]. Additionally, some frameworks address also domains like reflection, collaborative leadership, and patient-centredness. Most IPECP frameworks published worldwide are based on different theoretical approaches, such as team, communication, or systems theories. Regarding the educational part of the frameworks, most of them focus on aspects of constructivist and behaviourist theories of teaching and learning, considering both the learning process and the learning outcomes. Both theoretical strands (constructivist and behaviourist) are consciously and unconsciously included in the following frameworks. However, these two theories of learning are not fundamentally mutually exclusive. They simply have different emphases [21].

Where Are the Gaps?

The use of frameworks from the Anglo-Saxon world currently dominates the IPE landscape in Europe. This might be due to the more advanced developments in these countries in direct comparison to the European IPECP movement. However, the issue is that the healthcare systems in these countries are difficult to compare [26]. In addition, the training pathways for the health professions are very different. For example, in Germany, training for many health professions is not universally academic [20].

In addition, the development and existence of numerous frameworks contribute to a heterogeneous educational landscape and implementation in practice. While there is broad consensus on the need for IPCP, there is still disagreement on the implementation, design, and application of the content and recommendations set out in the frameworks. This becomes evident, for example, as non-standardised terminology is used [34]. Different definitions in relation to constructs that are central to IPCP, such as competency, and other related terms, such as intended learning outcomes. Currently, there is also a lack of standardised terminology, particularly in relation to what IPE and IPCP mean. This is aggravated by the fact that there is currently no consensus on the theoretical foundation of IPCP. Congruence can be seen in the individual frameworks, for example, in the theory-based selection of intended learning outcomes and the derivation of suitable teaching/learning methods [42]. However, awareness of various discrepancies and efforts to achieve congruence can be seen, for example, in the standardised communication objectives of the HPCC intended learning outcomes [5].

Overall, the objectives and competencies described in the frameworks often seem abstract and difficult to measure. Therefore, in terms of research activities, it has not been possible to agree and implement a single set of robust, empirically measurable criteria for IPECP across Europe. Clear definitions and congruent operationalisation of agreed and intended learning outcomes, including appropriate assessment instruments, within the European IPECP community would enable interprofessional competencies to be measured, promoted, and assessed in the context of empirical studies, thus supporting Europe-specific uniform standards of education and collaboration. This in turn would contribute to the evaluation of evidence of IPECP. A review of existing European frameworks for a differentiated comparison appears to be useful to facilitate decisions based on similarities and differences based on a theoretical background.

Synthesis of European IPECP Frameworks

To compare European IPECP frameworks, a literature search was conducted using the Medline database via PubMed. Articles in English and German, published between 2004 and 2024, were included.[1] This search identified 90 potential sources. After one of the authors (MW) screened the titles and abstracts, five sources were included. Additionally, IPECP experts were consulted informally and asked about frameworks they were familiar with. They identified three more sources. After

[1] The following search string was used: ("interprofessional education"[All Fields] AND "interprofessional collaboration"[All Fields] AND "framework*"[Title/Abstract] AND ("hasabstract"[All Fields] AND ("english"[Language] OR "german"[Language]) AND 2004/01/01:2024/01/01[Date - Publication])) AND (fha[Filter]).

full-text screening, one paper was excluded because it focused on interprofessional identity only. Finally, seven papers were eligible for analysis.

Based on these findings, the identified European frameworks for interprofessional teaching, learning formats, and collaboration were compared descriptively, using criteria based on a publication from Thistlethwaite et al. [42]. The identified frameworks are summarised in Table 1.

Table 1 Overview of European frameworks

Interprofessional capability framework Walsh et al. [45] I United Kingdom	
Brief description	The framework defines the capabilities that health professionals need in order to work together interprofessionally
Field of application	IPE, IPC
Objective(s)	The framework defines capabilities that health professions need to work together interprofessionally The framework has been developed to provide a model for teaching and assessing the capabilities required for a collaborative and practice-orientated health professional to work effectively and efficiently in an interprofessional team to deliver safe and high-quality services/care to patients, families, and communities
Addressed domains	The framework is based on the integration of core elements: client-centeredness, patient safety, and treatment quality, as well as collaborative practice. Necessary for this are five collaborative capabilities: • Communication • Team function • Role clarification • Conflict resolution • Reflection
Methodology (theoretical basis/ foundation) Reference theory	The basic theoretical framework was a mental health workforce development framework [41] Grounded theory based on all curricula in health and social care UK Empirically validated [42]
Terminology	Concept of ability according to Fraser and Greenhalgh [18]. Skill is the integrated application of knowledge in which the learner and practitioner can adapt to change, develop new behaviours, and continuously improve performance
Materials	n. a.
Other	n. a.
Interprofessional learning outcomes for health professions at Charité—Universitätsmedizin Berlin Behrend et al. [6] I Germany	
Brief description	The framework defines interprofessional learning outcomes and is intended to serve as the basis for standardised interprofessional training across all professions at Charité—Universitätsmedizin Berlin
Field of application	IPE

Table 1 (continued)

Interprofessional capability framework Walsh et al. [45] I United Kingdom	
Objective(s)	The framework developed aims to create a common understanding of interprofessionalism at Charité—Universitätsmedizin Berlin that is adapted to local needs in order to improve interprofessional education. The framework contains cross-faculty interprofessional education goals. The framework can be used for the development of interprofessional teaching/learning projects
Addressed domains	The focus of this framework is on four domains, which are differentiated with operationalised learning objectives for the areas of knowledge, skills/abilities, and attitude/attitude The domains are: • Professional roles and responsibilities in the IP team • Collaboration in the IP team • Dealing with conflicts in the IP team • Communication in the IP team
Methodology (theoretical basis/ foundation)/ Reference theory	2-stage process: Development of a draft (using the nominal group technique); followed by a Delphi process with own faculty members and students for validation. Theoretical basis is not mentioned
Terminology	n. a.
Materials	Validated training objectives and operationalisation; depicted in knowledge, skills/abilities, and attitude
Other	n. a.
INPRO competency framework—INPRO CF Aerts and De Weerdt [1] I Belgium	
Brief description	The INPRO competency framework is an adopted and adapted version of the WHO rehabilitation competency framework, and other existing interprofessional competency frameworks were integrated
Field of application	IPE, IPC
Objective(s)	The INPRO CF is an interprofessional competency framework developed to close the gap between education and practice The main objective of INPRO CF is to have one framework for all stakeholders during their lifelong learning process in health and social care. The use of International Classification of Functioning (ICF, WHO) learning outcomes is also included
Addressed domains	The focus of this framework is on five domains that centres around core values and beliefs. The domains are: • Interprofessional practice • Interprofessionalism • Learning and development • Management and leadership • Research These domains contain competencies, and each competency has learning outcomes on different levels
Methodology (theoretical basis/ foundation)/ Reference theory	Action-based research: Literature study, Delphi method, relevance-based research

(continued)

Table 1 (continued)

Interprofessional capability framework Walsh et al. [45] | United Kingdom	
Terminology	Interprofessional competencies are the observable abilities of a learner, integrating knowledge, skills, values, and attitudes that enable working together successfully across the professions and with a person and their family to improve health outcomes in specific care contexts. Competencies are durable, trainable, and, through the expression of learning outcomes, measurable. Personal characteristics such as motivation, self-confidence, willpower, and flexibility are part of a certain context
Materials	User guide INPRO CF competency book and movie (English, Finnish, German, Dutch) Operationalised learning objectives per domain Assessment and reflection guide (self- and peer-review) Suggestions of assessment tools for individual and group observation Examples of the use of INPRO CF in different contexts (education/internship/practice) [1]
Other	This work was supported by the ERASMUS+ [grant number 621428-EPP-1-2020-1-NL-EPPKA2-KA]
The EIPEN key competences for interprofessional collaboration EIPEN.eu [16] | Netherlands	
Brief description	The EIPEN framework defines five interprofessional competencies according to the European qualifications framework for Interprofessional Education (IPE) in health and social care. It also includes assessment forms for key competences
Field of application	IPE, IPC
Objective(s)	The aim of the framework is to stimulate and disseminate effective interprofessional education in European higher education and to improve cooperation in health and social care in Europe in order to optimise the quality of care and the quality of life of patients/clients
Addressed domains	The focus of the framework is on teaching and assessing five key competencies (behavioural indicators): • Consult and collaborate interprofessionally • Plan and manage interprofessionally • Refer and transfer interprofessionally • Handle issues and opportunities interprofessionally • Reflect and evaluate interprofessionally
Methodology (theoretical basis/foundation)/Reference theory	An EU-wide expert group developed the framework. Theoretical reference to team-based work, problem-based learning, and person-centred care according to the ICF model
Terminology	The concept of competencies is made up of the integration of the components knowledge, skills, and attitudes
Materials	Evaluation forms according to Interprofessional Practice & Education Quality Scales in English, Dutch, German, Finnish
Other	n. a.

Table 1 (continued)

Interprofessional capability framework Walsh et al. [45] I United Kingdom	
Framework for evaluation of interprofessional education and collaboration—FEIPEC Huber [23] I Switzerland	
Brief description	The FEIPEC framework defines an evaluation matrix for IPE and IPC and can support the planning of evaluations of interprofessional complex situations.
Field of application	IPE, IP-research
Objective(s)	The aim of the framework is to make complex interprofessional situations measurable and to visualise their process character in order to demonstrate the effective benefits of IPE and IPC. In addition, interactions between different process stages are visualised and can thus be included in an empirical analysis as additional influencing factors
Addressed domains	The FEIPEC proposes a basic grid with indicator variables for the evaluation of IPE and IPC: Input; implementation; output, outcomes, enabling factors, and impact Variables to be collected and empirical methodological approaches are proposed. The variables are to be adapted depending on the situation
Methodology (theoretical basis/ foundation)/ Reference theory	Expert panels and empirical validation Theoretical references are made on the basis of Cox et al. [11] regarding the learning continuum (input), to the model by D'Amour and Oandasan [12] (implementation) and model by Kirkpatrick and Kirkpatrick [29]. The 3-P model by Biggs [7] extended by Freeth and Reeves [19] and the impact model by Kaiser et al. [27] were used to depict the process character
Terminology	n. a.
Materials	Suggestions for empirical methods List of suggested questionnaires and variables to evaluate interprofessional aspects and psychometric data. These should not be considered independently of each other. It is important to define the variables with regard to the process and the analysis approach
Other	n. a.
FINCA—a conceptual framework to improve interprofessional collaboration in health education and care Witti et al. [50] I Germany	
Brief description	The FINCA framework conceptualises collaborative activities to improve interprofessional problem-solving skills in healthcare
Field of application	IPE, IPC, IP-research
Objective(s)	The FINCA framework provides definitions and operationalisations that enable empirical research studies to assess and subsequently promote collaborative problem-solving skills and practically integrate the results in different IPECP contexts

(continued)

Table 1 (continued)

Interprofessional capability framework Walsh et al. [45] I United Kingdom	
Addressed domains	At the Centre of the FINCA framework are observable collaborative activities that can be used to record the cognitive and social skills of individuals and reflect the process of interprofessional cooperation in a clinical context. These are: • Information sharing and grounding • Negotiating • Regulating • Executing interprofessional activities • Maintaining communication
Methodology (theoretical basis/ foundation)/ Reference theory	Iterative expert panel consisting of ILEGRA fellows, scientific supervisors, and international members of the ILEGRA Advisory Board The framework is based on a combination of three strands of theory from educational psychology and collaborative learning. These are: (1) fostering of diagnostic competencies, (2) collaboration scripts, and (3) collaborative problem-solving skills
Terminology	Collaborative activities according to Liu et al. [31]
Materials	n. a.
Other	Limitations: not yet empirically validated This work was supported by the Robert Bosch Stiftung (Graduiertenkolleg ILEGRA "Interprofessionelle Lehre in den Gesundheitsberufen—Vermittlung, evaluation, Prüfung", grant no. 32.5.A381.0058.0)
Applying landscapes of practice principles to the design of interprofessional education de Nooijer et al. [35] I The Netherlands	
Brief description	The framework uses an IPE team intervention (undergraduate, [44]) to explain the application and expansion of the "Landscapes of Practice" [44, 47] to include the aspects of professional identity and balance of the professions involved in the work process (IPE case) The body of knowledge of a profession is seen as a living landscape of practice; (inter)professional learning and all associated processes as social learning against the backdrop of constructivist learning theory It explains the complex system of several communities of practice, each of which comprises three dimensions: (1) the domain; (2) the community; and (3) the practice [46]
Field of application	IPE, IPC
Objective(s)	The framework includes the identification modes developed by Wenger-Trayner and Wenger-Trayner [47]: • Engagement ("how are we relevant to each other?") • Imagination ("who are we in our future professional context and in relation to one another?") • Alignment ("how do we align our activities and collaborate?") and • How these can be used in the context of IPE and contribute to identity development as a prerequisite for transcending one's own professional boundaries

(continued)

Table 1 (continued)

Interprofessional capability framework Walsh et al. [45] I United Kingdom	
Addressed domains	The framework focuses on three identification modes: • Engagement (how are we relevant to one another?) • Imagination (who are we in our future professional context and in relation to one another?) • Alignment (how do we align our activities and collaborate?)
Methodology (theoretical basis/ foundation)/ Reference theory	Social learning/landscape theory [47]: • Addresses identity and knowledge of one's own professional field • Three modes of identification to develop understanding (of self, other professions, and the systems in which they work) • Influences the view of collaboration. Learning thus takes place at the boundaries of different "professional landscapes" and enables the perception of differences (between professions), their interfaces, and interactions • IPE case [44]/constructivist learning [14, 15]
Terminology	Concept of knowledgeability IPE is often based on competency thinking: the contribution of the individual in a profession as a contribution to collaboration Landscape's concept, on the other hand, focuses on the ability to know and the ability to cross professional boundaries, i.e. interprofessional collaboration itself
Materials	n. a.
Other	Limitations: "A potential limitation of the proposed approach concerns the implementation, which requires coordination between different curricula" ([35], p. 213) Reservations on the part of teachers

Overall, the results depict a descriptive representation based on the available publications. The identified frameworks were published between 2004 and 2024. All frameworks cover aspects of IPE, but only a few focus explicitly on IPCP and/or research. Different, and in some cases inconsistent, terminology is used within the frameworks: While most of the frameworks have a broad (e.g. transnational) orientation [1, 16, 23, 35, 45, 50], one of the frameworks refers to a single institution [6]. Within the analysed domains addressed by the frameworks, there are overlaps as well as differentiations or extensions depending on its content focus. Therefore, the intended learning outcomes in the frameworks also differ. All the included frameworks address all health professions, including their educators, practitioners, and researchers.

What Does This Chapter Add?

This analysis provides a comprehensive overview of the currently published IPECP frameworks relevant to Europe. By selecting specific, literature-based criteria based on Thistlethwaite et al. [42], this study takes a comparative look at the various European frameworks.

Diversity and Objectives of the Frameworks

European frameworks for IPE are characterised by an impressive diversity, which is due to the different objectives and areas of application. The diversity ranges from the formalisation of specific IPE intended learning outcomes to the definition of relevant IPCP skills, competency areas, and observable activities. Each framework is based on different historical and cultural backgrounds, and pursues diverse goals that are either politically, research methodologically, or educationally motivated.

The differences in the frameworks are not surprising, given their origins. They are the result of specific local requirements in a dynamic and culturally diverse environment, which is characterised above all by different training paths and different structural and organisational perspectives on care. However, as suggested by Hean et al. [21] and Kaap-Fröhlich et al. [26] these differences could be partially resolved, at least in the IPE sector, to ensure more effective and coherent implementation in the IPE sector.

These different orientations are based on different theoretical foundations, contain different underlying terminologies and in some cases have different intended learning outcomes.

Theoretical Foundations and Terminological Differences

The discrepancies between the frameworks are reflected not only in their objectives and requirements, for example, in view of local needs, but also in the fundamental theoretical approaches and the resulting operationalisation. This diversity and the associated basic understanding of IPE have led to a complex conceptual and methodological landscape in long-standing discourses, which has been addressed and critically evaluated by several authors such as Reeves et al. [37] (see also [26, 33, 34, 48, 49]). In our view, this exemplifies the need for more standardised terminology in order to improve comprehensibility and comparability. This could be achieved, for example, by creating a cross-national glossary. A common understanding promotes the standardised use of terminology, facilitates/ensures communication between those involved, and is also the basis for targeted interprofessional patient care [22, 34].

Common Goals and Different Approaches

All frameworks pursue the overarching goal of (further) developing IPECP by addressing the competencies/skills to be educated and promoted—divided into different domains. However, this common objective becomes evident in a variety of approaches that reveal, for example, specific understandings of learning processes or of the interprofessional practitioners' role. While some overlaps between the competencies/skills that need to be developed in the defined domains can be recognised, there is often still a lack of transparent presentation of the learning theory associated with the respective framework and a uniform terminology. Possible research methodological approaches are desirable, leading to methodologically more transparent and comparable measurement instruments. A sound foundation for the promotion of interprofessional domains in the teaching and clinical setting therefore appears relevant. This requires an effort for coordination and standardisation of terminology and measurement approaches. The effectiveness and outreach of IPECP initiatives can thus be maximised and documented with corresponding evaluation results.

Standardisation and Organisational Perspectives

Standardisation, particularly with regard to measurement instruments, is desirable, but appears challenging in the European context due to language and cultural barriers. This must be considered when designing and adapting evaluation/measurement instruments. Regarding the applicability and usability of the frameworks, we believe that there are further perspectives that are relevant for research and health care practice. Looking at the frameworks from the perspective of organisational psychology could open up new perspectives, particularly with regard to team building (e.g. [43]) and open new approaches to integrating IPE measures into practice in the long term.

Outlook: Implications for the Effective Use of IPECP Frameworks

Two key implications for the use of interprofessional IPECP frameworks can be derived from our results.

First, Recognising Diversity

Despite their differences, all frameworks share the common goal of promoting IPECP through the development of relevant competency/skill domains. Recognising the diversity of European frameworks is a first step towards realising their full potential. By recognising the different historical, cultural, and theoretical backgrounds and core orientations (education, practice, research) of the frameworks as strengths, IPECP stakeholders can develop tailored approaches that enhance the quality of IPECP locally.

Second, Creating a Consistent Basis for Education, Practice, and Research

The domains defined in the respective frameworks should form the basis for the development of congruent and comprehensible teaching and intended learning outcomes. These intended learning outcomes must be translated into methodological and didactic approaches that both support the teaching of content and enable the assessment of learning progress. This is the prerequisite for the development of examination formats and measurement instruments that are specifically designed to effectively evaluate interprofessional domains. A standardised and consensual terminology and a clearly comprehensible theoretical foundation facilitate the systematic and comparative analysis of research results within Europe and in turn can contribute to the further development of research on the frameworks' effectiveness. These aspects are crucial to transparently demonstrate, measure, and evaluate the effectiveness of IPECP in professional practice.

Reflective Questions for the Reader

- Can frameworks truly promote and ensure the quality of IPECP?
- How should existing frameworks be updated to stay relevant?
- Is there a need for a standardised European IPECP framework?

Acknowledgements In Memory of Professor Hugh Barr. We are deeply saddened by the passing of Professor Hugh Barr in 2025, a pioneer of interprofessional health and social care education. His work has had a profound impact on the way health professionals learn and collaborate across disciplines. We had the privilege of benefiting from his expertise and vision when he contributed to our joint book chapter. His conviction that shared learning and practice among health professionals is not only possible, but also essential, will continue to inspire us. We have lost an influential voice and esteemed colleague, and his impact on research, education, and practice will continue to be felt. His lifelong commitment to collaboration in healthcare will remain both a legacy and a guiding light for the field.

References

1. Aerts I, De Weerdt C. INPRO competency framework: competencybook. 2023. https://www.inproproject.eu/wp-content/uploads/2023/11/4.5.d-INPRO-CF_ENG_competencybook.pdf.
2. Alderson A, Martin M. Outcomes based education: where has it come from and where is it going? Iss Educ Res. 2007;17(2):161–82.
3. Anderson ES, Lennox A. The Leicester model of Interprofessional education: developing, delivering and learning from student voices for 10 years. J Interprof Care. 2009;23(6):557–73. https://doi.org/10.3109/13561820903051451.
4. Babbie ER. The practice of social research. 15th ed. Cengage; 2021.
5. Bachmann C, Kiessling C, Härtel A, Haak R. Communication in health professions: a European consensus on inter- and multi-professional learning objectives in German. GMS J Med Educ. 2016;33(2):Doc23. https://doi.org/10.3205/zma001022.
6. Behrend R, Herinek D, Kienle R, Arnold F, Peters H. Development of Interprofessional learning outcomes for health professions at Charité - Universitätsmedizin Berlin - a Delphi-study. Das Gesundheitswesen. 2022;84(6):532–8. https://doi.org/10.1055/a-1341-1368.
7. Biggs JB. From theory to practice: a cognitive systems approach. High Educ Res Dev. 1993;12(1):73–85. https://doi.org/10.1080/0729436930120107.
8. Boulding KE. General systems theory: the skeleton of science. Manag Sci. 1956;2(3):197–208. https://www.jstor.org/stable/2627132.

9. CIHC – Canadian Interprofessional Health Collaborative. A national interprofessional competency framework. 2010. https://www.cihc.ca/files/CIHC_IPCompetencies_Feb1210.pdf.
10. Carron T, Rawlinson C, Arditi C, Cohidon C, Hong QN, Pluye P, Gilles I, Peytremann-Bridevaux I. An overview of reviews on interprofessional collaboration in primary care: effectiveness. Int J Integr Care. 2021;21(2):31. https://doi.org/10.5334/ijic.5588.
11. Cox M, Cuff P, Brandt B, Reeves S, Zierler B. Measuring the impact of interprofessional education on collaborative practice and patient outcomes. J Interprof Care. 2016;30(1):1–3. https://doi.org/10.3109/13561820.2015.1111052.
12. D'amour D, Oandasan I. Interprofessionality as the field of interprofessional practice and interprofessional education: An emerging concept. Journal of Interprofessional Care, 2005;19(sup1):8–20. https://doi.org/10.1080/13561820500081604.
13. Dörner D. Denken, Problemlösen und Intelligenz. Psychol Rundsch. 1984;35(1):10–20.
14. Dolmans DHJM. How theory and design-based research can mature PBL practice and research. Adv Health Sci Educ. 2019;24(5):879–91. https://doi.org/10.1007/s10459-019-09940-2.
15. Dolmans DHJM, De Grave W, Wolfhagen IH, Van Der Vleuten CP. Problem-based learning: future challenges for educational practice and research. Med Educ. 2005;39(7):732–41. https://doi.org/10.1111/j.1365-2929.2005.02205.x.
16. EIPEN.eu. The EIPEN key competences for interprofessional collaboration. 2021. https://www.eipen.eu/key-competences.
17. Ewers M, Schaeffer D. Interprofessionelles Lernen, Lehren und Arbeiten auf holprigen Wegen. In: Ewers M, Paradis E, Herinek D (Hrsg.). Interprofessionelles Lernen, Lehren und Arbeiten: Gesundheits- und Sozialprofessionen auf dem Weg zu kooperativer Praxis. Beltz Juventa; 2019.
18. Fraser SW, Greenhalgh T. Coping with complexity: educating for capability. BMJ. 2001;323(7316):799–803. https://doi.org/10.1136/bmj.323.7316.799.
19. Freeth D, Reeves S. Learning to work together: using the presage, process, product (3P) model to highlight decisions and possibilities. J Interprof Care. 2004;18(1):43–56. https://doi.org/10.1080/13561820310001608221.
20. German Science and Humanities Council & Geschäftsstelle/Head Office. HQGplus-Studie zu Hochschulischen Qualifikationen für das Gesundheitssystem - update. 2022. https://doi.org/10.57674/v8gx-db45.
21. Hean S, Craddock D, O'Halloran C. Learning theories and interprofessional education: a user's guide. Learn Health Soc Care. 2009;8(4):250–62. https://doi.org/10.1111/j.1473-6861.2009.00227.x.
22. Hollweg W, Heinzelmann B. Ein Kontinuum zur interprofessionellen Zusammenarbeit von Gesundheitsberufen: Vom Bedarf der Patient:innen über die Zusammenarbeit in der Praxis zur Auswahl geeigneter interprofessioneller Lehr-/Lernformate. In: Walkenhorst U, Fischer M, editors. Interprofessionelle Bildung für die Gesundheitsversorgung, Springer Reference Pflege – Therapie – Gesundheit. Springer-Verlag; 2024.
23. Huber M. Evaluation interprofessioneller komplexer Situationen. In: Walkenhorst U, Fischer M (Hrsg.). Interprofessionelle Bildung für die Gesundheitsversorgung, Springer Reference Pflege – Therapie – Gesundheit. Springer-Verlag; 2025.
24. IPEC – Interprofessional Education Collaborative. IPEC core competencies for Interprofessional collaborative practice: version 3. Washington, DC: Interprofessional Education Collaborative; 2023. https://www.ipecollaborative.org/assets/core-competencies/IPEC_Core_Competencies_Version_3_2023.pdf.
25. Jabareen Y. Building a conceptual framework: philosophy, definitions, and procedure. Int J Qual Methods. 2009;8(4):49–62. https://doi.org/10.1177/160940690900800406.
26. Kaap-Fröhlich S, Ulrich G, Wershofen B, Ahles J, Behrend R, Handgraaf M, Herinek D, Oberhauser H, Scherer T, Schlicker A, Straub C, Waury Eichler R, Wesselborg B, Witti M, Huber M, Bode SFN. Position paper of the GMA committee interprofessional education in the health professions - current status and outlook. GMS J Med Educ. 2022;39(2):Doc17. https://doi.org/10.3205/zma001538.

27. Kaiser L, Conrad S, Neugebauer EAM, Pietsch B, Pieper D. Interprofessional collaboration and patient-reported outcomes in inpatient care: a systematic review. Syst Rev. 2022;11(1):169. https://doi.org/10.1186/s13643-022-02027-x.
28. Kaiser S, Patras J, Martinussen M. Linking interprofessional work to outcomes for employees: a meta-analysis. Res Nurs Health. 2018;41(3):265–80. https://doi.org/10.1002/nur.21858.
29. Kirkpatrick JD, Kirkpatrick WK. Kirkpatrick's four levels of training evaluation. Association for Talent Development; 2016.
30. Körner M, Wirtz MA, Bengel J, Göritz AS. Relationship of organizational culture, teamwork and job satisfaction in interprofessional teams. BMC Health Serv Res. 2015;15:243. https://doi.org/10.1186/s12913-015-0888-y.
31. Liu L, Hao J, von Davier A, Kyllonen P, Zapata-Rivera J-D. A tough nut to crack: measuring collaborative problem solving. In: Rosen Y, Ferrara S, Mosharraf M, editors. Handbook of research on technology tools for real-world skill development (pp. 344–359). IGI Global; 2016. https://doi.org/10.4018/978-1-4666-9441-5.ch013.
32. Lutfiyya MN, Chang LF, McGrath C, Dana C, Lipsky MS. The state of the science of interprofessional collaborative practice: a scoping review of the patient health-related outcomes based literature published between 2010 and 2018. PLoS One. 2019;14(6):e0218578. https://doi.org/10.1371/journal.pone.0218578.
33. Mahler C, Gutmann T, Karstens S, Joos S. Terminology for interprofessional collaboration: definition and current practice. GMS J Med Educ. 2014;31(4):Doc40. https://doi.org/10.3205/zma000932.
34. Mitzkat A, Berger S, Reeves S, Mahler C. More terminological clarity in the interprofessional field - a call for reflection on the use of terminologies, in both practice and research, on a national and international level. GMS J Med Educ. 2016;33(2):Doc36. https://doi.org/10.3205/zma001035.
35. de Nooijer J, Dolmans DHJM, Stalmeijer RE. Applying landscapes of practice principles to the design of interprofessional education. Teach Learn Med. 2022;34(2):209–14. https://doi.org/10.1080/10401334.2021.1904937.
36. Popper K. The logic of scientific discovery. Hutchinson; 1959.
37. Reeves S, Fletcher S, Barr H, Birch I, Boet S, Davies N, McFadyen A, Rivera J, Kitto S. A BEME systematic review of the effects of interprofessional education: BEME guide no. 39. Med Teach. 2016;38(7):656–68. https://doi.org/10.3109/0142159X.2016.1173663.
38. Reeves S, Hean S. Why we need theory to help us better understand the nature of interprofessional education, practice and care. J Interprof Care. 2013;27(1):1–3. https://doi.org/10.3109/13561820.2013.751293.
39. Reichel K, Herinek D. Interprofessionelles Lehren und Lernen - Klärung und Orientierung. In: Ewers M, Reichel K (Hrsg.). Kooperativ Lehren, Lernen und Arbeit in den Gesundheitsprofessionen: das Projekt interTUT Working Paper No. 17-01 der Unit Gesundheitswissenschaften und ihre Didaktik; 2017.
40. Stachowiak H. Allgemeine Modelltheorie. Springer; 1973.
41. The Sainsbury Centre for Mental Health. The capable practitioner. SCMH; 2001.
42. Thistlethwaite JE, Forman D, Matthews LR, Rogers GD, Steketee C, Yassine T. Competencies and frameworks in interprofessional education: a comparative analysis. Acad Med. 2014;89(6):869–75. https://doi.org/10.1097/ACM.0000000000000249.
43. Tuckman BW. Developmental sequence in small groups. Psychol Bull. 1965;63(6):384–99. https://doi.org/10.1037/h0022100.
44. Van Lierop M, Van Dongen J, Janssen M, Smeets H, Van Bokhoven L, Moser A. Jointly discussing care plans for real-life patients: the potential of a student-led interprofessional team meeting in undergraduate health professions education. Perspect Med Educ. 2019;8(6):372–7. https://doi.org/10.1007/s40037-019-00543-6.
45. Walsh CL, Gordon MF, Marshall M, Wilson F, Hunt T. Interprofessional capability: a developing framework for interprofessional education. Nurse Educ Pract. 2005;5(4):230–7. https://doi.org/10.1016/j.nepr.2004.12.004.

46. Wenger E. Communities of practice: learning, meaning, and identity. 6th ed. Cambridge University Press; 1998.
47. Wenger-Trayner E, Wenger-Trayner B. Learning in a landscape of practice: a framework. In: Wenger-Trayner E, Fenton-O'Creevy M, Kubiak C, Hutchinson S, Wenger-Trayner B, editors. Learning in landscapes of practice: boundaries, identity, and knowledgeability in practice-based learning. Routledge; 2015. p. 13–29.
48. World Health Organization. Learning together to work together for health. 1988. https://apps.who.int/iris/handle/10665/37411.
49. World Health Organization. Framework for action on interprofessional education and collaborative practice. 2010. https://www.who.int/publications/i/item/framework-for-action-on-interprofessional-education-collaborative-practice.
50. Witti MJ, Zottmann JM, Wershofen B, Thistlethwaite JE, Fischer F, Fischer MR. FINCA - a conceptual framework to improve interprofessional collaboration in health education and care. Front Med. 2023;10:1213300. https://doi.org/10.3389/fmed.2023.1213300.

Matthias J. Witti is a nurse, nurse educator (B.A.), and educational scientist (M.A.). He gained practical experience in an anaesthesiological intensive care unit. His experience in nursing education was acquired through numerous teaching assignments. Before and during his doctorate, he also worked in an old people's home, where he was head of the nursing education department. Since 2018, he has been a research associate at the Institute for Didactics and Educational Research in Medicine at the LMU Hospital, LMU Munich, where he conducts research on interprofessional education and collaboration with a focus on interprofessional discharge planning and interprofessional patient handover.

He is a former scholarship holder of the Research College for Interprofessional Teaching in the Health Professions (ILEGRA). His dissertation on the topic: Interprofessional communication in discharge planning was completed in 2024. He has been a member of the extended board of the IP Health Association for 3 years and is a member of many other IPECP associations and networks.

Bettina Heinzelmann is a speech therapist (Teaching and Researchlogopaedics, RWTH Aachen, Germany), since 2011 a lecturer at various vocational schools and since 2017 also at universities of applied sciences. She is a former scholarship holder of the Interprofessional Teaching in the Healthcare Professions Research Training Group (ILEGRA) and is working on the design and evaluation of an interprofessional teaching/learning course for therapy professions with a focus on communication skills as part of her doctorate.

Claudia De Weerdt is a researcher at AP UAS, Antwerp (Belgium). She graduated as a Master physiotherapist in 2018 and completed the master's degree in Management and Policy in Healthcare in 2019. She works as a physiotherapist in a hospital and has experience as a physiotherapist in the primary care. She was involved in the INPRO project with specialism in interprofessional competencies which led to the development of the INPRO Competency Framework.

Ingrid Aerts is a lecturer and researcher at the Nutrition and Dietetics programme at AP UAS, Antwerp (Belgium). She graduated as a dietician in 1987 and specialised in sports nutrition in 2001. She has been working for the Food and Dietetics programme since 2004. In 2019, she completed the master's degree in training and education sciences as a working student. Since 2008, she has been involved in IPCIHC in Antwerp (InterProfessional Collaboration in Healthcare) as a tutor and steering committee member, and since then she has deepened her understanding of interprofessional collaboration. As part of her master's thesis, she investigated the tutors' perceptions of evaluating the interprofessional collaboration of a learning group. Within the INPRO project (Interprofessionalism in action!) she was responsible for the workpackage of developing interprofessional competencies and the assessment of them.

Hugh Barr Following 4 years as a probation officer in the English Midlands, Hugh was seconded for 3 years to the London-based Home Office Research Unit to join its newly established interdisciplinary probation team. Setting aside career prospects in criminology or a return to the probation service, he opted to lead a pioneering project recruiting "voluntary associates" supported by probation officers to befriend ex-prisoners. He was then appointed as an Assistant Director of the newly established Central Council for Education and Training in Social Work (CCETSW) where his responsibilities included developing research strategies, information services, and extensive education programmes for untrained and undertrained residential, day, and domiciliary care workers. Opting for early retirement, he responded to calls to advise and support the development of interprofessional education in and between health and social care in the UK and increasingly abroad to further collaborative practice.

Marion Huber 's main research interests are interprofessional competence development, collaboration and task shifting. Her scientific track provides vast results focusing on competencies for interprofessional collaboration and suitable teaching formats. Moreover, she took part in the development and analysis of large quantitative studies assessing student mental health during the COVID-19 pandemic. She is also in the lead of the long-term evaluation of the Zurich Interprofessional Clinical Training Ward (ZIPAS), which is designed as a sequential nested mixed-methods study.

Doreen Herinek is a physiotherapist with a Bachelor of Science in Health Sciences and a Master of Science in Health Professions Education. She is working at the Institute of Health and Nursing Science of the Charité—Universitätsmedizin Berlin, holding a Dr.-cand. position. She conducts research on interprofessional peer-assisted learning and is a Co-editor of the first German-speaking book about IPECP in social and health professions. She has been Vice Chair of the IP Health Association for 3 years and is a member of many other associations and networks for IPECP in the DACH-region.

Evaluation, Quality Improvement, and Research in Interprofessional Education and Collaborative Practice

Veronica O'Carroll, Lisa-Christin Wetzlmair-Kephart, Noreen O'Leary, and Marion Huber

Abbreviations

ENQUIRE	Evaluation, Quality Improvement, and Research
IPC	Interprofessional Collaboration
IPE	Interprofessional Education
IPECP	Interprofessional Education and Collaborative Practice
PDSA	Plan, Do, Study, Act
QI	Quality Improvement

Introduction

Interprofessional education and collaborative practice (IPECP) is well considered for tackling many health and social care challenges, such as the shortage of specialists, poor teamwork and ineffective communication. IPECP is well positioned to help meet increasing global health complexities and inequalities [20]. Proof of the

V. O'Carroll (✉)
School of Medicine, University of St Andrews, Fife, Scotland, UK
e-mail: vo1@st-andrews.ac.uk

L.-C. Wetzlmair-Kephart
Gleville State University, Glenville, WV, USA

N. O'Leary
Health Professions Education Centre, RCSI, 118 St Stephen's Green, Dublin 2, Ireland

M. Huber
Center of Interprofessional Learning and Practice, Institute of Public Health at the Department of Health Sciences, Zurich University of Applied Sciences, Zurich, Switzerland

A. Xyrichis et al. (eds.), *Building Bridges: A European Perspective on Interprofessional Education, Practice, Policy and Research*,
https://doi.org/10.1007/978-3-032-23222-9_3

effectiveness of IPECP concerning health outcomes, patient safety and quality of care, on the other hand, is still hard to show. Why is there little evidence of effectiveness? Does it always have to be a research study? These are time-consuming and require resources. Or, you may think, "I'm a practitioner and not a researcher, and I do not want to do a research study". It doesn't always have to be research. Evaluation and quality improvement can be valuable alternatives to show the impact of IPECP. Often, the people who are best placed to identify the most pressing needs for a service or education programme are those working at the frontline. However, these are often the people with the least time to engage with the evaluation of IPECP. In this chapter, we discuss and signpost to supports and tools that you can use to show the value of IPECEP through evaluation, quality improvement or research (ENQUIRE).

Throughout this chapter, we explore the practicalities you can apply to conduct impactful ENQUIRE that can be used in academic, health or social care settings to advance IPECP. The main aim is to raise awareness of the value of these approaches and to help you, as the reader, consider relevance to your contexts. The objectives of this chapter are intended to enable you to:

- Reflect on your understanding of IPECP.
- Define ENQUIRE within the context of IPECP.
- Consider the context-specific factors driving the need for the research of evaluation or quality improvement related to IPECP.
- Illustrate the application of ENQUIRE frameworks and models to IPECP.
- Consider opportunities within your contexts for the ENQUIRE in IPECP.

Your IPECP Positioning

Before we delve into this chapter, it is worth reflecting on the questions below. These questions will help you understand your position concerning IPECP and the positions of others in your context. This reflection can be a useful starting point for using ENQUIRE in IPECP. ENQUIRE aims to generate momentum and encourage you to reflect on your motivations for IPECP and potential areas for change in your context. We encourage you to write down your thoughts, which may support your thinking and serve as a starting point for your journey through IPECP ENQUIRE.

Self-Reflective Questions:

- What does IPECP mean to you within your context?
- How do you and others perceive the value of IPECP in your context?
- How do you know if your current IPECP activities affect education and practice?
- What areas of IPECP could be better understood in your context or could benefit from further exploration?

What Is ENQUIRE in the Context of IPECP?

While there are many commonalities between ENQUIRE, there are also some key differences (Table 1). Understanding these will help you decide the most suitable approach for your context.

Evaluation

Evaluation is "a routine, systematic, deliberate gathering of information to uncover and identify what contributes to the "success" of the program and what actions need

Table 1 Key features of ENQUIRE

Evaluation	Quality improvement	Research
Mainly used to understand how well an intervention (in education, health or social care practice) reaches its intended outcomes	Mainly used to judge, measure or observe provision, performance or improvement of a service	Mainly used to generate new knowledge
Can follow a recognised evaluation framework or tool to investigate the impact	Follows a recognised QI methodology, e.g. plan, do, study, act (PDSA) cycle	Follows recognised research methodology to address a defined research aim, question(s) and objectives
Usually, there are no hypotheses	Hypotheses can be flexible	Hypotheses used depend on the research approach, e.g. quantitative research. Hypotheses, if present, are fixed
Data is usually generated in the evaluation process	Usually, it involves the analysis of an existing dataset with the aim of optimising this data	Data is usually generated during the research process but can be used in existing datasets, e.g. secondary data analysis, to address a specific research question
Usually internally funded but can be externally funded, e.g. a specific funding call to evaluate a service	Usually internally funded	Usually externally and internally funded
Ethics approval may be needed, particularly if intending to publish findings	It may or may not involve human participants (involvement is low risk). Usually, it does not require ethics approval	It may or may not involve humans as participants (involvement can be low to high risk). Usually, it requires ethical approval
Usually, the impact is local and related to individuals, groups, organisations or departments	The impact is usually local and related to individuals, groups, organisations or departments	The impact can be related to individuals, groups, organisations or departments, but it can also be a local or wider impact
Limited oversight of the process to safeguard against bias	Minimal oversight of the process to safeguard against bias	Numerous safeguards and measures are in place to limit bias

to be taken to address the findings of the evaluation process" [7]. Evaluations are not confined to educational programs or interventions and can be used to evaluate health and social care services. Furthermore, evaluations can also be used to determine the outcomes or impact of a program or intervention, and therefore, this approach is suitable for evaluating IPECP. Anderson [1] and Reeves and Barr [18] are seminal papers highlighting important considerations for robust evaluation processes in IPECP.

Quality Improvement

The primary goal of Quality Improvement (QI) is to optimise existing activities, programmes or processes in local health and social care or healthcare education [5]. QI is a core component of health and social care whereby practitioners can use data from their settings to improve practice [13]. Those improvements are achieved by a combined effort of professionals in the health, social care and educational settings, service users (e.g. patients, families, caregivers), researchers and governmental stakeholders [3, 5], indicating the collaborative nature of QI [15]. QI uses concepts and methods from theories such as change management, communication strategies and plan-do-study-act cycles. The outcomes that QI seeks to improve include patient outcomes, key performance indicators of systems and professional development [3]. QI can address these three outcomes by seeking to improve health and social care through IPECP activities.

Research

Research can be described as the systematic generation of new knowledge to answer a specific research question by collecting data in a transparent and replicable way. In IPECP, research can be used to develop a new understanding of the impact, effectiveness or experience of an IPECP initiative occurring in an academic, health or social care environment with undergraduate and postgraduate pre-licensure students or post-licensure health or social care professionals. Research is a process that follows a stepwise approach [8] and comprises the identification of a gap in existing knowledge, the selection of a research approach and data collection, the analysis of the gathered data and the dissemination of the findings [8, 15]. The findings can be applied to a broader context [15]. The research cycle is analogous to clinical reasoning on the individual professional and patient levels. Knowing that there are different approaches to clinical reasoning, research can also be approached in many ways.

Why Is ENQUIRE in IPECP Important?

We continue to face various challenges in the realm of IPECP. A global workforce shortage needs to be counteracted with effective, efficient and high-quality interprofessional collaboration (IPC) [12]. However, despite an increase in the reporting of IPECP initiatives, the high methodological quality of the evidence highlighting the positive impact of IPECP on health outcomes, patient safety and quality of care in the European region is limited [4, 19]. How interprofessional education (IPE) can be successfully transferred into IPC practice and what constitutes successful IPC remains somewhat unclear [4]. Therefore, investigating both educational and practice activities is essential to understanding the interplay between both or how one may influence the other.

Investigating IPECP can be challenging due to limited time and resources or lack of knowledge and expertise. Enabling learning from other colleagues and sharing expertise locally, nationally and internationally can be valuable for professionals who do not have the resources or confidence to conduct ENQUIRE. When IPECP does happen, we must raise awareness to continue to build evidence of its impact. Both successful and unsuccessful IPECP activities need to be disseminated. Only then can we learn how to advance, improve and implement IPECP to impact health and social care.

Examples of ENQUIRE Previously Used in IPECP

Numerous examples of IPECP initiatives have been reported and published. Table 2 provides an overview of a few European examples where ENQUIRE have been used to investigate IPECP.

Table 2 Examples of IPECP ENQUIRE

Approach	IPE	IPC
Research	Svobodová et al. [21]. Czech Republic Investigated efficiency of simulation-based team training on door-to-needle time (DNT) for intravenous thrombolysis. Team training improved DNT	Kyriacou Georgiou et al. [12] Cyprus Investigated health professionals' perceptions of patient safety and teamwork. Teamwork was perceived more positively compared to perceptions of patient safety
Evaluation	Mileder et al. [14]. Austria Evaluated the impact of in situ simulation training interventions on latent safety threats. Sustained effect of IPE in situ simulation on patient safety	De Bruin et al. [6] Netherlands A cross-European multiple case study design. Provides an overview of the SUSTAIN project to evaluate integrated care for older people living at home
Quality improvement	Tully et al. [22] Scotland An interprofessional student-led QI project within a clinical environment. The QI project centred around improving the medication reconciliation for individuals prescribed insulin. The IPE activity involved pharmacy and medical students	Glover Williams et al. [9] England Examined implementation of a perinatal care bundle (PERIPrem) to reduce injury in preterm birth and measured impact on psychological safety and teamwork. Implementation of PERIPrem had a positive impact on team function, situation monitoring and team communication

Getting Started and Building Momentum

Different factors can contribute to the desire or need to conduct ENQUIRE. Before getting started, consider what lies behind your motivation. Examples are (but are not limited to):

- The theoretical motivation can be based on identified gaps in the literature.
- Personal motivation, such as issues arising in your working context.
- Leadership initiatives that are challenging current practices.
- Societal motivation includes problems that affect the health of the population, access to healthcare and health economics.

Tools for Generating Momentum

To undertake any project, be it research, evaluation or QI, requires momentum. Frontline health and education may not have access to literature outlining frameworks and tools which can inform ENQUIRE projects or may not have time to identify frameworks or theories. However, within an organisation, there may be resources such as an evaluation toolkit or quality improvement personnel specific to your area. The task then becomes explaining the issue you see in such a way that will help you identify an appropriate approach and framework. Communications teams can help you identify a suitable medium for communicating your findings and delivering them in such a way as to engage the people you want to listen to your message. For example, how you present QI findings to a service manager would differ from how you would present them to a policymaker.

For managers and senior leaders, the task is to create space and opportunity for frontline staff to reflect on the issues they see in practice and generate ideas for ENQUIRE.

Levers for change can also help generate momentum for change. Professional regulation and requirements for evidence of IPECP can act as a powerful lever across education and healthcare services.

Momentum can also be generated and maintained through joining relevant groups and networks. Many European countries, such as the United Kingdom, have national IPECP bodies, such as the Centre for the Advancement of IPE (CAIPE). At a European level, the European Interprofessional Education Network works to influence educational and healthcare policy. Collaboration is key to ENQUIRE, where collaboration is the core topic. Consider who your key collaborators are.

Selecting an Appropriate Approach and Considerations for Using ENQUIRE

ENQUIRE share similarities in that they follow a systematic approach. Each approach will have different vulnerabilities, and a little risk is fine as long as the safety of those undertaking the work and those participating is assured. QI, like evaluation, is often perceived as of less value than research, which is frequently due to a lack of understanding or confusion around how these approaches can be used in or benefit education and health or social care services. To shed light on this and avoid confusion, the flowchart in Fig. 1, inspired by several authors [3, 5, 10, 15, 18], will help you to decide which approach suits your endeavour. The steps outlined in the ENQUIRE Roadmap (Fig. 2) will help you consider your project's key activities. Throughout these steps, it is important to bring a range of stakeholders or individuals involved in different roles on board.

Step 1: The Question
ENQUIRE has to start with a clear objective. Are you interested in IPECP at the individual, organisation/institution or societal levels? The many potential areas or topics you could look at need to be narrowed down to a focused question. This approach is similar to setting learning outcomes in education or intervention goals in clinical practice. What do you want to know by the end of the process? This might take a while to refine, and it is worth getting input from colleagues to ensure you have a well-defined question before beginning any further work. Otherwise, you may find yourself drawn in all kinds of interesting directions but ultimately not answering the question you set out to answer. You may find it helpful to incorporate one central question and multiple sub-questions. The questions will depend on your motivation and your aim to undertake ENQUIRE [2].

Step 2: Resources
Once you have refined your question, it is useful to read around the topic and check if someone else has not previously answered some or all of your questions. You can find relevant information in national/regional health policies, websites of Special Interest Groups, e.g. CAIPE, and scientific journals. This information can also help you craft your rationale or argument for your proposed ENQUIRE, which you may need for steps 3 (approval) and 6 (dissemination).

Step 3: Approval
Firstly, determine if your ENQUIRE project requires ethical approval. Find out if you need approval from the Head of Department or Line Manager.

Step 4: Theory
According to Reeves et al. [19], thinking about or exploring theories that might help frame your ENQUIRE can be helpful. It is not essential to use theory in ENQUIRE, but it can help you better understand why something is or is not working or position

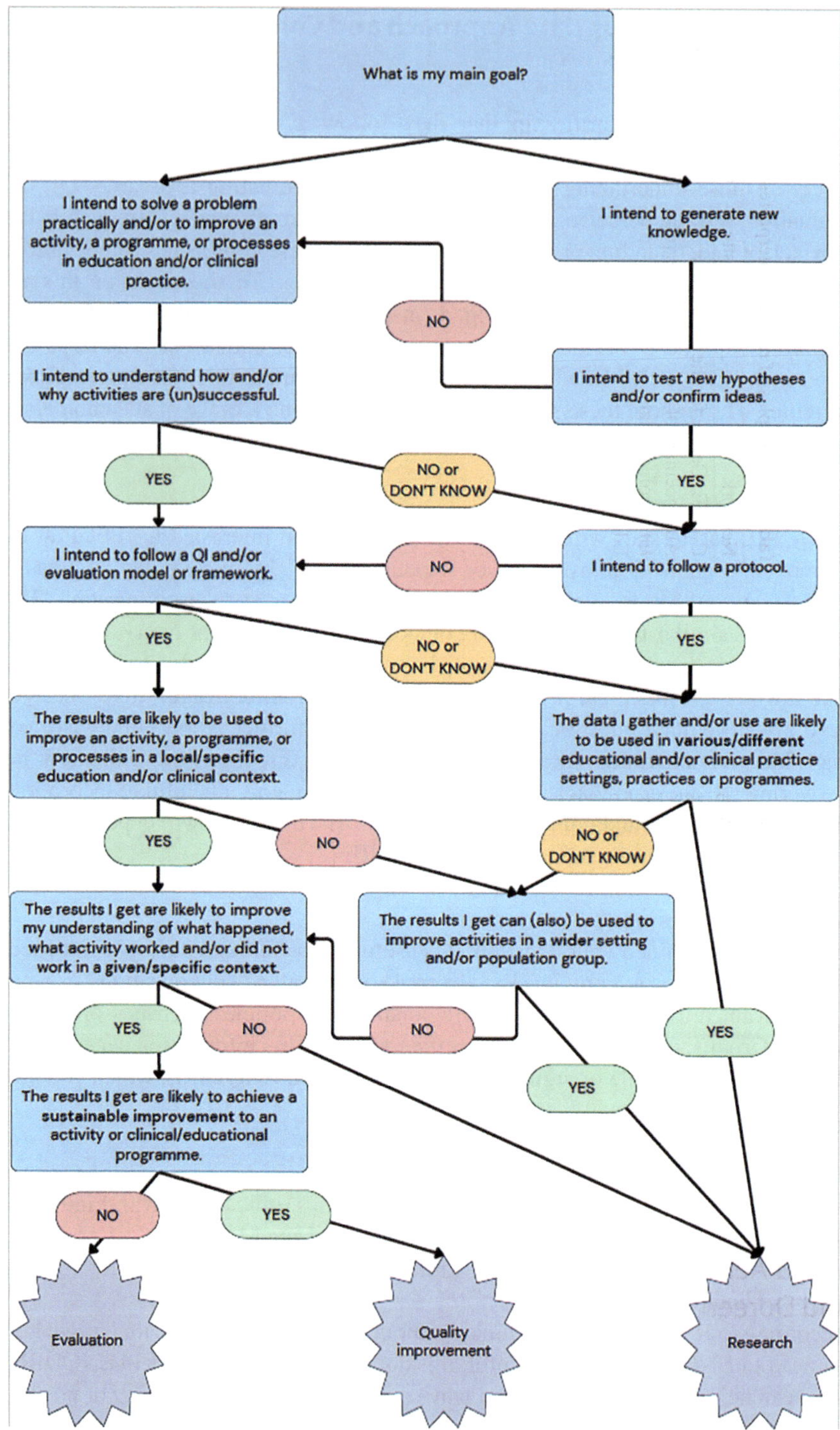

Fig. 1 ENQUIRE flowchart. *Note*. The flowchart serves as a decision-making tool for the selection of the appropriate methodological approach. (The figure was developed by the authors)

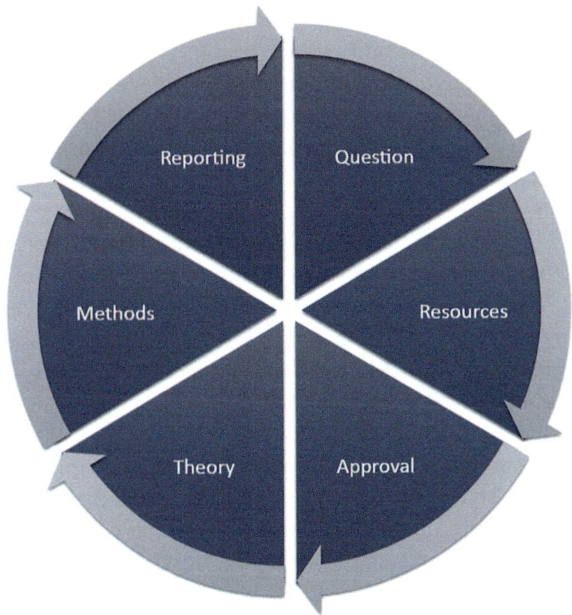

Fig. 2 ENQUIRE roadmap

what is happening in your area in a broader context. For example, the Kirkpatrick Model [11] has often been used in evaluations looking at IPE.

Step 5: Methods

This is where you decide what you will do to research, evaluate or improve the area you are interested in. IPECP ENQUIRE often involves asking students or staff for their opinions after an IPECP activity, e.g. surveys or interviews. This type of self-reported data can be useful, but it does not allow us to examine the impact of IPECP as we do not have a baseline from before the IPECP activity. If you want to measure the impact or the effect, you need before and after data and, ideally, data from a group that was not part of the IPECP activities (control group). In research studies, randomly assigning participants to groups is best practice. Ideally, you measure a third time, some weeks or months later, to determine the sustainability of impact.

You also need to be clear on what you are measuring, which could be knowledge, attitudes and skills, as well as efficacy measures or health outcome measures for patients, such as the IPECP activity. The methods chosen rarely include patients (Xyrichis et al., [24]). However, a core aim of all ENQUIRE is to improve patient experiences and quality of care. With this in mind, it is worth considering how you might involve patients in ENQUIRE. IPECP is also seeking to improve collaboration and teamwork. Therefore, it can be appropriate to measure interprofessional team functioning. Once you have decided what you are measuring, you may use existing tools, such as a survey, or you might develop your tool, i.e. questions to ask staff or students.

Step 6: Reporting

You do not necessarily have to publish your "findings" in scientific journals to disseminate them. Findings might be published in report form or shared with local service managers on regional/national health organisations/government websites. If you are considering publishing in scientific journals, reporting guidance may help apply findings, relate or transfer findings beyond the local context and improve the quality of ENQUIRE reporting overall.

For readers interested in carrying out IPECP QI projects in health and social care settings, the Standards for Quality Improvement Reporting Excellence (SQUIRE 2.0) guidelines [16] following reporting tools can be useful for planning and reporting purposes. The Standards for Quality Improvement Reporting Excellence in Education (SQUIRE_EDU) [17] may also be helpful for reporting on QI projects within an educational setting.

Using these guidelines enhances the quality and transparency of your QI project. It allows others to replicate your project and see if their findings are similar or different. They can also improve the likelihood of the project being accepted for publication or conference presentation, which publicises your work and may address similar questions that others in the IPECP field have.

Conclusion

Ultimately, it may not seem so relevant whether you are evaluating, improving quality or researching. What may be more important to consider is that in the context of IPECP, all approaches intend to enhance the quality of care. What matters is that the outputs from ENQUIRE endeavours need to be disseminated to enable professionals and policymakers to understand better how interprofessionalism can improve health and social care.

Each approach can offer benefits and opportunities to investigate IPECP. Regardless of the approach, high-quality ENQUIRE is achievable as long as key principles associated with each approach are adhered to.

Reflective Questions for the Reader

- What IPECP activities are you engaged in within your contexts?
- What IPECP questions, issues or outcomes do you want to investigate?
- Can you address the question or issue through ENQUIRE?
- Who can you collaborate with?
- What resources do you need to undertake ENQUIRE?
- If a tool is required, what tool can help you with ENQUIRE?
- How will you share your findings, and who will you share them with?

References

1. Anderson ES. Evaluating interprofessional education: an important step to improving practice and influencing policy. J Taibah Univ Med Sci. 2016;11(6):571–8., ISSN 1658-3612. https://doi.org/10.1016/j.jtumed.2016.08.012.
2. Barroga E, Matanguihan GJ. A practical guide to writing quantitative and qualitative research questions and hypotheses in scholarly articles. J Korean Med Sci. 2022;37(16):e121. https://doi.org/10.3346/jkms.2022.37.e121.
3. Batalden PB, Davidoff F. What is "quality improvement", and how can it transform healthcare? Qual Safety Health Care. 2007;16(1):2–3. https://doi.org/10.1136/qshc.2006.022046.
4. Bowman C, Paal P, Brandstötter C, Cordina M. Evidence of successful interprofessional education programs—models, barriers, facilitators and success: a systematic review of European studies. J Health Organ Manag. 2023;37(8):526–41. https://doi.org/10.1108/JHOM-04-2022-0115.
5. Brown A, Grierson L. There are two sides to the same coin: quality improvement and program evaluation in health professions education. J Eval Clin Pract. 2022;28(1):3–9. https://doi.org/10.1111/jep.13598.
6. De Bruin SR, Stoop A, Billings J, Leichsenring K, Ruppe G, Tram N, et al. The SUSTAIN project: a European study on improving integrated care for older people living at home. Int J Integr Care. 2018;18(1):61–12. https://doi.org/10.5334/ijic.3090.
7. Durning SJ, Hemmer PA. Program evaluation. In: Ende J, editor. ACP teaching internal medicine. Philadelphia: American College of Physicians; 2010.
8. Green J, Thorogood N. Qualitative methods for health research. 4th ed. Sage Publications; 2018.
9. Glover Williams A, Tuvey S, McBain H, et al. Perinatal excellence to reduce injury in preterm birth (PERIPrem) through quality improvement. BMJ Open Quality. 2022;11:e001904. https://doi.org/10.1136/bmjoq-2022-001904.
10. Jones B, Vaux E, Olsson-Brown A. How to get started in quality improvement. BMJ. 2019:k5408. https://doi.org/10.1136/bmj.k5437.
11. Kirkpatrick JD, Kirkpatrick WK. Kirkpatrick's four levels of training evaluation. Alexandira: ATD Press; 2016.
12. Kyriacou Georgiou M, Merkouris A, Hadjibalassi M, et al. Correlation Between Teamwork and Patient Safety in a Tertiary Hospital in Cyprus. Cureus 13(11). 2021. e19244. https://doi.org/10.7759/cureus.19244.
13. Lackie K, Murphy GT. The impact of interprofessional collaboration on productivity: important considerations in health human resources planning. J Interprof Educ Pract. 2020;21:100375. https://doi.org/10.1016/j.xjep.2020.100375.
14. Lynn J, Baily M, Bottrell M, Jennings B, Levine R, Davidoff F, Casarett D, Corrigan J, Fox E, Wynia M, Agich G, O'Kane M, Speroff T, Schyve P, Batalden P, Tunis S, Berlinger N, Cronenwett L, Fitzmaurice J, James B. The ethics of using quality improvement methods in health care. Ann Intern Med. 2007;146:666–73. https://doi.org/10.7326/0003-4819-146-9-200705010-00155.
15. Mileder LP, Schwaberger B, Baik-Schneditz N, et al. Sustained decrease in latent safety threats through regular interprofessional in situ simulation training of neonatal emergencies. BMJ Open Qual. 2023;12:e002567. https://doi.org/10.1136/bmjoq-2023-002567.
16. Newhouse RP, Pettit JC, Poe S, Rocco L. The slippery slope: differentiating between quality improvement and research. J Nurs Adm. 2006;36(4):211–9. https://doi.org/10.1097/00005110-200604000-00011.
17. Ogrinc G, Davies L, Goodman D, et al. SQUIRE 2.0 (standards for QUality improvement reporting excellence): revised publication guidelines from a detailed consensus process. BMJ Qual Saf. 2016;25:986–92.
18. Ogrinc G, Armstrong GE, Dolansky MA, Singh MK, Davies L. SQUIRE-EDU (standards for QUality improvement reporting excellence in education): publication guidelines

for educational improvement. Acad Med. 2019;94(10):1461–70. https://doi.org/10.1097/ACM.0000000000002750. PMID: 30998575; PMCID: PMC6760810
19. Reeves S, Barr H. Twelve steps to evaluating interprofessional education. J Taibah Univ Med Sci. 2016;11(6):601–5., ISSN 1658-3612. https://doi.org/10.1016/j.jtumed.2016.10.012.
20. Reeves S, Boet S, Zierler B, Kitto S. Interprofessional education and practice guide no. 3: evaluating interprofessional education. J Interprof Care. 2015;29(4):305–12. https://doi.org/10.3109/13561820.2014.1003637.
21. Ruebling I, Eggenberger T, Frost JS, Gazenfried E, Greer A, Khalili H, et al. Interprofessional collaboration: a public policy healthcare transformation call for action. J Interprof Educ Pract. 2023;33:100675. ISSN 2405-4526. https://doi.org/10.1016/j.xjep.2023.100675.
22. Svobodová V, Maršálková H, Volevach E, et al. Simulation-based team training improves door-to-needle time for intravenous thrombolysis. BMJ Open Qual. 2023;12:e002107. https://doi.org/10.1136/bmjoq-2022-002107.
23. Tully V, Al-Salti S, Arnold A, Botros S, Campbell I, Fane R, Rowe I, Strath A, Davey P. Interprofessional, student-led intervention to improve insulin prescribing to patients in an acute surgical receiving unit. BMJ Open Qual. 2018;7(2):e000305. https://doi.org/10.1136/bmjoq-2017-000305.
24. Xyrichis A, Reeves S, Zwarenstein M. Examining the nature of interprofessional practice: An initial framework validation and creation of the InterProfessional Activity Classification Tool (InterPACT). J Interprof Care. 2018;32(4):416–25. https://doi.org/10.1080/13561820.2017.1408576.

Veronica O'Carroll a qualified nurse, is a Senior Lecturer and Director of Postgraduate Teaching at the School of Medicine, University of St Andrews, Scotland. Since 2007, she has led the design and implementation of several initiatives to develop interprofessional education for the health and social care workforce, as well as for students learning within the practice placement settings. Her research relates to interprofessional education and collaborative practice. She is an Associate Editor for the *Journal of Interprofessional Care* and a board member of the Centre for Advancement of Interprofessional Education (CAIPE).

Lisa-Christin Wetzlmair-Kephart a qualified occupational therapist, worked in an Austrian secondary care setting before completing her PhD at the School of Medicine, University of St Andrews, Scotland, in 2023. Her main research areas involve digital health and experiences with interprofessional education and collaborative practice. Applying mixed methods and a phenomenological research design, Lisa explores how patient experiences can facilitate the co-development of a digital health curriculum for healthcare professional students. She is the Vice-President of Finance for the Council of Occupational Therapists for the European Countries (COTEC).

Noreen O'Leary a qualified speech and language therapist, completed her PhD at the School of Allied Health, University of Limerick, in 2021. Her research relates to practice-based interprofessional education and is influenced by principles of Public Patient Involvement. Noreen works in the Health Professions Education Centre at the Royal College of Surgeons in Ireland, cultivating an interest in women's and maternal health. Other research interests include professional identity formation, pedagogical theories and qualitative research methodologies.

Marion Huber is a qualified Physiotherapist, Psychologist and Neuroscientist. She leads the Interprofessional Learning and Practice Unit of the Institute of Public Health at the Department of Health Sciences at the Zurich University of Applied Sciences.

Her research focuses on competence development for interprofessional collaboration and the competence development of teachers who design interprofessional learning settings, both classroom-based and clinical settings. Methodologically, the focus is on mixed-method designs.

Making Healthcare Safer: Improving Outcomes for Service Users

Elizabeth Anderson and Ane Johannessen

Abbreviations

CAIPE	Centre for the Advancement of Interprofessional Education UK
CP	Collaborative Practice
GPs	General Practitioners
HEIs	Higher Education Institutions
HVL	Western Norway University of Applied Sciences
IPE	Interprofessional education
IPL	Interprofessional learning
IPP	Interprofessional practice
JET	Joint Education Team
QI	Quality Improvement
SEIPS	System Engineering Iitative for Patient Safety
TVEPS	Centre for Interprofessional Workplace Learning (*Norwegian acronym for Senter for tverrprofesjonell samarbeidslæring)*
UiB	University of Bergen
WHO	World Health Organization

E. Anderson (✉)
Leicester Medical School, School of Medical Sciences, University of Leicester, Leicester, UK
e-mail: esa1@leicester.ac.uk

A. Johannessen
Department of Global Public Health and Primary Care, University of Bergen,
Bergen, Norway
e-mail: Ane.Johannessen@uib.no

A. Xyrichis et al. (eds.), *Building Bridges: A European Perspective on Interprofessional Education, Practice, Policy and Research*,
https://doi.org/10.1007/978-3-032-23222-9_4

Introduction

When planning interprofessional education (IPE), educational designers focus heavily on bringing students together to learn about the roles and responsibilities of the caring professions, considering learning with, from and about each other [11]. They may fail to focus on the final section of the definition of IPE which states that this learning should aim to '…improve the quality of care' [11] or 'to improve health outcomes' [40]. Learning to be an interprofessional practitioner is learning about how to collaborate. Collaborative practice (CP) results in better patient outcomes, because all practitioners work in a connected way with the patient and family at the centre of care plans and delivery.

In this chapter, we share European contributions on IPE that focus on the final stage of the definition of IPE and seek to improve safety outcomes for patients. We are mindful of the WHO directives, which state that all training healthcare practitioners should receive learning on patient safety [40, 41]. Interprofessional learning (IPL) for interprofessional teamwork and communication was perceived as essential across pre- and post-registration curricula;

> *At the heart of IPE is the preparation of future practitioners for effective team-based practice, by bringing students from different disciplines together during their undergraduate education to learn from and with each other. This helps students learn to appreciate and respect the different roles of health professionals before they have joined specific professional groups themselves* ([40], p. 147).

These WHO directives draw attention to the complexity of modern team-based health and social care delivery. Working in teams is challenging because it involves many highly trained individuals from different backgrounds and perspectives, yet together, they must coordinate care delivery. In the main, they are asked to do this within a complex social network. This can be hard when working in the same clinical environment, but often the immediate patient team is separate from the wider collaborative team or network [36]. Team working lies at the heart of excellent patient care [38]. As well as working effectively to deliver care, team members are required to support and care for each other if team working is to flourish [18, 27]. Effective team working and its component of interprofessional communication are now seen as causal factors for unsafe care leading to serious errors [15]. These mistakes are understood to relate to *human factors,* or human fallibility, sometimes caused by challenges in the work environment, and to *systems* failures which prevent excellent practice [14, 39].

Bringing students together for a deeper understanding of the role of collaboration in quality and safe care remains an important objective for IPE. Here, we share examples of IPE designed to advance interprofessional safe practice to inspire IPE leaders to have more conversations about learning that improves the quality outcomes for service users. At the same time, this learning helps students appreciate that team working is not easy, giving them insights into the realities of complex everyday practice.

We share: (i) Patient safety context relevant for IPE, and (ii) European examples of where safe practice is advanced through IPE.

Patient Safety and Interprofessional Education

Background and Context of Patient Safety Learning

Improving the safety of patients is a fundamental requirement and responsibility of all those who work in health and social care. Although medical error has been described and studied for centuries, it is only in the last twenty years that we have begun to focus on contributory factors. In 1999, a report from the USA sent shock waves worldwide. This report highlighted the extent of possible error in everyday healthcare delivery, stating that at that time 10% of all care could result in error or harm [21]; this figure remains similar [28, 31]. At the same time, in the UK, the report 'An organisation with a Memory', described a similar picture of persistent patient safety error [17].

Reports of unsafe care continue across Europe [7, 13, 16, 30, 37]. In the UK, following the Francis report in 2013, Don Berwick set out a plan for improving patient safety in which better learning for collaborative working was emphasised, along with greater-patient involvement, improved leadership and collaborative networks to promote safety [9]. The emergence of IPL in the UK was propelled 20 years ago by a report on poor teamworking and hierarchical systems at Bristol Royal Infirmary neonatal surgical unit and sadly has been emphasised again more recently within maternity care [22, 30]. In a recent study across emergency departments in 26 European countries, the need for well-functioning teamwork with efficient collaboration was emphasised as the major factor to improve patient safety [32].

Learning about patient safety remains central to pre- and post-registration curriculum and for continuous professional development. Much of this learning should be delivered interprofessionally or at the very least as shared or common learning [3, 24]. The content of key knowledge and theory can only be fully understood from within practice. This is because everyday practice has many competing pressures and understanding these can only come from immersion into the realities of delivering care, whether in the community or acute care setting.

Patient safety is described in the academic literature as having two vantage points, namely 'Safety I' and 'Safety II':

First, *Safety I* relates to learning from mistakes, looking back at what has happened and asking 'why?'. This analytical approach was underpinned by the seminal work of James Reason and the Swiss Cheese Model [34]. The model refers to errors as '*Active Failures*' illustrated as the holes in the layers of a Swiss cheese.

Each hole is caused by incorrect human actions, for example, slips, lapses, mistakes and violations, which erode through the protective barriers put in place to prevent error. In the main, small isolated errors are containable, but it is when several errors (holes) align that serious incidents occur. Alignment is seen to arise because of '*Latent Conditions*' in the design of a system, such as poor training, inadequate supervision, ineffective communications, inadequate staffing, equipment and machinery design. The work of 'Safety I', has led to a greater appreciation of the following:

- *Human factors*, the science that explains how errors involving human actions occur. It applies to understanding human limitations in a working context. In drawing upon relevant concepts and considering their alignment to IPE, we draw our readers' attention to the System Engineering Initiative for Patient Safety (SEIPS) Model, a framework for understanding outcomes within complex socio-technical systems (Table 1) [19, 20]. These principles for learning directly relate to the core values of interprofessional practice and collaborative working as they are relational, patient-centred and are concerned with how practitioners work together.
- *Systems thinking*, exploring the context of care delivery. The systems approach to safety focuses not on the performance of individual members of staff, but the way work is constructed, managed and supported. Many argue that if we work in flawed systems, then it is the system that contributes to error [14]; however, this does not mean that practitioners are not individually accountable for their actions.

Table 1 Human factors[a] system engineering imitative for patient safety SEIPS model

Interpersonal aspects of human factors	
Human factors collective	*Implication for interprofessional learning*
Team working and its constituents—be kind, care, respect others, welcome different perspectives, communication, listen, think about how you send and receive messages Interprofessional communication is an aspect of how people work in a team and share relevant information with each other, and importantly with the patient and their family Leadership is another constituent of team working, and today we ask for people to have collaborative or collective leadership competence to lead across professions	Team working is the medium for collaboration. Teams differ in structure depending on the type of work. In learning situations, each profession or team member learns how to work with the other, share and navigate roles to support patient outcomes. In addition, teams require to have effective mechanisms for oral, written and electronic information sharing and for wider team debate and discussion. Interprofessional communication is important for safe practice and an important driver for IPL. Leaders today are expected to be collaborative, collective and compassionate, seeing and valuing the connections between and across professions
Human factors personal characteristics	*Implication for interprofessional learning*

(continued)

Table 1 (continued)

Psychological state: tired, unwell, lacking sleep or food, stress—must be managed and understood Personal preferences: behavioural responses Cognitive processes: decision making and bias, the tricks our brains can play on us, memory, attention! Doing the task: all must complete profession-specific work	Different differences must be understood and considered within relational work. Learning theories on personality and team working roles and attributes help learners to understand the challenges for these human factors. Hierarchy that impacts effective working must be removed
Environment aspects of human factors	
Human factors—the context of where	*Implication for interprofessional learning*
Physical layout: design of equipment Ambient environment—lighting, temperature Culture: the environment for effective working together Clutter, tidiness, clean	Working with others depends on shared values adopted by all the team and open cultures where everyone feels safe (psychological safety). Together teams can play a huge role in enabling practitioners to feel safe to speak up for optimal effective working
Doing the job aspects of human factors	
Human factors—policy, procedures and doing the right job	*Implication for interprofessional learning*
Difficulty Complexity Sequence Competence Tools and technology	Within the era of integrated care job role substitution, workforce pressures might mean several practitioners function at the same level or work space and within a learning context. Students need to understand how to make the team function, welcome new members to the team and negotiate roles
Human factors—system/organisation	
Human factors—interactional within the system	*Implication for interprofessional learning*
Time, space, resource, scheduling, staffing, training, organisational values, communications infrastructure, roles and responsibilities, etc.	While reforming the workforce is policy driven in today's era of integrated care, students must learn what this means to practice within a system. Team negotiated working might find new solutions for improving the outcomes for patients. Asking is there another way to do this? And so on…

[a]We acknowledge the SEIPS Model:
Holden and Carayon [20]

Rarely are serious patient safety incidents the result of just one error from a single profession. They mostly involve a set of situations, linking human factors with systems factors in the working environment. Reason's work sought to align human factors in the midst of systems factors.

To overcome these errors, modern care seeks to implement Quality Improvement (QI), whereby all practitioners are asked to constantly seek and implement improvements in the services they provide. The responsibility for QI should not lie with one group of healthcare professionals but should be a shared responsibility across professions. It is now an imperative that all practitioners have a strong understanding of QI and its application in health and social care delivery. Batalden, one of the forefathers of QI in healthcare, aptly stated, '*In healthcare everyone has two jobs: to do your work and to improve it*' p. 3 [8]. We would advocate for IPE aligned to QI projects.

Second, Safety II looks forward and focuses on how everyday clinical work, for the vast majority of care delivery, is safe. Safety II starts by understanding how care usually goes right, instead of searching for specific causes that only explain when care has failed [10]. Developing a culture of respect and psychological safety is essential for Safety II, as it relies on practitioner support and a positive culture where concerns can be shared. Systems thinking also applies in Safety II; however, this is more about adjusting work done prior to, during or following a clinical moment. People make sensible adjustments according to the demands of the situation and as systems continue to develop and introduce more complexity to the clinical context, these adjustments become increasingly important to maintaining acceptable and safe performance. This allows for variability rather than bimodality as practitioners can be flexible and adaptive, rather than following precisely what was expected. Complex Adaptive Systems rely on *Workarounds* and *Trade-offs* because the working environment is increasingly unpredictable. This means that the routines that work well today may not work well tomorrow, and we should pay attention to how things work well. Understanding Safety II requires an understanding of the realities of everyday clinical practice.

Safety I and Safety II offer a plethora of possible IPL opportunities to propel safe practice.

Summary

Patient safety curriculum content offers huge potential for IPL. These may be from QI projects, or from shared exploration of the constituents of safe practice, effective communication, team working, role exchange functioning and so on. Despite patient safety having roots in the values of IPL and CP, immersing healthcare students in real-world complexity remains rare in Europe (see Table 2). Our findings exclude

Table 2 Patient safety examples of interprofessional learning in Europe

Patient safety issue	Summary of the IPE	Pre or post registration	Country	Publication details
Patient-centred care: Teams and role functions	Students improved their understanding of role functioning and professional identity and contributed together to patient-centred care	Pre-registration	Sweden and Denmark	Jakobsen D. An overview of pedagogy and organisation in clinical interprofessional training units in Sweden and Denmark. J Interprof Care. 2016;30(2):156–64. https://doi.org/10.3109/13561820.2015.1110690
Collaborative practice	Students supported for delivery care in a real clinical environment, advancing their understanding of collaborative practice	Pre-registration	Denmark	Jakobsen F, Hansen J. Spreading the concept: an attempt to translate an interprofessional clinical placement across a Danish hospital. J Interprof Care. 2014;28(5):407–12. https://doi.org/10.3109/13561820.2014.900479
Quality improvement	A programme to encourage action-learning based on applying quality improvement's methodology to make changes to improve practice	Post-registration	UK	Slater BL, et al. Training and action for patient safety: embedding interprofessional education for patient safety within an improvement methodology. J Contin Educ Health Prof. 2012;32(2):80–89
Patient-centred care: teams and role functioning	Students contribute together to run a post-operative ward in which patients report improved care. Contributions to all aspects of ward functioning for safe delivery of care	Pre-registration	Sweden	Hallin K, et al. Effects of interprofessional education on patient perceived quality of care. Med Teacher. 2011;33(1):e22–6. https://doi.org/10.3109/0142159X.2011.530314

(continued)

Table 2 (continued)

Patient safety issue	Summary of the IPE	Pre or post registration	Country	Publication details
Communication	Communication training for doctors and nurses in a cancer care ward to improve the outcomes for patients	Post-registration	Netherlands	Visser A, Wysmans M. Improving patient education by an in-service communication training for health care providers at a cancer ward: communication climate, patient satisfaction and the need of lasting implementation. Patient Educ Counsell. 2010;78:402–8
Team working collaborative competence Ability to manage clinical work	Learning to work in a team and run a ward	Pre-registration	Sweden	Hallin K, Kiessling A, Waldner A, Henriksson P. Active interprofessional education in a patient-based setting increases perceived collaborative and professional competence. Med Teacher. 2009;31(2):151–7. https://doi.org/10.1080/01421590802216258
Team working skills: Patient facing clinical work	Students work together to run a ward in a client-facing experience: Realistic experiences of collaboration in a clinical real-world legitimate environment	Pre-registration	Sweden	Lidskog M, Löfmark A, Ahlström G. Learning through participating on an interprofessional training ward. J Interprof Care. 2009;23(5):486–97. https://doi.org/10.1080/13561820902921878
Team functioning	A facilitated team development programme for clinical teams to advance their understanding of effective teamworking	Post-registration	UK	Watts F, et al. Introducing a post-registration interprofessional learning programme for healthcare teams. Med Teacher. 2007;29(5):443–9. https://doi.org/10.1080/01421590701513706

simulated learning as this is the focus of a different chapter. We note that simulation can be rooted in safety practice [1]. This type of learning may not immediately impact patient outcomes, although students may go on to practice more safely because of this learning.

European Examples of Interprofessional Education Advancing Patient Outcomes

We share two models of IPE designed to impact on patient outcomes and help students learn about the challenge of providing safe and complex care. These models unpack teamwork, interprofessional communication, roles and responsibilities, and systems thinking, and can lead to deeper appreciation of the value of interprofessional practice (IPP).

The UK-Leicester Model of Practice-Based Interprofessional Learning

The Leicester Model arose from the early beginnings of modern interprofessional community health and social care centres in the UK. In the late 1990s, these new centres were seen as essential to tackle the challenges of care delivery, especially in areas of disadvantage where populations were experiencing inequity. The emergence of specifically designed new community centres to bring together many health and social care practitioners was seen as the way forward and became widely adopted as best practice. Learning to help students to understand how to work in these new interprofessional centres followed; initially understood as multiprofessional learning. The first iterations of the Leicester Model arose from co-creation of the learning with students, clinical faculty and the local population where it was first applied [25].

From these early beginnings and following further understandings of IPL, a learning model for practice-based IPL evolved. The model was first adopted in the community and then applied within acute care settings [5, 26]. While the initial learning outcomes were focused on appreciation of interprofessional solutions to tackle poverty and disadvantage, later adoptions of the model focused on team working in mental health, understanding discharge processes and the management of safe prescribing. In essence, the model can be applied into any clinical setting where a team of practitioners make shared decisions in the midst of complexity and for bringing the patient and family to the centre of team working, for example, in stroke recovery [2]. Complexity here refers to patients with many comorbidities requiring constant healthcare management, but also where the patient may also require social care support.

What Does the Model State

Placing IPE into a practice setting requires support and commitment by all those involved. The following points are integral to the model's success and for anyone seeking to adapt or adopt this IPL model. These include the following:

- High-level stakeholder partnerships for sustainability, resource allocation and support.
- An organisational infrastructure, including new practice-aligned teaching roles. These coordinators go between and liaise with clinical practice teams and the Higher Education Institutions (HEIs).
- An understanding of IPE by the clinical team hosting and supporting the interprofessional student learning teams, including appreciation of how IPL occurs with alignment to pedagogic theory.
- Active engagement with ethical principles to support patients who commit to being partners and engage with the IPL.
- An ability to seek understandings of real-world clinical contexts, seeking authenticity for all the different relevant practitioner students involved.
- Time-tabled support within each profession's curriculum.
- The willingness of the actual practice team to ensure the cycle of learning takes place and is completed, enabling improvements to patient outcomes to be highlighted, understood and taken forward, even where they as practitioners might have missed important pieces of clinical work.
- Sign up by all participating health and social care schools to the same assessment methods applicable to all students [2].

The first step is to identify clinical teams where students can be enabled to learn together. The clinical team receiving the student team must be aware that their clinical work will be scrutinised and be willing to work with student challenges to their practice. The student findings are likely to lead to improvements in care and benefit the patient. In some instances, the clinical teams will need to support the student teams' nativity when the students identify concerns that are in fact good practice. The practice team, therefore, needs to be sensitive, patient and willing to help students learn about everyday team-based practice issues. All of this requires that the clinical team identify time to come alongside the student team to support their learning. This might also mean identifying suitable patients for the students to work with, which might take time as the patients need to be consented to participate. Clinical placement leads must work out authenticity issues, concerning which students should be aligned to the learning and at which stage in their mid-to-late training. The students require some understanding of what their own profession contributes to care delivery.

The steps of the learning cycle can be seen in Fig. 1. The students who take part could be working in the chosen clinical area, for example, on a mental health placement, or could be directed to join students who are learning in this clinical site (for example, in one iteration, pharmacy students are directed to be with medical

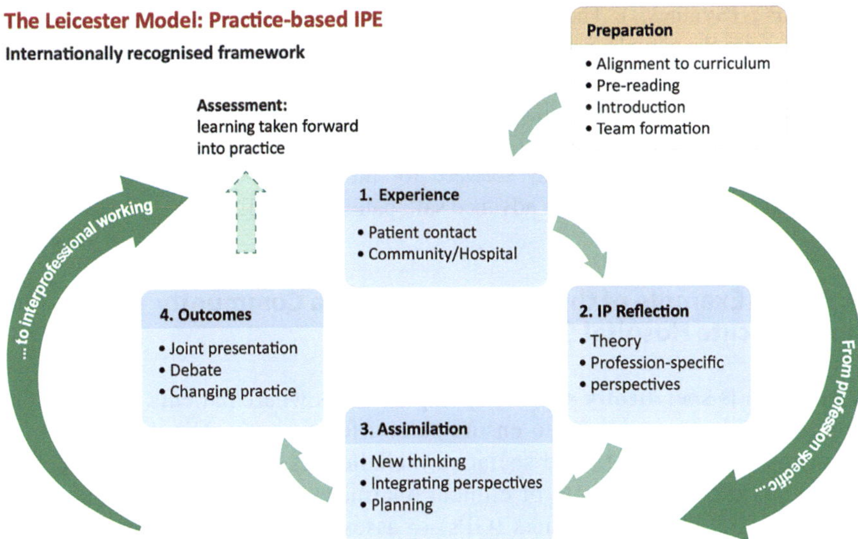

Fig. 1 Leicester model. (Leicester model drawn by ES Anderson)

students who are based and learning in primary care). Students often complete pre-course work accessible to them on their university online learning platforms or suitable repositories for learning materials. The aim and learning outcomes are aligned to interprofessional clinical aspects of care delivery. To start the process, students are brought together in training rooms adjacent to the clinical area where they are given time to understand what they will be doing together and to get to know each other, forming a working student team. They then progress through the cycle as follows:

- STEP 1 (Experience): Meeting and working with their allocated patient to complete their clinical task. This may be an analysis of the patient's prescription and the discharge plan, or assessing a patient to design or update a care plan. Once they have worked through the task with the patient, the student team analyses what the actual clinical team is doing for their patient. This might lead them to read and understand the patient notes and clinical record or to interview and discuss the patient with the relevant clinical team members.
- STEP 2 (Analysis): Together, the students have to make sense of the clinical communication they have undertaken. They need to see the issue through the eyes of the patient and the care professionals, and apply their own thinking drawing upon their profession-specific knowledge. They may do this away from the clinical setting, in a nearby room or in a corner of the ward, and they may go back to check any information, such as patient data, they have missed and subsequently realise they need.

- STEP 3 (Synthesis): The students then have to prepare their findings ready to share with the actual clinical team. This might mean agreeing a new way forward and clarifying any changes to care delivery that are required.
- STEP 4 (Feedback): In an interactive feedback session, members of the clinical team come to hear the student feedback on their work and engage in debate and discussion to agree the way forward for the patient. Often students identify changes that are required to advance safe patient care [6].

A Recent Example of the Model Applied in a Community and an Acute Hospital Setting

The model is specifically suited to complex cases where patients require input from multiple practitioners to ensure safe, effective care. These patients may present with both health and social care challenges. A recent UK application highlights the evolving role of clinical pharmacists in primary care, working alongside General Practitioners (GPs) to assess complex prescriptions. Since 2018, a new IPE initiative has brought together medical and pharmacy students at health centres. Typically working in pairs, but occasionally in groups of three or four, students engage in pre-course preparation to refresh their knowledge of STOPP/START tools and prescription reconciliation. The program begins with a classroom session before students travel to the primary care health centre. The healthcare team identifies and obtains consent from patients awaiting medication reviews, allowing the student team to visit them at home. During these visits, students assess the patient's understanding of their medications, how they manage and store them, and collaborate with the GP and other team members while reviewing patient records. The student team then evaluates whether the current prescription is appropriate or requires adjustments. After thorough analysis, they present their findings to the GP and clinical team (Anderson, Sanders, & Lakhani, in press). A similar adaptation has also been implemented in hospitals [4].

Outcomes from This Learning: Advancing Care

A Best Evidence Medical Education (BEME) review examined the impact of IPE against the six levels of the Kirkpatrick framework—Reaction, attitudes/perceptions, knowledge and skills, behaviour, organisational practice, benefits to patients/clients to identify forty-six papers [23, 35]. The Leicester Model paper was included as one of the few papers reaching the highest levels of the Kirkpatrick framework because patient care was improved as a result of the students' interprofessional work. In most versions of the model, various aspects of care are enhanced—for example, preventing poor patient discharges, adjusting prescriptions, and updating and improving care plans. Student learning is highly enriched, offering first-hand exposure to the complexities of clinical care, collaborative teamwork and the integration of clinical teams to improve care practices. More importantly, students feel valued and take pride in helping patients receive the best possible care while engaging in interprofessional learning. Assessment methods, as outlined in the referenced papers, include presentations and case study analyses.

The Norway: Bergen Model (TVEPS)

The Centre for Interprofessional Workplace Learning (TVEPS, an acronym based on the Norwegian words tverrprofesjonell samarbeidslæring) is a collaboration among several faculties at the University of Bergen (UiB) (Faculty of Medicine; Faculty of Psychology; Faculty of Law; and Faculty of Fine Art, Music and Design), Western Norway University of Applied Sciences (HVL) (Faculty of Health and Social Sciences, Faculty of Engineering and Science, and Faculty of Education, Arts, and Sports) and the municipalities of Bergen and Øygarden. The Higher Education Institutions (HEIs) contribute funding for the centre, while the municipalities provide practice placements for the students.

During its first years, TVEPS offered elective workplace-based interprofessional collaboration learning to students from the health and social care study programs at both HEIs and included approximately 40 students a year. In 2017, however, the Norwegian Ministry of Education and Research introduced a new regulation on a joint curriculum for health and social care education. In the new regulation, interprofessional collaboration is included as one of 12 compulsory learning outcomes that students must achieve during their studies. In 2018, UiB and HVL agreed that the TVEPS centre would align with this national regulation, and TVEPS-practice was consequently made compulsory for all final year health and social care students in the Bergen area, while remaining elective for students from law and teaching.

TVEPS currently encompasses 17 different study programs at UiB and HVL, with approximately 1000 students completing TVEPS-practice each year in one of more than 110 different workplaces within the municipal health and social care sector. Figure 2 provides an overview of the study programs and the workplaces included in TVEPS. The remainder of the TVEPS description will focus on workplace collaboration learning in nursing homes and home nursing services for the

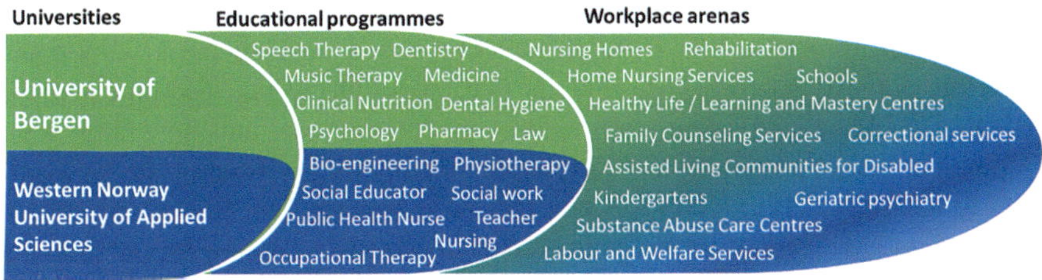

Fig. 2 Educational programs and workplaces included in TVEPS. (Designed by TVEPS)

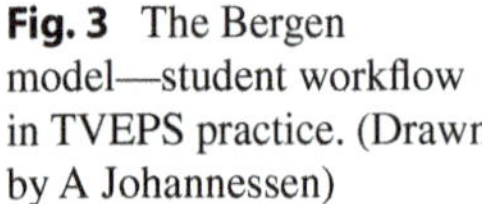

Fig. 3 The Bergen model—student workflow in TVEPS practice. (Drawn by A Johannessen)

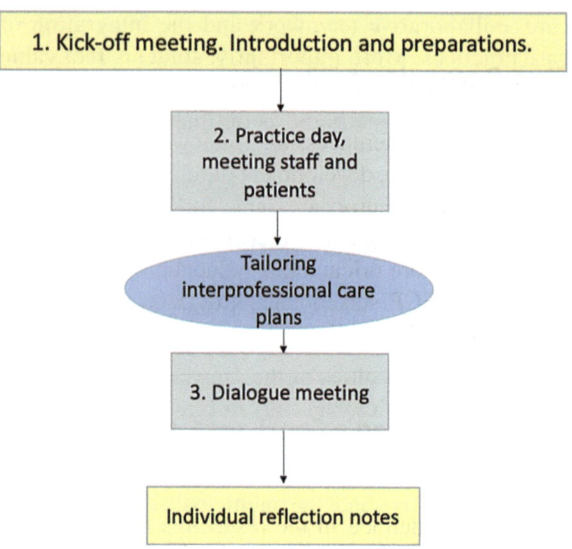

elderly. The TVEPS practice follows the same design for most workplace genres as outlined in Fig. 2, with the exception of schools and kindergartens where the students work with pedagogical tasks rather than individual patients and service users.

The TVEPS practice flow in primary healthcare workplaces is illustrated in Fig. 3. During TVEPS-practice, students are dispatched to nursing homes, home nursing services, and other primary health and social services within the municipality in interprofessional groups consisting of 4 to 5 students each. During one day in the workplace, the students meet two patients or healthcare service users. Based on background information from the workplace staff and in-depth conversations with each patient, as well as observations from the patients' domestic surroundings, students develop interprofessional care plans specifically tailored for each patient. Each plan offers a holistic assessment of the patient's life situation and proposes specific measures that the students believe will improve the patient's daily life, enhance the patient's sense of life mastery and increase their quality of life. One week after they talk to the patients, the students present their proposed care plans to the staff at the workplace, with a facilitator from TVEPS present. In this dialogue meeting, students bring fresh theoretical perspectives that intersect with the staff's experience-based knowledge, creating a dynamic learning environment where everyone benefits. After the meeting, the students revise the care plans based on suggestions for improvements that arose during the meeting, and the patients later benefit from the plans as they are incorporated into their care when TVEPS-practice is completed. The dialogue meeting in TVEPS has been referred to as a 'natural exam', yielding more permanent learning than classic classroom examination [33]. In this formative exam, the objective is not simply to test that students' have internalised their curriculum, but rather to allow them to demonstrate competencies while engaging in critical reflection and active mutual learning with the health personnel at the workplace. In times with increasing use of artificial intelligence in the production of written products, also among students, this kind of competency evaluation is also very well suited to minimise the risk of cheating—even if students have used artificial intelligence in the writing of the care plans, they will learn from it and maintain a sense of ownership of the included information as they are challenged to present and reflect upon each component together with the workplace staff.

Nisbet and co-workers have previously underlined the importance of IPE in real-life settings in a paper entitled 'untapped opportunity for learning and change' [29]. This was further emphasised in a report from the American Institute of Medicine [12]. However, despite the increasing consensus that IPE in real-life workplace settings is of particular value with its additional potential for beneficial impacts on patients and workplace staff, TVEPS-practice is one of few large-scale IPE initiatives in real-life workplace settings within primary healthcare in Europe.

The IPE model used in TVEPS provides students with interprofessional collaboration skills while simultaneously holding tangible societal value. Through TVEPS-practice, students gain practical insights, equipping them with collaboration skills to address future challenges in the health and social care sector. This IPE model aligns closely with the WHO's strategy of enhancing interprofessional collaboration to improve health services.

Workplace-based IPE in primary healthcare enhances patient safety both in the short and long term. In the long term, it equips future healthcare providers with the interprofessional insights and perspectives needed to deliver 'optimal health services', as described by the WHO. In the short term, it helps identify potential gaps in patient safety within the workplace during their TVEPS practice. Research from the TVEPS centre is ongoing in this regard, but we would like to highlight three examples here as preliminary results.

The first example is a TVEPS student group in the home nursing services that discovered how a sudden weight loss and reluctance to eat for an elderly woman was caused by an acute inflammation in the gums due to bacterial growth on her dental prosthesis. As home nursing services seldom have the luxury of having dental hygienists or dentists as part of their staff, students from these fields of study can provide observations of particular value in this type of workplace. Another example is a TVEPS student group that tailored interprofessional recommendations for preventing falls in an elderly nursing home resident with high risk of falling. As a third, more general example, TVEPS student groups often conduct comprehensive medication reviews for selected patients in the workplace, ensuring the absence of harmful drug interactions.

These examples show the potential value of workplace-based IPE from a patient safety perspective. Indeed, the primary healthcare workplaces involved in TVEPS frequently select their most complex patients/healthcare service users for the students for this very reason. Furthermore, the diversity of study programs plays a crucial role in enhancing patient safety within this interprofessional context. Involving students from diverse study programs—both those outside the workplace staff's typical competency areas and those commonly represented—enriches the workplace with fresh insights and recommendations on complex patient cases. This approach integrates knowledge from different fields while also incorporating recent theoretical updates from students trained in the staff's own disciplines. This is a win-win situation for all stakeholders, as the students at the same time learn interprofessional collaboration for the benefit of future healthcare.

Discussion

We have shared two models of practice-based IPE, which are patient-focussed and authentic in that students are preparing for the work they will be doing when qualified. The models can be adapted for both pre- and post-registration students. These types of interventions require supportive infrastructure and committed practice teams who support students to learn alongside them.

IPE requires students to learn about the roles and responsibilities of all the health and social care practitioners with appreciation of the realities of every-day complex team working. Patient safety is directly linked to complexity and human factors, including team working, and these are internationally recognised practice concerns. Ultimately, effective CP cultivates compassionate patient-centred team working, and CP improves the quality of care delivery. Practice-based IPE that can immerse students into everyday care helps students to appreciate these complexities and can result in better outcomes for the people and populations.

Recommendation and Reflection

Patient safety is closely aligned to team working and therefore IPE. This is because working together in teams is the way in which modern professional care delivery is framed. Team working is now the expected norm for all care delivery. IPE beyond the classroom must develop practice-based models that reveal the challenges for effective team working and highlight how and why interprofessional working impacts on patient care. While we offer the templates for two successful practice-based models, we understand that they will need modifications to be replicated in other contexts, we recommend these approaches for pre- post-registration curriculum.

Reflective Questions

1. In what ways can IPE help future healthcare practitioners in your context develop the skills necessary for effective team working and patient safety?
2. How might the Leicester, UK, and TVEPS Norway, models contribute to improving patient safety in everyday practice, and what challenges might arise when attempting to implement these models in different healthcare settings?

3. What are some key examples from the chapter that demonstrate how interprofessional student teams positively impact patient care outcomes, and how could these examples be applied to your own practice or education setting?
4. How can the integration of students from diverse healthcare fields enhance patient safety, and what are the potential opportunities and challenges of this approach in your setting?
5. In your opinion, what are the key factors that make IPE effective in shaping safe practice, and how can these factors be maximised in clinical environments?

References

1. Anderson ES, Bennett S. Taking a closer look at undergraduate acute care interprofessional simulations: lessons learnt. J Interprof Care. 2020;34(6):772–83. https://doi.org/10.1080/13561820.2019.1676705.
2. Anderson ES, Ford J, Kinnair DJ. Interprofessional education and practice guide no. 6: developing practice-based interprofessional learning using a short placement model. J Interprof Care. 2016a;30(4):433–40. https://doi.org/10.3109/13561820.2016.1160040.
3. Anderson ES, Gray R, Kim P. Patient safety and interprofessional education: a report of key issues from two interprofessional workshops. J Interprof Care. 2016b;31(2):154–63. https://doi.org/10.1080/13561820.2016.1261816.
4. Anderson ES, Lakhani N. Interprofessional learning on polypharmacy. Clin Teach. 2016;13:291–7. https://doi.org/10.1111/tct.12485.
5. Anderson ES, Lennox A. The Leicester model of interprofessional education: developing, delivering and learning from student voices for 10 years. J Interprof Care. 2009;23:557–73. https://doi.org/10.3109/13561820903051451.
6. Anderson ES, Thorpe LN. Students improve patient care and prepare for professional practice: an interprofessional community-based study. Med Teach. 2014;36:495–504. https://doi.org/10.3109/0142159X.2014.890703.
7. Aranaz-Andrés JM, Aibar C, Limon r, Mira JJ, Vitaller J, Agra Y, Terol E. A study of the prevalence of adverse events in primary healthcare in Spain. Eur J Pub Health. 2011;22(6):921–5. https://doi.org/10.1093/eurpub/ckr168.
8. Batalden PB, Davidoff F. What is "quality improvement" and how can it transform healthcare? Editorial BMJ Qual Saf. 2007;2007(16):2–3. https://www.ncbi.nlm.nih.gov/pmc/articles/PMC2464920/
9. Berwick D. A promise to act, a commitment to learn. Improving the safety of patients in England. The advisory Group on the Safety of Patient in England. Department of Health; 2013. https://assets.publishing.service.gov.uk/media/5a7cc74540f0b6629523bc31/Berwick_Report.pdf
10. Braithwaite J, Wears RL, Hollnagel E. Resilient health care: turning patient safety on its head. Int J Qual Health Care. 2015;27(5):418–20. https://doi.org/10.1093/intqhc/mzv063.
11. CAIPE. Interprofessional education – a definition. 2002. www.caipe.org
12. Cox M, et al. Measuring the impact of IPE on collaborative practice and patient outcomes. Institute of Medicine, 2015. J Interprof Care. 2016;30(1):1–3.
13. Deilkås ET, Bukholm G, Lindstrøm JC, et al. Monitoring adverse events in Norwegian hospitals from 2010 to 2013. BMJ Open. 2021;2015(5):e008576. https://doi.org/10.1136/bmjopen-2015-008576.
14. Dekker S, Leveson N. The systems approach to medicine: controversy and misconceptions. BMJ Qual Saf. 2015;24:7–9. https://doi.org/10.1136/bmjqs-2014-0031067.

15. Dixon-Woods M, Baker R, Charles K, et al. Culture and behaviour in the English National Health Service: overview of lessons from a large multimethod study. BMJ Qual Saf. 2015;23:106–15. https://doi.org/10.1136/bmjqs-2013-002471.
16. Francis R. The report of the mid Staffordshire NHS foundation trust public inquiry; executive summary. London: The Stationery Office; 2013. https://assets.publishing.service.gov.uk/media/5a7ba0faed915d13110607c8/0947.pdf
17. Donaldson L. An organisation with a memory. Department of Health. London. The stationery Office. 2000. https://psnet.ahrq.gov/issue/organisation-memory-report-expert-group-learning-adverse-events-nhs-chaired-chief-medical
18. Gittell JH, Godfrey M, Thistlethwaite J. Interprofessional collaborative practice and relational coordination: improving healthcare through relationships. J Interprof Care. 2013;27(3):210–3. https://doi.org/10.3109/13561820.2012.730564.
19. Holden RJ, Carayon P, Gurses AP, Hoonakker P, Schoofs Hundt A, Ozok AA, Rivera-Rodriguez AJ. SEIPS 2.0: a human factors framework for studying and improving the work of healthcare professionals and patients. Ergonomics. 2013;56(11):1669–86.
20. Holden RJ, Carayon P. SEIPS 101 and seven simple SEIPS tools. BMJ Qual Saf. 2021;30:901–10.
21. Institute of Medicine (US) Committee on Quality of Health Care in America. In: Kohn LT, Corrigan JM, Donaldson MS, editors. To err is human: building a safer health system. Washington, DC: National Academies Press (US); 2000. https://doi.org/10.17226/9728. PMID: 25077248.
22. Kennedy I. Learning from Bristol: the report of the public inquiry into children's heart surgery at the Bristol Royal Infirmary 1984–1995. London: Command Paper: CM 5207: The Stationery Office; 2001. https://www.gov.uk/government/publications/the-department-of-healths-response-to-the-report-of-the-public-inquiry-into-childrens-heart-surgery-at-the-bristol-royal-infirmary
23. Kitto S, Wondwossen Fantaye A, Davies N, McFadyen AK, Rivera J, Birch I, Barr H, Fletcher S, Fournier K, Xyrichis A. The evidence base for interprofessional education within health professions education: a protocol for an update review. J Interprof Care. 2023;37(3):515–8. https://doi.org/10.1080/13561820.2022.2097651.
24. Ladden MD, Bednash G, Stevens DP, Moore GT. Educating interprofessional learners for quality, safety and systems improvement. J Interprof Care. 2006;20(5):497–505. https://doi.org/10.1080/13561820600935543.
25. Lennox A, Petersen S. Development and evaluation of community based, multi-agency course for medical students: descriptive study. Br Med J. 1998;316:596–9.
26. Lennox A, Anderson ES. The Leicester Model of Interprofessional Education. A practical guide for implementation in health and social care. Higher Education Academy, Subject Centre Medicine, Dentistry and Veterinary Medicine Special Report 9. 2007. Access: retrieved 5th February 2024 https://www.advance-he.ac.uk/knowledge-hub/leicester-model-interprofessional-education
27. Mannion R, Smith J. Hospital culture and clinical performance: where next? BMJ Qual Saf. 2017. Published Online First: [please include Day Month Year]. https://doi.org/10.1136/bmjqs-2017-007668.
28. Nauman J, Soteriades ES, Hashim MJ, Govender R, Al Darmaki RS, Al Falasi RJ, Ojha SK, Masood-Husain S, Javaid SF, Khan MA. Global incidence and mortality trends due to adverse effects of medical treatment, 1990–2017: a systematic analysis from the global burden of diseases, injuries and risk factors study. Cureus. 2020;12(3):e7265. https://doi.org/10.7759/cureus.7265.
29. Nisbet G, Lincoln M, Dunn S. Informal interprofessional learning: an untapped opportunity for learning and change within the workplace. J Interprof Care. 2013;27(6):469–75. https://doi.org/10.3109/13561820.2013.805735.
30. Ockenden D. Findings, conclusions and essential actions from the independent review of maternity services at the Shrewsbury and Telford Hospitals NHS Trust. The Stationery Office;

2022. https://www.ockendenmaternityreview.org.uk/wp-content/uploads/2022/03/FINAL_INDEPENDENT_MATERNITY_REVIEW_OF_MATERNITY_SERVICES_REPORT.pdf
31. Panagioti M, Khan K, Keers RN, Abuzour A, Phipps D, Kontopantelis E, Bower P, Campbell S, Haneef R, Avery AJ, Ashcroft DM. Prevalence, severity, and nature of preventable patient harm across medical care settings: systematic review and meta-analysis. BMJ. 2019;366:l4185. https://doi.org/10.1136/bmj.l4185.
32. Petrino R,·Biondi C,·Castrillo LG. Healthcare professionals' perceptions of patient safety in European emergency departments: a comparative analysis of survey results. Internal Emerg Med. 2023. https://doi.org/10.1007/s11739-023-03523-1
33. Raaheim A. The exam revolution. Oslo: Gyldendal Akademisk; 2016. p. 178. ISBN: 9788205525146 [only available in Norwegian]
34. Reason J. Human error: models and management. BMJ. 2000;320:768–70. https://doi.org/10.1136/bmj.320.7237.768.
35. Reeves S, Fletcher S, Barr H, Birch I, Boet S, Davies N, et al. A BEME systematic review of the effects of interprofessional education: BEME 2016 Guide No. 39. Medical Teacher. 2016;38(7):656e668. https://doi.org/10.3109/0142159X.2016.1173663.
36. Reeves S, Xyrichis A, Zwarenstein M. Teamwork, collaboration, coordination, and networking: why we need to distinguish between different types of interprofessional practice. J Interprof Care. 2018;32(1):1–3. https://doi.org/10.1080/13561820.2017.1400150.
37. Roux B, Bezin J, Morival C, Noize C, Laroche M. Prevalence and direct costs of potentially inappropriate prescriptions in France: a population-based study. Expert Rev Pharmacoecon Outcomes Res. 2022;22(4):627–36. https://www.tandfonline.com/doi/full/10.1080/14737167.2021.1981863
38. Salas E, Shuffler ML, Thayer AL, Bedwell WL, Lazzara EH. Hum Resour Manag. 2015;54(4):599–622.
39. Waterson P, Catchpole W. Human factors in healthcare: welcome progress, but still scratching the surface. BMJ Qual Saf. 2016;25:480–4. https://doi.org/10.1136/bmjqs-2015-005074.
40. World Health Organization (WHO). Framework for action on interprofessional education and collaborative practice (WHO/HRH/HPN/10.3). Geneva: World Health Organization; 2010.
41. World Health Organization (WHO). Global competency framework for universal health coverage. Geneva: World Health Organization; 2022. https://www.who.int/publications/i/item/9789240034686

Elizabeth Anderson is Professor of Interprofessional Education at Leicester Medical School in the UK. She trained and worked as a nurse, midwife and health visitor before pursuing an academic career. She has led interprofessional education in the Midlands UK and has widely published in interprofessional education, patient safety and patient involvement. She is currently the Joint Chair of CAIPE (UK Centre for the Advancement of Interprofessional Education) and a Non-Executive Director of a UK NHS Trust.

Ane Johannessen is Professor of Epidemiology and head of TVEPS (Centre for Interprofessional Workplace Learning) at the Department of Global Public Health and Primary Care, University of Bergen, Norway. She has a particular research focus on interprofessional collaboration and workplace learning. She researches interprofessional collaboration both from a pedagogical perspective, investigating learning outcomes for students and health personnel, and from a public health perspective, investigating the potential value of interprofessional collaboration in the health and social care services for patients and society.

Interprofessional Healthcare and Workforce Policy

Christoph Golz, Mirjam Körner, and Andreas Xyrichis

Abbreviations

EIPEN	European Interprofessional Practice and Education Network
EU	European Union
HEROES	European Union-funded Joint Action on HEalth woRkfOrce to meet health challEngeS
ICM	International Confederation of Midwives
IPE	Interprofessional Education
IPECP	Interprofessional Education and Collaborative Practice
NHS	National Health Service
NIPNET	Nordic Interprofessional Network
OECD	Organization for Economic Co-operation and Development
UK	United Kingdom
WCP	World Confederation for Physical Therapy

C. Golz (✉)
Applied Research and Development in Nursing, School of Health Professions, Bern University of Applied Sciences, Bern, Switzerland
e-mail: christoph.golz@bfh.ch

M. Körner
Institute for Collaborative Practice and Leadership in Healthcare, Bern University of Applied Sciences, Bern, Switzerland
e-mail: mirjam.koerner@bfh.ch

A. Xyrichis
Faculty of Nursing, Midwifery, and Palliative Care, King's College London, London, UK
e-mail: andreas.xyrichis@kcl.ac.uk

A. Xyrichis et al. (eds.), *Building Bridges: A European Perspective on Interprofessional Education, Practice, Policy and Research*,
https://doi.org/10.1007/978-3-032-23222-9_5

Introduction

Health workforce policy is an essential part of general health policy. It is the bedrock upon which effective interprofessional education (IPE) and collaborative practice (IPCP) are built. This chapter delves into the complexities of health workforce policies across European countries, exploring how these policies shape and are shaped by the principles of IPE and IPCP. By examining variations in policies, training requirements, and regulatory frameworks, we aim to illuminate the critical connections between macro-level policy decisions and the micro-level realities of interprofessional collaboration in healthcare delivery. Understanding these connections is essential for fostering resilient, adaptable, and equitable health systems that prioritize team-based care and optimize patient outcomes through effective interprofessional practice.

The healthcare workforce includes physicians, nurses, midwives, physiotherapists, dieticians, and many more. They form the backbone of any healthcare system [31]. A well-formulated health workforce policy is crucial for the efficient functioning of the healthcare system and the provision of high-quality care [25]. Such a policy can cover key aspects such as education and training, recruitment and retention, licensing and accreditation, distribution and migration, and the working conditions of the health workforce. It also outlines strategies to address workforce shortages and ensure that the health system can adapt to the changing health needs of the population. Essentially, the health workforce policy sets out the mechanisms by which the health workforce is trained, regulated, and supported to deliver the services outlined in broader health policy [20]. Without sound health workforce policies, even the best-intentioned health policies can fail in their implementation, underscoring the importance of these policies, which are interdependent and inextricably linked.

Health and Health Workforce Policies Across European Countries

The diversity of health workforce policies in European countries reflects the diversity of languages, cultures, and administrative systems that make up the continent. Europe, with its 44 sovereign states, is subdivided into four distinct regions: eastern, western, southern, and northern Europe. Each of these regions and their respective countries exhibits a level of autonomy in their health policy formulation, reflecting the diversity of their sociopolitical landscapes. The absence of a universal health policy or a standardized health workforce policy for the entire continent is indicative of the sovereign authority of individual states, which operate independently at the national level. However, within this complex milieu, certain European nations have some similarities in terms of linguistic, cultural, and political paradigms. These similarities create fruitful ground for the potential development of uniform workforce policies. This pursuit of commonality is perhaps most evident within the confines of the European Union (EU).

The EU is currently an economic and political consortium of 28 member countries. It has its own health policy, and the policy's aim is to improve public health across member nations through financial support, legislative measures addressing transnational health threats, safeguarding patient rights in cross-border healthcare scenarios, promoting disease prevention, and fostering an overall culture of good health [9]. This intense focus on public health can be traced back to the EU's early efforts in the 1980s to combat health crises such as cancer, AIDS, and substance abuse [12]. It is essential to recognize that the EU's role in health policy primarily supplements national policies. The responsibility for implementation ultimately lies with the individual member states. Therefore, despite a shared commitment to public health within the EU, both the overarching health policy and the specific health workforce policy can vary significantly from one member state to another. This array of policies across Europe reflects the delicate balance between shared objectives and individual sovereignty that characterizes the region's approach to health workforce policy. This coexistence of two interests must be taken into account in any future efforts to find cross-border solutions.

Several factors contribute to the differences in health workforce policies among European nations, and one key aspect is the degree to which the policy is centralized or decentralized. Centralized health policy, as predominantly practiced in the United Kingdom (UK) and France, has the central government playing a significant role in setting health policies and administering health services. In the UK, the National Health Service (NHS) is a government-run entity that oversees health services across its countries [17]. Despite some regional variances, the overarching policies are coordinated at a central level, and funding is allocated from the central government's budget. Similarly, France's healthcare system is highly centralized, with policy and funding flowing from the central government. In contrast, countries with a federal structure, such as Germany, have a more decentralized approach to health policy. Each of Germany's 16 states has considerable autonomy in governing their health systems, with the central government playing a facilitating role. Consequently, health workforce policies can vary among states in Germany, reflecting unique local needs and conditions. This flexibility can be an advantage in responding to regional health challenges but can also lead to inconsistencies in healthcare provision across the country [26]. Since the 1990s, several countries have acknowledged the advantages of decentralized health systems and have introduced reforms by keeping relevant aspects centralized [23].

Another significant factor is the cultural and societal norms of each country [6]. Northern European countries, such as the Netherlands, Denmark, and Sweden, have traditionally placed a high value on social welfare and have developed healthcare systems that reflect this priority [2, 15, 28]. Their workforce policies often emphasize work-life balance, preventative healthcare, and strong social support mechanisms. In contrast, Southern European countries such as Italy and Greece, with their own cultural norms and economic challenges [27], may prioritize different aspects of their workforce policies, such as ensuring healthcare accessibility in rural areas or coping with higher levels of informal employment.

In summary, the diversity of health workforce policies in Europe is a reflection of the varied political structures, societal norms, and historical contexts of each country. Recognizing this diversity is crucial when considering pan-European health policy initiatives and understanding their implementation at the national level.

Health System Challenges Across European Countries

Despite the considerable disparities in health workforce policies among European countries, they share common challenges concerning their healthcare human resources. These challenges span the spectrum of recruitment, retention, and demographic shifts, as highlighted in a comprehensive 2022 report by the World Health Organization [31]. The current and anticipated workforce shortage is of great concern across many European nations. Projections suggest an escalating demand for healthcare professionals, accelerated by two primary factors. First, an aging population coupled with medical advancements results in an increase in longevity and a corresponding rise in complex, chronic health cases. The healthcare workforce must expand to keep pace with these evolving healthcare needs. Second, the retention of healthcare professionals is currently hampered by unappealing employment and working conditions. With the strain of long hours, high stress levels, and often inadequate remuneration, many health professionals are leaving the sector or choosing not to enter it first. These conditions erode job appeal and contribute to a shortage of new recruits entering the field. Furthermore, health disparities and accessibility issues add another layer of complexity. The uneven distribution of healthcare professionals between urban and rural areas, along with cross-border migration, presents additional challenges to maintaining a robust and evenly dispersed health workforce.

It is not without reason that the search for solutions to the recruitment of healthcare professionals and possible measures for improved job retention have increased significantly in recent years. Here, too, however, it is clear that experiences between EU countries are not being sufficiently exchanged, and each country is trying to respond to the challenges on its own [14]. However, the COVID-19 crisis forced countries to improve their cross-border cooperation. Countries have learned from this, and it seems that there is now a growing understanding of the need for cooperation, as European health ministers' conclusions are promising summarized with the title "A Europe that cares, prepares, protects: Strengthening the EU Health Union" of a recently published issue in the Journal EuroHealth [10].

In this context, interprofessional collaboration has been discussed as one of the "promising solutions" for responding to human resources for health crises, which led to the development of a Framework for Action on Interprofessional Education & Collaborative Practice by the World Health Organization [29]. One intention of the framework was to "provide policy-makers with ideas on how to implement interprofessional education and collaborative practice" ([29], p. 7). A decade has passed since the publication, and the question is now to what extent the recommendations have been recognized or implemented.

In conclusion, while there are clear differences in health workforce policies across European countries, there are also significant opportunities for learning and collaboration. By examining and understanding these differences and similarities, policymakers can develop more effective strategies to address the common challenges facing Europe's healthcare systems.

National Measures and Cross-National Initiatives

Policy, law (macro-level), organization/team (meso-level), and workforce (micro-level) policies influence the care approach as well as collaborative practices. As the need for interprofessional collaboration is undisputed, practical implementation lags behind. Among other issues, there is a lack of political and organizational incentives for collaborative practice. However, in Europe, there are a variety of regional or national efforts to implement interprofessional education and collaborative practices in healthcare.

Approach

For a European overview, we scanned the websites of political instances and institutions, e.g. ministries in the European Countries for collaborative practice and interprofessional care, to analyse the political base for collaborative practice in healthcare. The search terms used were: interprofessional healthcare policy, interprofessional collaboration / cooperation healthcare, interdisciplinary / multidisciplinary healthcare policy, interdisciplinary collaboration /cooperation healthcare, integrated care policy, multiprofessional team healthcare, healthcare policy, and healthcare centre policy. We divided the results into three categories: (1) explicitly (interprofessional care, collaborative practice) and (2) implicitly mentioned (e.g. integrated care, cooperation), as well as (3) no programs found. We do not claim to be exhaustive with our description. A systematic analysis would go beyond the scope of this chapter, and therefore, examples from different countries are given. The findings of the search can be accessed here: https://osf.io/m5kdg. The results are visualized in Fig. 1.

Interprofessional collaboration is explicitly mentioned in policy papers or statements in the following countries: Denmark, Norway, Sweden, Iceland, Belgium, Ireland, the Netherlands, Lithuania, Portugal, Switzerland, the UK, Luxembourg, and Malta. The Danish Health Quality Program states that interdisciplinary, intersectional, and coordinated care for specific chronic diseases is needed. Norway concentrated especially on interprofessional education to strengthen the interdisciplinary approach in healthcare. Better cooperation and coordination of healthcare professionals is planned through primary healthcare reform in Sweden. Belgium, Ireland, the Netherlands, Lithuania, Portugal, Luxembourg, and Malta write that providing healthcare requires a multi/interdisciplinary team approach. In the UK, the NHS promotes interprofessional collaboration as a key component of delivering

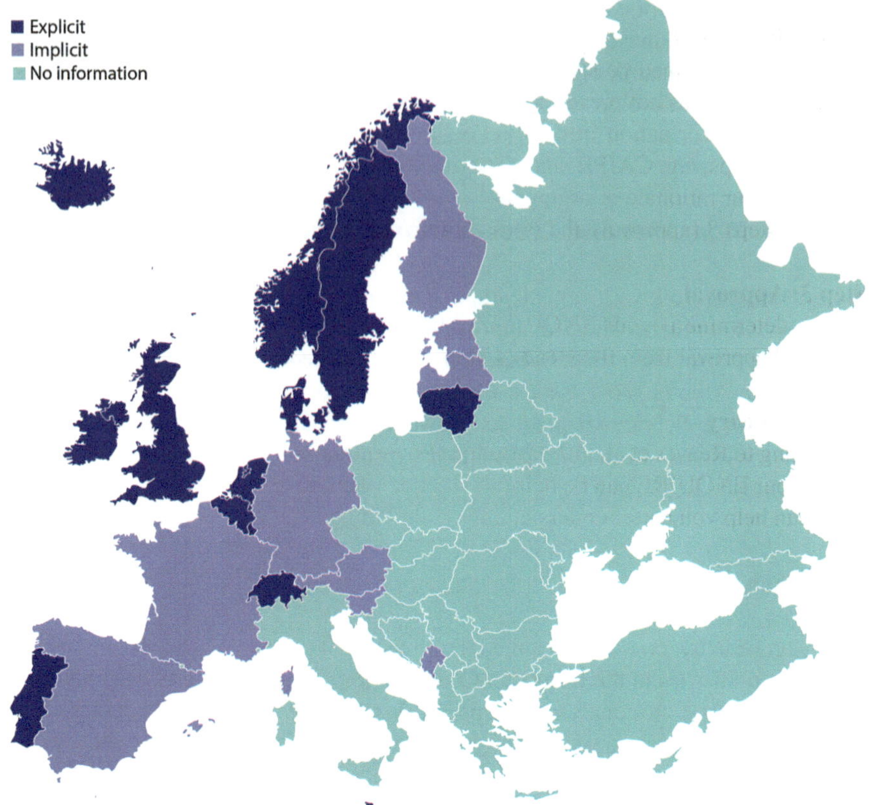

Fig. 1 Overview of European countries categorized with regard to the indication of interprofessional collaboration

integrated care. Various workforce strategies and frameworks emphasize the importance of working across professional boundaries to improve patient outcomes. The Department of Health and Social Care stated in a policy paper that it is important to enable "different parts of the health and care system to work together effectively, in a way that will improve outcomes and address inequalities" [7].

Various committees, such as professional associations, patient organizations, and health insurance companies, have acknowledged the negligence of interprofessional collaboration and the demand for sustainable implementation in practice [1]. Thus, reforms are being implemented with currently predominantly mono-professional focus on medical processes, neglecting allied-health professionals' processes [24]. There is currently no national concept for the implementation and realization of interprofessional education and collaboration. In the report of the German Council of Economic Experts of Developments in the Health Care System, the main issue is the resilience of the healthcare system. Overall, the report calls for a structural, legal, and organizational strengthening of interprofessional collaboration as a central element of sustainable healthcare. However, the focus is mainly on nurses and public health services. [3]. In their report of 2024, the interprofessional collaboration is also described as a crucial basis for quality and efficiency in care—especially in primary care and in the care of patients with multiple illnesses. Interprofessional collaboration is therefore repeatedly recommended to the Federal Minister of Health [4].

Countries such as Finland, Estonia, Latvia, Germany, France, Montenegro, Austria, Slovenia, and Spain mentioned only interprofessional collaboration implicitly. In their policy papers, they write about integrated care, health service centres, integration, and cooperation of health professionals.

This indicates that the challenge of Europe-wide measures arises from the inconsistent use of various concepts in the context of interprofessionalism, such as interdisciplinary, collaboration, integration, teamwork, or interprofessional concepts [21]. In this context, it seems that some political efforts to describe integrated care imply but do not directly mention interprofessional collaboration. However, collaboration and integration are not interchangeable concepts. Collaboration is a precondition for integration, but integration entails a more comprehensive approach that includes organizational and systemic coordination beyond collaborative practices among healthcare professionals [5]. This undifferentiated use of terms in relation to interprofessionality already describes a barrier in a Europe-wide consensus.

In addition to the various challenges, initiatives are already emerging that could form a promising basis for Europe-wide measures.

Initiatives to Strengthen Interprofessional Education and Collaborative Practice

The increasing attention and priority given to wider health workforce issues and policy in Europe is evident in the significant investment by the European Commission in the HEROES Joint Action, the largest-funded project of its kind to date. Its significance lies in the comprehensive approach taken to health workforce planning, overcoming past siloed approaches addressing individual professions in isolation.

HEROES is a European Union-funded Joint Action on HEalth woRkfOrce to meet health challEngeS, granted by the European Health and Digital Executive Agency (HaDEA) under the powers delegated by the European Commission. The grant amounts to 8.7 million € across 3 years (2023–2026), funding 51 partners across 19 countries.

The project aims to improve state-level capacity to plan for the states' health workforce. This is critical to ensure accessibility, sustainability, and resilience of healthcare services. European-funded initiatives have already paved the way for discussions about healthcare workforce planning and forecasting, with the EU Joint Action on Planning and Forecasting (JAHWF) and the SEPEN joint tender unfolding in the last decade. Other projects have also addressed the healthcare workforce, for instance, focusing on task shifting or medical deserts.

The effort of HEROES is not a solitary one. It is a collaborative endeavour, building on the existing knowledge and expertise on healthcare workforce planning to deliver actual change in national and sub-national planning and forecasting systems. The project seeks to foster cross-country learning and expertise sharing, for instance, by supporting the creation of policy or practice communities. In particular, HEROES aims to improve three areas: data, models, and skills related to healthcare workforce planning and forecasting. First, each participating country will assess the status quo in healthcare workforce planning. The project builds on existing knowledge developed in previous collaborative efforts and will update the available information based on changes that occurred in past years. Subsequently, each of these areas will be addressed in a national list of objectives to precisely define the system changes that are needed and hoped for. Finally, national action plans will be drafted to define the implementation steps and to closely monitor the signs of progress.

HEROES provides an opportunity to advance interprofessional workforce planning in Europe, with implications for workforce preparation and training, although its success remains to be seen.

In addition to this promising European collaboration, various international organizations and collaborations, such as the International Confederation of Midwives (ICM), International Council of Nurses (ICN), and World Confederation for Physical Therapy (WCPT), work to promote interprofessional collaboration globally. These organizations often develop guidelines for policies that support collaborative practice.

In response to the absence of comprehensive policies on interprofessional collaboration, various initiatives aimed at bridging these gaps have been created. The European Interprofessional Practice & Education Network (EIPEN) promotes the development and sharing of best practices in interprofessional education and collaborative practice throughout Europe. EIPEN's activities serve as a platform for professionals and educators in healthcare to exchange knowledge, thereby fostering a culture of collaboration across different health professions. This network has been important in advocating for the integration of interprofessionalism into both curricula and the clinical context, highlighting the need for a change in the health system to support collaborative practice [8]. Additionally, the INPRO project, cofunded by the European Union, exemplifies a direct action towards enhancing interprofessional collaboration within healthcare teams. This initiative focuses on creating and implementing innovative educational resources and methods to support the interprofessional development of health professionals. By doing so, INPRO aims to improve patient care outcomes through enhanced teamwork and understanding among different healthcare professionals [13]. Another initiative is the Nordic Interprofessional Network (NIPNET), which is dedicated to advancing interprofessional education and collaboration in the Nordic region. Their efforts emphasize the importance of creating preconditions for health professionals that allow them to efficiently address the complex needs of patients. NIPNETs' activities include organizing conferences, workshops, and collaborative research projects that bring together educators, practitioners, and policy makers to share experiences and strategies for successful interprofessional practice [19].

The Federal Office of Public Health in Switzerland had 2017–2020 a support programme for "interprofessionality in healthcare", which was intended to improve interprofessional cooperation in the healthcare system and increase efficiency. This is based on the assumption that interprofessional education and interprofessional practice are necessary for a changing society and healthcare system. In Germany, Robert Bosch adopted a similar approach from 2013 until 2022. With the program Operation Team and other projects, Robert Bosch Stiftung has been continuously promoting the development of interprofessional collaboration in healthcare [18]. Three 2-year periods of supporting projects allowed several teaching and continuous training projects to be completed. Furthermore, with the support of Robert Bosch Stiftung, the first interprofessional training wards in a clinical environment in Germany based on the Scandinavian model were designed and implemented in Germany. The Institute for Medical and Pharmaceutical Examination Questions (IMPP) developed a model curriculum with the aim of promoting interprofessional teaching in medical state examinations and thus its permanent curricular implementation in compulsory teaching at all medical faculties in Germany; this, however, is not yet in place. Finally, 2018–2022 doctoral scholarships to young academics for the further development of interprofessional teaching were funded by the Robert Bosch Foundation.

These initiatives, driven by the recognition of the crucial role of interprofessional collaboration in improving healthcare outcomes, underscore efforts to compensate for the lack of formal policies at the national or EU level. These examples not only highlight the innovative approaches being taken to promote interprofessional education and practice but also point to a future where collaborative care becomes the norm rather than the exception. As these networks and projects progress, they provide valuable insights that can support the development and implementation of healthcare policies.

Recommendations for a European-Wide Approach to the Development of Interprofessional Workforce Policy

As discussed in the preceding sections, workforce policy is increasingly recognized as a top priority by health decision-makers at both the European and national levels. As of January 2024, the Belgian presidency of the Council of the EU has made the health workforce one of its top priorities. To address the growing and complex health needs of Europe's citizens, interprofessional collaboration, education, training, and care delivery are emphasized as key strategies.

While European healthcare systems vary, there are also many similarities and common challenges, such as aging populations, increasing chronic diseases, and limited resources. These common concerns could be addressed more effectively and sustainably through enhanced cross-national collaboration and European coordination, which would allow for the sharing of best practices, the development of joint initiatives, and the pooling of resources.

In this section, we consolidate the preceding arguments and highlight the intricate interplay among national context, cultural factors, and healthcare system design in shaping European interprofessional health workforce policy. By examining the diversity and complexities of existing workforce policies in Europe, with a particular focus on interprofessionalism, we aim to contribute to a deeper understanding of the current landscape. Furthermore, we seek to establish principles that can guide the development of context-specific recommendations for resilient health workforce policies across Europe. This approach acknowledges the unique challenges and opportunities that exist in different countries and healthcare systems, ensuring that policies are tailored to effectively address the specific needs of each context.

Policy Framework

Internationally, the interprofessional education and collaborative practice (IPECP) space is shaped by the complexity of the socio-economic and political landscape of different countries. This has been acknowledged by Girard [11], who reflected on two conceptual models for sustainable IPECP implementation. The author combined the model of Mulvale et al. [16], which distinguished between micro-, meso-, and macro-levels. The model describes factors that can be influenced by policy makers, organizational managers, interprofessional teams, and the individual health professional. The second model is the WHO health labour market framework, which offers a more systematic approach by applying a comprehensive policy and law perspective [30]. The model Fig. 2 by Girard [11] outlines the complex process from education to practice, emphasizing policy influences at different levels, including the micro (individual), meso (institutional), and macro (systemic) levels. This model serves to facilitate a comprehensive view of IPECP from both a clinician and managerial perspective, highlighting the need for systemic approaches to foster

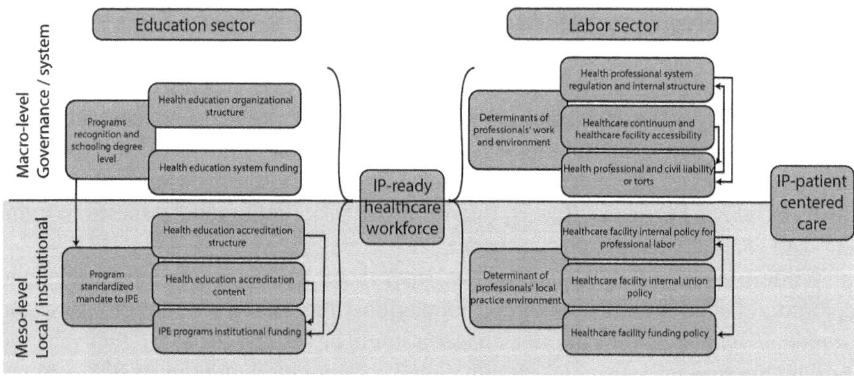

Fig. 2 Adaptation of the conceptual model by Girard [11] with focus on governance. The greyed-out area meso-level is not the focus of this chapter. IP, interprofessional; IPE, interprofessional education

collaborative practice and education among healthcare professionals. As this chapter is about the interprofessional healthcare and workforce policy, we focus on the macro-level, in which fields of action for political governance are described (Fig. 2).

Differences and Commonalities

As we pointed out earlier in this chapter, "The diversity of health workforce policies in European countries reflects the diversity of languages, cultures, and administrative systems that make up the continent". Indeed, some countries, such as France and the UK, have centralized health policies, where the central government plays a significant role in setting health policies and administering health services. In contrast, countries with a federal structure, such as Germany, have a more decentralized approach to health policy.

Another significant factor that contributes to the different approaches to health workforce policy is the cultural and societal norms of each country. Northern European countries, such as Denmark and Sweden, have traditionally placed a high value on social welfare and have developed healthcare systems that reflect this priority. Their workforce policies often emphasize work-life balance, preventative healthcare, and strong social support mechanisms. In contrast, Southern European countries such as Italy and Greece, with their own cultural norms and economic challenges, may prioritize different aspects of their workforce policies, such as ensuring healthcare accessibility in rural areas or coping with higher levels of informal employment.

There are a variety of regional and national efforts to implement interprofessional education and collaborative practice in healthcare, but there is no one-size-fits-all approach. Some countries, like Denmark, Norway, and Sweden, have explicit policies in place that support interprofessional collaboration. Others, like Finland, Estonia, and Latvia, only mention interprofessional collaboration implicitly in their policy papers. Still others, like Germany, have no national concept for the implementation and realization of interprofessional education. A key challenge to interprofessional collaboration is the inconsistent use of terms in the context of interprofessionalism. Words like interdisciplinary, collaboration, integration, teamwork, and interprofessional are often used interchangeably, which can lead to confusion and misunderstanding. Misuse of the terms in policy documents further contributes to the confusion, such as conflating teamwork, collaboration, coordination, and networking [22]. Language barriers and different translations of key terms and literature may compound these challenges.

The Opportunity

Despite the aforementioned challenges, there is a significant opportunity for countries in Europe to work together in addressing some of their common challenges. The development of national networks for IPE is a promising way forward, as is their coordination at a European and Global level through the European IPE Network (EIPEN) and the Global Confederation for IPE (Interprofessional.Global). An important development is the formation of the Pan European Academy for Interprofessional Science (henceforth, the Academy), the members of which initiated the current book.

The Academy is well-positioned to play a key role in coordinating and advancing interprofessional workforce policy across Europe through:

- Networking and Collaboration: The Academy can foster a collaborative environment where educators, researchers, clinicians, and policymakers can exchange information and ideas. This allows for a comprehensive understanding of challenges and opportunities in interprofessional practice across Europe.
- Knowledge Sharing: Through publications, summer schools, and targeted research projects, the Academy can disseminate best practices and research findings from across Europe. This knowledge base can inform policymakers on effective strategies for workforce development.
- Capacity Building: The Academy focuses on building the capacity of interprofessional scientists through professional development programs and mentorship. This can create a critical mass of experts who can advocate for and implement interprofessional policies within their respective countries.
- Pan-European Platform: By providing a platform for open communication and exchange across professions and countries, the Academy can help identify common challenges and solutions for workforce policies. This can lead to a more standardized and effective approach to interprofessional care across Europe.

Through developing a stronger network between interprofessional practitioners, policy advocates, and scientists, significant advancements could be made towards interprofessional workforce policies in Europe. The Academy, alongside other stakeholder groups, can contribute to this goal via convening working groups with policymakers and stakeholders to develop principles for policy making in this space. Moreover, education, training, and information resources to aid such working groups could be developed systematically with pan-European input on implementing interprofessional workforce models.

Awareness raising, through public education campaigns, is another important consideration, especially among the general public but also health professionals and policy makers in areas less familiar with interprofessional science. A further step in the right direction would be to encourage consistent use of interprofessional terms; examples exist in English and German languages, which could be developed in other languages. Ultimately, these and other initiatives would help to encourage dialogue among stakeholders in Europe about advancing interprofessional science, workforce policy, education and training, and ultimately interprofessional collaboration in practice.

Need for Systematic Knowledge Exchange

Effective policy making in the realm of professional workforce development requires a comprehensive understanding of successful strategies and solutions implemented across different European countries. However, as we have demonstrated, despite the interconnectedness of economies and the shared challenges faced by European countries, there exists a notable gap in the systematic sharing and exchange of best practices in Europe. While individual countries have developed innovative approaches to address specific workforce issues, these insights often remain localized, hindering the potential for broader impact and cross-country learning.

To address this gap, European collaboration and networking funds could be leveraged to prioritize systematic knowledge exchange as a cornerstone of future research efforts. By establishing platforms for sharing and exchanging best practices, policymakers and stakeholders can harness the wealth of diverse experiences and perspectives present across Europe. Then, through collaborative initiatives, such as cross-national research projects and policy forums, countries can learn from each other's successes and challenges, ultimately driving the development of more effective and sustainable workforce policies. Moreover, fostering a culture of knowledge sharing can foster greater cohesion and solidarity among European nations, facilitating collective efforts to tackle common workforce challenges and promote inclusive economic growth.

Proposed Principles for Interprofessional Workforce Policy

Based on our analysis of the current landscape, including the limitations and opportunities for the future, we propose a set of guiding principles for advancing interprofessional workforce policy that can be adapted to suit the unique context and needs of individual countries: Flexibility, Equity, Sustainability, and Accountability.

Flexibility stands as the paramount principle, recognizing that what works in one European country may not necessarily be applicable elsewhere. Policymakers must have the agility to tailor strategies and solutions to their country-specific challenges while drawing inspiration from successful practices implemented elsewhere. By embracing flexibility, countries can foster innovation and experimentation, paving the way for tailored approaches that maximize impact and sustainability.

Equity emerges as another fundamental principle for advancing professional workforce policy. Ensuring fair and inclusive policies is not only a matter of social justice but also a prerequisite for economic prosperity. Policymakers must strive to address disparities in access to education, training, and employment opportunities, particularly among marginalized and underrepresented groups. By promoting equity in interprofessional workforce development, countries can unlock the full potential of their health workforce, potentially fostering greater productivity and resilience in the face of economic uncertainty.

Sustainability serves as a critical pillar for advancing interprofessional workforce policy. Policies and initiatives must be designed with long-term viability in mind, ensuring that they not only address immediate challenges but also lay the groundwork for enduring success. Sustainable interprofessional workforce development requires strategic investment in education, training, and career advancement opportunities, as well as the creation of supportive environments that promote lifelong learning and skill development through IPE.

Accountability rounds out our proposed principles, specifically for establishing robust mechanisms for evaluation and improvement to ensure the effectiveness and efficiency of interprofessional workforce initiatives. Policymakers must set clear goals and benchmarks for workforce growth and development, regularly monitoring progress and outcomes to identify areas for refinement and optimization.

Conclusion

In conclusion, we identify a need for a more coordinated approach to interprofessional workforce policy in Europe. The diversity of health workforce policies in European countries reflects the diversity of languages, cultures, and administrative systems that make up the continent. This diversity, however, should not be a barrier to collaboration. To address the common challenges facing European health systems, such as aging populations, increasing chronic diseases, and limited resources, it is essential to develop interprofessional workforce policies that are tailored to the specific needs of each country.

Great opportunities lie ahead in Europe for developing inclusive and transferable interprofessional workforce policies. Through this chapter, we sought to raise awareness of current best practice initiatives as well as challenges to encourage further debate and dialogue. Our purpose was not to be exhaustive but rather to provide a snapshot in time from which we and others can build on. We caution that interprofessional educators, practitioners, and researchers must remain up-to-date with the latest policy developments in their specific region, as healthcare policies can evolve rapidly, and new initiatives could be introduced to enhance interprofessional collaboration.

Looking forward, we expect our messages, recommendations, and proposed principles for interprofessional workforce policy development to provide the springboard for European discussions, projects, and other collaborative initiatives. As we have argued throughout this chapter, there are opportunities for European countries to learn from each other's experiences and to collaborate on common challenges. We miss these opportunities to our peril.

Reflective Questions for Readers

- Current State Assessment: Where Does Your Country Stand?
  - Reflect on the current state of interprofessional workforce policy in your country. What are the key strengths and weaknesses?
  - Identify any gaps or areas for improvement in existing policies and practices. What challenges are hindering progress in advancing your interprofessional workforce development goals?
- Identification of Gaps: What Areas Need Improvement?
  - Reflect on the alignment between workforce policy objectives and on-the-ground realities. Are there discrepancies or disconnects that need to be addressed?
  - Examine disparities in access to education, training, and employment opportunities for the different professions. How can these disparities be mitigated to promote greater equity and inclusivity?
- Future Direction: How Can Lessons from Other Countries Inform Policy Development?
  - Explore some of the examples shared in this chapter of interprofessional workforce initiatives implemented in other countries. What lessons can you learn from these experiences?
  - Consider the potential for cross-country collaboration and knowledge exchange in advancing workforce policy goals. How can your country benefit from international partnerships and best practice sharing?
- Stakeholder Engagement: Who Should Be Involved in Shaping Interprofessional Workforce Policy?
  - Identify key stakeholders and partners with a vested interest in interprofessional workforce development in your country, including government agencies, employers, educators, and community organizations.
  - Reflect on the importance of inclusive and participatory decision-making processes in shaping workforce policy. How can you and other stakeholders collaborate effectively to co-create interprofessional workforce solutions that meet the needs of diverse populations?

References

1. Amelung V, Eble S, Sjuts R, Ballast T, Hildebrandt H, Knieps F, Lägel R, Ex P. Stand und Zukunft der inter-professionellen Zusammenarbeit in Deutschland. Medizinisch Wissenschaftliche Verlagsgesellschaft; 2020.
2. Anell A, Glenngard AH, Merkur SM. Sweden: health system review. Health Syst Transit. 2012;14(5):1–159.
3. Barth S, Böning S-L, Franke J, Groß V, Hinkler J, Hinneburg J, Hower KI, Meisel N, Müller-Rehm R, Niggemeier F, Wehrt D. Resilienz im Gesundheitswesen. Wege zur Bewältigung künftiger Krisen. Gutachten 2023. Sachverständigenrat zur Begutachtung der Entwicklung im Gesundheitswesen; 2023. https://www.svr-gesundheit.de/fileadmin/Gutachten/Gutachten_2023/Gesamtgutachten_ePDF_Final.pdf.

4. Barth S, Böning S-L, Franke J, Groß V, Hinkler J, Klaßen P, Müller-Rehm R, Niggemeier F, Räker M. Fachkräfte im Gesundheitswesen. Nachhaltiger Einsatz einer knappen Ressource. Sachverständigenrat zur Begutachtung der Entwicklung im Gesundheitswesen; 2024. https://www.svr-gesundheit.de/fileadmin/Gutachten/Gutachten_2024/2.__durchgesehene_Auflage_Gutachten_2024_Gesamt_bf_2.pdf.
5. Boon HS, Mior SA, Barnsley J, Ashbury FD, Haig R. The difference between integration and collaboration in patient care: results from key informant interviews working in multiprofessional health care teams. J Manip Physiol Ther. 2009;32(9):715–22. https://doi.org/10.1016/j.jmpt.2009.10.005.
6. Borisova LV, Martinussen PE, Rydland HT, Stornes P, Eikemo TA. Public evaluation of health services across 21 European countries: the role of culture. Scand J Public Health. 2017;45(2):132–9. https://doi.org/10.1177/1403494816685920.
7. Department of Health and Social Care. Integration and innovation: working together to improve health and social care for all—CP 381. The Department of Health and Social Care's legislative proposals for a Health and Care Bill; 2021. https://assets.publishing.service.gov.uk/media/60251afb8fa8f5037e13c418/integration-and-innovation-working-together-to-improve-health-and-social-care-for-all-web-version.pdf.
8. EIPEN. European Interprofessional Practice & Education Network. EIPEN; 2024. https://www.eipen.eu/.
9. European Council. EU health policy. European Council; 2023. https://www.consilium.europa.eu/en/policies/eu-health-policy/.
10. European Observatory on Health Systems and Policies. A Europe that cares, prepares, protects: strengthening the EU Health Union. European Observatory on Health Systems and Policies; 2023. https://eurohealthobservatory.who.int/publications/i/a-europe-that-cares-prepares-protects-strengthening-the-eu-health-union-(eurohealth).
11. Girard M-A. Interprofessional education and collaborative practice policies and law: an international review and reflective questions. Hum Resour Health. 2021;19(1):9. https://doi.org/10.1186/s12960-020-00549-w.
12. Greer SL, Rozenblum S, Fahy N, Brooks E, Jarman H, de Ruijter A, Palm W, Wismar M. Everything you always wanted to know about European Union health policies but were afraid to ask. World Health Organization. Regional Office for Europe; 2022.
13. INPRO. INPRO - Interprofessionalism in action. INPRO; 2024. https://www.inproproject.eu/.
14. Kroezen M, Dussault G, Craveiro I, Dieleman M, Jansen C, Buchan J, Barriball L, Rafferty AM, Bremner J, Sermeus W. Recruitment and retention of health professionals across Europe: a literature review and multiple case study research. Health Policy. 2015;119(12):1517–28. https://doi.org/10.1016/j.healthpol.2015.08.003.
15. Meijer M, Brabers A, De Jong J. Social context matters: the role of social support and social norms in healthcare solidarity. Eur J Pub Health. 2022;32(Supplement_3):ckac129.164. https://doi.org/10.1093/eurpub/ckac129.164.
16. Mulvale G, Embrett M, Razavi SD. 'Gearing up' to improve interprofessional collaboration in primary care: a systematic review and conceptual framework. BMC Fam Pract. 2016;17(1):83. https://doi.org/10.1186/s12875-016-0492-1.
17. NHS. What we do. NHS; 2023. https://www.england.nhs.uk/about/what-we-do/.
18. Nock L. Interprofessionelles Lehren und Lernen in Deutschland–Entwicklung und Perspektiven. Stuttgart: Robert Bosch Stiftung; 2020.
19. Interprofessional Global. Nordic Interprofessional Network of Europe. Interprofessional Global; 2024. https://interprofessional.global/scandinavia/.
20. OECD. OECD health policy studies. In: Health workforce policies in OECD countries. Right jobs, right skills, right places. OECD Publishing; 2016. https://www.oecd.org/publications/health-workforce-policies-in-oecd-countries-9789264239517-en.htm.
21. Perreault K, Careau E. Interprofessional collaboration: one or multiple realities? J Interprof Care. 2012;26(4):256–8. https://doi.org/10.3109/13561820.2011.652785.

22. Reeves S, Xyrichis A, Zwarenstein M. Teamwork, collaboration, coordination, and networking: why we need to distinguish between different types of interprofessional practice. J Interprof Care. 2018;32(1):1–3. https://doi.org/10.1080/13561820.2017.1400150.
23. Saltman R, Busse R, Figueras J. Decentralization in health care: strategies and outcomes. McGraw-Hill Education; 2006.
24. Schaeffer D, Hämel K. Kooperative Versorgungsmodelle. In: Kriwy P, Jungbauer-Gans M, editors. Handbuch Gesundheitssoziologie. Springer Fachmedien Wiesbaden; 2020. p. 463–80. https://doi.org/10.1007/978-3-658-06392-4_26.
25. Scheffler RM, Arnold DR. Projecting shortages and surpluses of doctors and nurses in the OECD: what looms ahead. Health Econ Policy Law. 2019;14(2):274–90. https://doi.org/10.1017/S174413311700055X.
26. Sreeramareddy CT, Sathyanarayana T. Decentralised versus centralised governance of health services. Cochrane Database Syst Rev. 2019;2019:CD010830. https://doi.org/10.1002/14651858.CD010830.pub2.
27. Toth F. Is there a Southern European healthcare model? West Eur Polit. 2010;33(2):325–43. https://doi.org/10.1080/01402380903538963.
28. Vrangbæk K, Christiansen T. Health policy in Denmark: leaving the decentralized welfare path? J Health Polit Policy Law. 2005;30(1–2):29–52. https://doi.org/10.1215/03616878-30-1-2-29.
29. World Health Organization. Framework for action on Interprofessional Education & Collaborative Practice. World Health Organization; 2010. https://www.who.int/publications/i/item/framework-for-action-on-interprofessional-education-collaborative-practice.
30. World Health Organization. National health workforce accounts: a handbook. World Health Organization; 2017. https://iris.who.int/bitstream/handle/10665/259360/9789241513111-eng.pdf.
31. World Health Organization. Health and care workforce in Europe: time to act. World Health Organization Regional Office for Europe; 2022. https://www.who.int/europe/publications/i/item/9789289058339.

Christoph Golz is a senior researcher at the Bern University of Applied Sciences, School of Health Professions. He leads a research team that studies working conditions and occupational health among health professionals. One main focus is developing, evaluating, and implementing effective measures during education or after graduation at work on an individual and organizational level, particularly leadership.

Mirjam Körner is the Head of the Institute for Collaborative Practice and Leadership in Healthcare as well as the Co-Head of the study program Master of Science Healthcare Leadership at Bern University of Applied Sciences, School of Health Professions. As a senior researcher, she focuses on interprofessional teamwork and team development in healthcare. Her main research area is organizational health services research. She is on the extended board of IP-Health.

Andreas Xyrichis is a Reader in Interprofessional Science at the Florence Nightingale Faculty of Nursing, Midwifery and Palliative Care, King's College London. An intensive care nurse by background, he researches interprofessional practice-based interventions for quality, safety, and equity, working with collaborators across and beyond Europe. Andreas is a Trustee of the UK Centre for the Advancement of Interprofessional Education (CAIPE), co-founder of the European Academy for Interprofessional Science, and Editor-in-Chief of the Journal of Interprofessional Care, the leading international journal in interprofessional science.

Focus on Patient Voices: Benefits for Learners and Experienced Health Professionals in Everyday Practice in Interprofessional Healthcare Settings

Andrea Glässel, Katrin Kunze, and Frank Clasemann

Abbreviations

BDO	Federal Association of Organ Transplant Recipients—Bundesverband der Organtransplantierten e. V.
DGPPN	German Society for Psychiatry and Psychotherapy, Psychosomatics & Neurology—Deutsche Gesellschaft für Psychiatrie und Psychotherapie, Psychosomatik und Nervenheilkunde e. V.
DIPEx	Database of Individual Patients' Experiences
EDP	Everyday Practice
EPF	European Patients' Forum
EX-IN	Experienced Involvement
FOPH	Federal Office of Public Health—BAG (Bundesamt für Gesundheit, Schweiz)

A. Glässel (✉)
Institute of Public Health (IPH), Interprofessional Education and Collaborative Practice Unit, Zurich University of Applied Sciences (ZHAW), Winterthur, Switzerland

Institute of Biomedical Ethics and History of Medicine (IBME), University of Zurich, Zurich, Switzerland

Digital Health Design Living Lab – DHD LL, Zurich, Switzerland
e-mail: andrea.glaessel@zhaw.ch; https://www.zhaw.ch/gesundheit; https://www.ibme.uzh.ch/en/Biomedical-Ethics/Team/Research-Fellows/Andrea-Gl%C3%A4ssel.html

K. Kunze
Bielefeld University of Sciences and Arts, Bielefeld, Germany
e-mail: katrin.kunze@hsbi.de; https://www.hsbi.de/personenverzeichnis/katrin-kunze

F. Clasemann
Patient Representative Switzerland & Germany and Physiotherapist Coach, Glarus, Zurich, Switzerland; https://www.physiotherapie-beratung-coaching.com/

A. Xyrichis et al. (eds.), *Building Bridges: A European Perspective on Interprofessional Education, Practice, Policy and Research*,
https://doi.org/10.1007/978-3-032-23222-9_6

HERG	Health Experience Research Group
HEXI	Health Experiences International
HP	Health Professionals
ICF	International Classification of Functioning, Disability and Health
IPC	Interprofessional Collaboration
IPE	Interprofessional Education
LiHPs	Learners in Health Professions
RCT	Randomized Controlled Trial
SAMW	Swiss Academy of Medical Sciences—Schweizer Akademien der Medizinischen Wissenschaften
SPO	Swiss Patient Organization
WHO	World Health Organization
ZHAW	Zurich University of Applied Sciences—Zürcher Hochschule für Angewandte Wissenschaften
ZHdK	Zurich University of Art—Zürcher Hochschule der Künste

Introduction

This chapter highlights the importance of incorporating the viewpoints of patients and their families in interprofessional collaboration (IPC) in practice and education for health professionals (HPs) from a nursing and educational perspective. This perspective frequently serves as a pivotal nexus for collaboration among diverse HPs.

Collaborative healthcare practice, according to the World Health Organization [59], occurs when multiple healthcare professionals from different professional backgrounds provide comprehensive services by working with patients, their families, caregivers, and communities to achieve the highest quality of care across settings. Achieving this standard requires developing a mindset that integrates the perspectives of patients and family members as users of healthcare. Additionally, fostering an awareness of interprofessional collaboration should begin early in HP education. Interprofessional education (IPE), traditionally centered on learning from, with, and about other professions, can be expanded to a user-integrated approach, recognizing the contributions of patients and families to care strategies and outcomes. While coordination among HPs is essential, considering the perspective of patients and family members is the decisive factor for patient- or person-centered healthcare. This approach should be embedded in both (a) HPs' everyday practice (EDP) and (b) in theoretical training for learners in healthcare professions (LiPHs).

To truly realize interprofessional collaboration (IPC), it is crucial to involve patients in the learning process not only as passive recipients of care, but also as active participants and co-educators. The chapter starts from the premise that education plays a central role in enabling this change and emphasizes the need to integrate patients as part of the healthcare team. Involving patients in educational settings for health professionals can enhance learners' understanding of real-world complexities, foster empathy, and promote the skills needed for effective IPC. In this sense, there is a call for interprofessional education to evolve to systematically incorporate lived patient experiences into interprofessional learning environments, thus strengthening the collaborative skills needed for high-quality, person-centered care. There is evidence that involving patients in the training of healthcare professionals can improve communication skills, professional attitudes, and willingness to work in teams [53], making it an essential component of interprofessional education and collaboration.

This chapter outlines best practice models based on patient, family, and patient representative experiences, providing a foundation for IPE and IPC. Reflection, a core methodological and didactic approach in the healthcare profession, serves as the central focus. Written from an interprofessional perspective—including Occupational Therapy, Physiotherapy, and patient representation—the chapter on patient voices and their meaning for IPE refers to educational, structural, and professional policies in Germany and Switzerland. Based on this context, recommendations for action are derived for initial and continuing education and training.

The purpose of this chapter is to show how LiHPs, and HPs experienced in EDP, are allowed to question the leitmotifs of their professional thinking, actions, and understanding of their role from the experiences and reports of those affected and to reflect on them in the context of interprofessional care to (further) develop their professional self-concept [47]. The starting point for LiHPs is formed by considerations and results from the interprofessional reflection of real patient voices from an interprofessional perspective. From this, initial impulses for action can be derived for healthcare practice and for learning from, about, and with one another. The key question for LiHPs is "How does the conscious inclusion of patient and family perspectives change my view of the care situation and my professional actions in my role as an HP, also in the context of intra- and interprofessional collaboration?" The chapter focuses on the perspective of patients and includes their relatives and the surrounding social environment. The term "patient-centeredness" is used as a theoretical concept. In recent years, the focus has shifted toward "person-centeredness," which engages patients in the care process as individuals with unique needs and fosters a spirit of partnership. This approach also includes HPs involved in care [41]. Besides widespread international use of person-centered questionnaires [56], open discourse enables HPs to find treatments aligned with patients' needs [25]. Since the 2000s, networks in some countries have made it possible to present patient experiences in narrative form on the Internet, thus collecting patient- or person-centered information. As indicated by Légaré et al. [34], these experiences facilitate improved communication between patients, persons, and HPs, thereby enhancing decision-making. Implementing person-centered care also requires strong communication skills [16]. The chapter addresses both students and HPs in EDP across professions like nursing, occupational and physiotherapy, speech therapy,[1] midwifery, and health promotion. Medical professionals, while part of healthcare, are not explicitly included due to differing professionalization histories. HPSs span various qualification levels and stages within lifelong learning.

[1] In Germany, speech therapy is a health profession, and in Switzerland, it is a pedagogical profession and is included in this amount in the healthcare setting under the term health professionals.

Background

Current developments in healthcare also place increasingly complex demands on the healthcare professions, such as the increase in mental disorders, changing disease spectrums, pandemics, migration, fragmentation of the healthcare system, and digitalization [37, 61, 62]. Unlike their counterparts in European and intercontinental countries, the nursing and therapy professions in Germany and Switzerland have created new opportunities for independent development through academization and professionalization. This shift has enabled them to recognize the challenges of person-centered healthcare and address them through IPC. In Germany, the academization process began about 30 years ago and is still ongoing. Less than 5% of HPs currently have a bachelor's degree [57]. In Switzerland, the health professions of nursing and therapy have been almost fully academized since 2006. This change in training also takes up an increasingly demanded goal in healthcare, namely, to strengthen person-centered care. The introduction of the International Classification of Functioning, Disability, and Health (ICF) also played a pivotal role in this regard. The underlying biopsychosocial model of the ICF prioritizes resources over deficits, incorporating individual, environmental, and participation factors [58]. This is reflected both in HP interprofessional training as explained by Moran et al. [39] and in research in both countries [4, 47]. Given the life-changing consequences for patients and their relatives, incorporating the individual, real experiences of those affected, based on their descriptions, into the care and treatment setting is becoming increasingly important [61]. Subjective narratives provide critical insight into subjective experiences, fostering HPs' reflective processes and shaping their professional self-concept [13, 20, 21].

The WHO presented the global action plan at the 74th Assembly (2021) and defined the goal for the current decade as proactively incorporating patients' perspectives and knowledge to design safe and effective healthcare. Five strategies have been formulated to prevent healthcare-triggered risks and harm to patients. The first two strategies are as follows:

(a) Involving patients, families, and civil society organizations in the joint development of policies, plans, strategies, programs, and guidelines to make healthcare safer.
(b) Learning from the experiences of patients and their families who have been exposed to unsafe care to maintain an understanding of the course of the injury and to promote the development of more effective solutions. Healthcare institutions such as clinics and doctors' offices can benefit directly from the experiences of patients and their families. Possible applications of patient involvement include improving safety-related educational materials, adapting treatment procedures, and making physical infrastructure more accessible. Barriers such as funding and resource management require resolution, and a cooperative attitude is required on both sides. International examples, such as patient advisory boards in clinical institutions, already exist. In Germany, however, a comprehensive inventory of activities and measures to promote patient safety through

patient involvement in healthcare institutions is still lacking. Placing patients at the center of healthcare systems, together with the HPs who treat them, is crucial to ensuring the quality of healthcare and patient safety. The WHO's Model Curriculum for Patient Safety highlights the relevance of patient involvement and underscores its importance as a previously underestimated resource for training in medicine and health professions [60], which was translated for the German-speaking countries (D-A-CH-Region) of Germany, Austria, and Switzerland in 2018 [11]. ICF provides the theoretical framework for a comprehensive understanding of functioning and disability from a person's perspective, which means "patients first," their families, and HPs [39].

Self-Help Organizations and Patient-Centeredness

Self-help organizations in Switzerland have a long tradition in providing support and resources for individuals facing health and social challenges. Typically structured as associations or foundations, they operate locally and focus on specific needs. Patient representatives play an important role in decision-making processes, advocating for affected persons. The Swiss Patient Organization (SPO) acts as an umbrella organization and promotes exchange between self-help organizations. The Federal Office of Public Health (FOPH) provides guidelines and support for self-help as part of the national health strategy. In research and healthcare education, self-help organizations offer valuable insights and support the development of needs-oriented programs [9].

In addition, patient organizations markedly contribute to the development and shaping of healthcare by articulating the voices and interests of patients at the political level and bringing about change. Historically, the first patient movements can be traced back to the 1960s, when organizations such as the "Deutsche Rheuma-Liga" and the "Bundesverband der Organtransplantierten e. V." (BDO) were founded in Germany. In Switzerland, similar organizations such as the "Swiss Rheumatism League" were founded in the 1970s. At the European level, patient movements began to gain importance in the 1980s, with the emergence of umbrella organizations such as the "European Patients' Forum" (EPF) in 2003, which represents the interests of patients at the European level. Internationally, patient organizations began their work even earlier, for example, with the founding of the "National Association for Retarded Citizens" in the USA in the 1950s, which campaigned for the rights of people with intellectual disabilities. Understanding patient's experiences is key to person-centered care and high-quality healthcare. However, patient experiences are multifaceted and include individual stories about illness and healthcare that complement epidemiological and health policy evidence. Interview-based research on accumulated experiences, based on narratives and possibly delivered through low-threshold digital tools or audiovisual media, as in DIPEx, can provide compelling evidence. These findings can influence policy and practice and support person-centered care [40]. To this end, staff must be sensitized to the experiences and perspectives of people with disabilities and trained to involve them in the care process. High-quality healthcare goes beyond purely medical measures, requiring empathetic, reflective communication to uphold ethical principles and address individual needs [24].

Dialogue-oriented approaches, such as active listening and empathic attitudes, support patients to actively participate in the care and decision-making process and to contribute their own experiences with their illness in partnership [14]. Comprehensible communication is crucial to conveying medical information and explaining treatment options more clearly [21], which not only leads to more accurate diagnoses and therapies but also empowers patients [36, 45]. Scholl et al.'s [45] integrated model of person-centeredness combines the following key aspects:

- Provide information to patients as a starting point to strengthen their self-empowerment.
- Offering physical and psychological support in addition to biological and medical aspects.
- Consider and consciously reflect on doctor-patient communication and the related relationship.

Interprofessional collaboration depends on fostering these principles among all healthcare disciplines, as purposeful communication strengthens therapeutic relationships and enhances patient satisfaction and treatment outcomes [31, 52], while ineffective communication can lead to misunderstandings, jeopardizing patient safety [19]. Dialogue between patients and HPs goes beyond the mere transfer of information and combines professional expertise with individual needs.

The aspects described in the integrated model suggest how to develop a basic attitude toward the patient, which must be initiated and shared among the professions involved as a starting point for successful interprofessional care. In addition, the models for person-centered action demonstrate the central role that conscious and reflective communication plays in both professional and interprofessional action. Studies have shown that purposeful communication supports therapeutic relationships, positively influences treatment outcomes, and increases patient satisfaction [31, 52], but ineffective communication can lead to misunderstandings while jeopardizing patient safety [19]. Dialogue between patients and HPs goes beyond the mere transfer of information and combines professional expertise with individual needs. Epstein and Street [21] revealed that reflective communication is the key to person-centered care that focuses on individual values and preferences. The ability to communicate purposefully and reflectively is also a key skill for interprofessional competence in practice. The same can be said for the education of interprofessional competence. This is because communication and reflection skills are also required as fundamental components in the design of IPE for health professions.

Person-centeredness has been a guiding principle of inpatient rehabilitation in both countries for many years and, in some cases, has been implemented and further developed in specific settings. As early as the mid-1990s, admission interviews were conducted jointly with patients in interprofessional teams. The aim is to spare patients repeated questions about their medical history or the course of their illness and instead to start their rehabilitation in a coordinated, collaborative, and patient-oriented manner. In contrast, only a few successful models for person-centered implementation in acute and outpatient care exist, attributed to numerous reasons. Thanks to digitalization and concept development, the first approaches are emerging, such as the pilot project on reference therapy in cooperation with the patient organization "Schlaganfall-Ring" [42]. Patient- and person-centered healthcare can also be found in some international competency frameworks for interprofessional teaching, learning, and working, including the Curtins University Interprofessional Capability Framework [7], the Canadian Interprofessional Competency Framework [10], and the Framework for Action on IPE and Collaborative Practice [59]. Some of these frameworks are interrelated and are often used to guide or conceptualize IPE [33]. To date, comparable framework recommendations or overarching concepts for the realization and implementation of IPE in health profession education in German-speaking countries remain lacking [32, 44]. Even in 2024, the active, equal, and appropriate inclusion of patients with their experiences, expectations, needs, and demands as partners in the interprofessional care team is still not commonplace, even in highly specialized and differentiated care settings such as those in Switzerland and Germany.

In summary, this chapter demonstrates the importance and deliberate inclusion of patient voices using the reflection approach as a starting point for IPE in the health professions and for experienced HPs in EDP. This is presented in an application-oriented manner using best-practice examples that were applied in an interprofessional elective module.

Approach of Reflection as Method for Lifelong Learning

In this part of the chapter, the methodological approach to including patient voices in IPE and EDP will be highlighted. Focused reflection as a method provides a basis and can be considered a didactic element for the lifelong learning of HPs. Frenk et al. [23] stated that reflection is a key competence that needs to be developed as part of education to be effectively applied in EDP. Reflection is still an ongoing element in the EDP of healthcare. Reflection offers advantages for all parties involved. Students who engage in reflection with practitioners in their work benefit directly from their experience. Practitioners, in turn, also benefit from joint reflection with students based on their questions and discussions of current knowledge from the literature.

The deliberate inclusion of patient voices in different IPE situations and formats offers great potential for the IPE and EDP of experienced HPs. While it prepares students for reality in an authentic, first-hand, perspective-rich, and at the same time blunt or sometimes "unsparing" way, it has the advantage that learners can reflect on the reports of those affected and/or their relatives and exchange ideas without having to have an immediately available and competent course of action at hand.

In his work "The Reflective Practitioner," Schön [46] emphasizes how reflection occurs in professional practice to solve problems and expand professional competence. "Reflection in action" and "reflection about action" differ. The former is a competence that comes into play in professional, case-related actions. It can be initiated and learned through "reflection on action." "Reflection on action" can be didactically accompanied in the training context and tested in various teaching–learning arrangements. In this way, the ability to reflect on action can be prepared and (further) developed [48]. Experience in training practice shows that many learners are initially somewhat perplexed and sometimes overwhelmed when they are asked to "reflect." This is because they have often not learned what exactly is meant by it and what it is supposed to achieve (ibid.). For this reason, preparing learners for reflection should be facilitated by experienced HPs in the EDP. To this end, a theory-based discussion of (self-)reflexivity can take place together with learners [17]. In addition, reflection can be incorporated into didactic teaching–learning arrangements, such as through methods that encourage reflection and reflection-based assessments. Jointly guided reflection on patient voices or experiences in the healthcare context trains learners to change their perspectives and is practical and directly relevant to their actions. This makes learning through reflection more accessible to the learners, as it is directly relatable to them, as opposed to theory-based action.

Reflection's ability to promote critical thinking makes it a crucial method of skill acquisition for LiHPs. Through reflective practice, students can gain a deeper understanding of their actions, attitudes, and values, which in turn improves their professional development and the quality of patient care [8]. Reflection is also an important tool for personal development and professional improvement, enabling active engagement with one's own experiences and beliefs. Various methods of reflection include journaling, critical (self-) discussion, or self-reflection using guiding questions. In addition to honesty and the ability to be self-critical, effective reflection requires awareness and attentiveness [38]. To engage in reflection, especially in the context of teaching and, or learning opportunities, certain framework conditions, such as time and space, are also conducive. Learning or practicing reflection requires a protected environment that is free from pressure to act and time constraints [28]. For access to reflection, the path of experience-based teaching and lifelong learning is also recommended, in which action and reflective tasks are linked to tangible practical value [5, 46].

Authentic Experiences Based on Narratives as a Starting Point for Learning from Best Practice Models

The following section presents a selection of exemplary best practice models that adopt various approaches to amplifying the voices of those affected. These examples are unified by their common approach representing authentic experiences, perspectives, and guiding principles of experts with first-hand experience in the roles of affected individuals, patients, and family members navigating the complexities of health and illness. They offer invaluable insights into the nuances of shared care and the potential for incorporating this perspective into healthcare to enhance person-centeredness [39]. The early inclusion of individual patient voices in education demonstrates added value in connection with the ability to reflect as a didactic element and an integral part of health profession education and for experienced HPs in EDP. The approach is based on the following leading perspective: How do patients' experiences alter the learner's perspective of the care situation? Among other things, the reference to prerequisites, framework conditions, responsibilities, and one's own professional identity can be reflected. The patient experiences presented can serve to reinforce or prepare for future experiences in a care setting.

Anderson et al. [2] also showed that patient involvement "is central to the values of IPE" (p. 216). Patients can support the teaching–learning process in different ways. Anderson et al. [2] suggested using them as co-tutors and mentors. Supportive infrastructure and the careful preparation of students can also enable patients to fulfill their roles in an appropriately educational and constructive manner. Overall, further research is needed to intensively explore the benefits of patient involvement and to provide a further theoretical underpinning for the inclusion of patients in training [2, 3].

EXperienced INvolvement (EX-IN): An Example of Persons' Voices from the Field of Peer Support

The EX-IN movement focuses on the psychosocial field. Its goal is to qualify people who have experienced crises and their relatives so that they can help shape mental healthcare as experts by experience. Specifically, specific training is offered to people with psychiatric experience so that they can work as recovery counselors or peer counselors in psychiatric services or as trainers in education and training. They can help others in a complementary way and in the sense of a trialogue (affected persons, relatives, and professionals) and positively influence the social image of people with psychiatric experience [22]. This is because "the use of peers has become a symbol and an instrument of change in psychiatric practice" [55, p. 276].

EX-IN emerged from a European pilot project. The movement is now widespread in the DACH region (Germany, Austria, Switzerland) and supports the development of certified qualifications in many locations, as well as the introduction of recovery coaches in other European countries [22]. The one-year training focuses on reflecting on one's own experience and acquiring skills and knowledge to work from an experiential perspective. Concepts such as salutogenesis, experience and participation, recovery, trialogue, and empowerment form the basis of the basic course [18, 54]. Apart from benefiting those affected, peer work is assumed to promote the general therapeutic climate in treatment and care facilities and to support the fight against the stigmatization and discrimination of mentally ill people [35]. Several studies have shown that involving people with experience in psychiatry in research, training, and psychiatric services can markedly contribute to improving services [1, 54]. However, the current evidence is by no means consistent. Due to the high heterogeneity of individual studies, the data in reviews can rarely be reconciled with each other. Overall, the evidence base is still considered insufficient to recommend peer work as a clear standard of care in the treatment and care of people with severe mental illnesses, even if individual studies indicate positive effects [18].

In the field of psychosocial support, the role of peer support has become increasingly significant in recent years, both within Europe and beyond. In this context, the work of UPSIDES ("Using Peer Support in Developing Empowering Mental Health Services") is worthy of note. The UPSIDES project is an international research initiative with partners in Africa, Asia, and Europe. Its objective is to enhance the global reach of peer support (cf. [27]).

Two peer mentors from Germany provide the following account: Understanding the role and responsibilities of a peer mentor is crucial. The peer counselor is part of a team that includes psychiatrists, psychologists, and more. It is crucial to refrain from encroaching upon the domain of the other person, which entails avoiding therapeutic discussions, medication advice, and trauma-related content. These matters are the purview of the professionals, as they fall within the scope of their expertise [27, p. 17].

> [...] I consider this space for open, in-depth discussions beyond therapy and without a compelling focus on solutions to be very valuable. [...] (I.H. in ibid.)

Another voice on the importance of peer work from an EX-IN recovery coach:

> The other day a peer told me that you would think I had no crisis experience. You could talk to me normally. And I thought to myself, well, they did back then, but in the clinics, you usually only find out about people when they're in bad shape. I also see it as my job to
> to sensitize people: To help the staff understand the patients, and vice versa, to help the staff understand the patients because they are just people doing their job.
> are just people doing their job. I try to mediate between the chairs.
> Mediate. (N. L. in an interview on the blog locating-your-soul. https://locating-your-soul.de/experten-durch-erfahrung-ich-bin-hoffnungstraegerin-interview-mit-einer-ex-in-genesungsbegleiterin/, 21.12.25)

DIPEx: Database for Individual Patient Experiences—An Example of Personal Voices from the Field of Academia

Nowadays, authentic patients' experiences are shared as narratives online, as accessible by DIPEx ("Database of individual Patients' Experiences") as one example of options. This database allows patients to share their illness experiences, encompassing diagnosis, treatment, and emotional, social, and psychological aspects, thus enhancing patient–professional dialog and supporting care decisions [34]. DIPEx contributes to person-centered care design [16] and serves as a valuable, quality-assured resource for patients, HPs, researchers, educators, and the public. Websites like www.hexi.ox.ac.uk/, www.healthtalk.org, https://dipex.ch/, or www.krankheitserfahrungen.de offer interview extracts in video, audio, or text. The DIPEx network spans 14 countries, including England, Germany, and the US, and covers over 100 health topics worldwide. The DIPEx network was recently renamed Health

Experiences International "HEXI" www.healthexperiencesinternational.org/ and is an association of academic and non-profit groups from around the world committed to improving understanding of health and illness experiences globally.

Founded at the University of Oxford in 2000, DIPEx uses an established qualitative research methodology outlined by the Health Experience Research Group [29, 30, 63, 64]. As a freely accessible resource, DIPEx supports patients, families, HPs, trainees, educators, and researchers, bringing real-world experiences into educational settings and enhancing practical learning from both professional and interprofessional perspectives. DIPEx brings real-world experience to learners and experienced HPs in EDP almost unfiltered, bringing first-hand insights into the classroom. Patient experiences presented as audio, video, or text are shared with learners on a theme-based basis and are accessible, understandable, and transferable to their understanding of their actions from both a professional and interprofessional perspective.

Examples are shown as a quote from a patient in a rehabilitation clinic who would have found it helpful to take her by the hand during this process to find her way around the complex setting of rehab more easily (P = Patient—I = Interviewer).

> P: "Yes, I think I can help myself, but it would have been nice to have been taken by the hand. Because otherwise you often feel a bit left alone. And I think life is a struggle anyway. But then fighting this illness is just a bigger battle. And the fact that I had to take care of everything myself was a bit annoying."
>
> I: "That means someone who would have taken you by the hand and guided you through these offers, through this variety?"
>
> P: "Yes, that's right. Because, let me tell you, I could see on this prescription that there were a thousand applications. But then I could guess: Can I only choose from the oncology group, or can I also choose from the heart group or the back group, or something? Yes, these are things like that." (Source: B.L. https://www.krankheitserfahrungen.de/module/medizinische-reha/personen/brigitte-lenz, 21.12.25)

Example of a patient's experience interacting with HPs:

> Yes, listen. Listen for a moment. And maybe even look at the patient. You also have to look each other in the eye. Listen and look into their eyes and say, okay, what do they want? Not doing other things on the side or just sitting in front of the thing and typing and typing and typing. And you sit there and talk and then he listens, he writes, he listens, but he doesn't see your facial expressions, he doesn't look you in the face, he doesn't perhaps recognize how desperate you are. You can say that, yes, but the face or the eyes also play a role. That's the case, I'll say now, with my GP today. (Source: R.S. https://www.krankheitserfahrungen.de/module/prostatakrebs/personen/reinhard-stockmann/meine-erfahrungen-9, 21.12.25)

Message from a patient to other patients in dealing with illness:

> Well, my message would be: Everyone should first come to terms with their illness themselves. Understand it deeply. And then they will surely come to the decision that they can live with it if they consider certain things. That might be my message. I mean, sure, you could also say that I should have gone for regular check-ups earlier. But I don't want to be arrogant, so everyone has to judge that for themselves. (Source: S.S. https://www.krankheitserfahrungen.de/module/darmkrebs/personen/sebastian-siemens/meine-erfahrungen, 21.12.25)

A person-centered approach is a collaborative process that actively engages the person in the consultation process to explore their narrative [25]. It uses the person's knowledge and experience to guide the interaction with HPs, thereby softening the authoritarian stance of professionals and shifting the focus to the person's autonomy.

Statement from a Patient Representative: An Example of a Patient's Voice

The following subchapter takes the form of a narrative experience report and adopts the perspective of an affected person, a patient representative, a physiotherapist, a "systems expert," a co-researcher, and an author ("At the border you reinvent yourself!"). This position on the role of patient voices in the care setting with learners and experienced therapists is presented in the form of a narrative experience report that incorporates aspects of learning and EDP.

My experiences as a patient with a permanent handicap are shaped by different perspectives: those of a therapist, coach, book author, and, of course, as a patient—or should I say, as a person.

To elucidate a scenario from my everyday life as a patient, I alternate between my various roles to compare these disparate perspectives or highlight their inconsistencies. I engage in introspective reflection. This has resulted in numerous discussions with therapists in a coaching capacity, with medical practitioners as a patient, and, not least, as a member of an ethics committee. It has enhanced my professional development as a therapist and my personal growth as an individual.

As a physiotherapist who has become a patient with a permanent disability and thus requires ongoing treatment, I have had the opportunity to engage in communication with numerous therapists in professional and interprofessional settings. Each of the aforementioned therapists exhibited a unique combination of human qualities and professional attitudes. "Meeting the patient where they are" is a core competency that should not be underestimated. However, what does it mean to "meet the patient where they are"? To respond to this question, it is first necessary to ascertain the patient's status. This necessitates an understanding of how the patient is physically and emotionally coping with their suffering, as well as their capacity to comprehend the consequences of their suffering on their life in its full complexity. To contextualize the aforementioned information, it is necessary to direct the conversation deliberately and filter out irrelevant information. The most fruitful source of information is open dialogue, yet it is also the most challenging form of communication for eliciting targeted information.

It has been my experience that open dialogue is the most effective method for clarifying my situation. Such an approach engenders a sense of being treated and recognized as an individual, in stark contrast to the experience of processing a checklist or questionnaire. Moreover, statements from the scientific community that lacked a clear connection to my circumstances also appeared to be too general and impersonal. The skepticism and generalized treatment, which is a rather negative experience, were further reinforced by the standard statements and queries.

Both the therapist and the patient bear responsibility for the efficacy of the therapy. It was often assumed that I was held to a high standard of responsibility and capability once I disclosed my professional title. This is a misperception. The capacity to assume responsibility is not solely contingent upon educational attainment; it is also influenced by an individual's emotional state. Frequently, I was emotionally depleted to the extent that I was unable to fulfill the level of responsibility expected of me. This resulted in challenging and occasionally untenable circumstances in which the therapist was taken aback or even disheartened, despite the lack of justification for such reactions. Navigating this predicament was challenging and, at times, an impossible task for both parties involved. It is detrimental when a therapist assumes that an individual lacks motivation or is faking.

Over time, I have developed the practice of addressing this matter promptly and openly to prevent any potential misunderstandings. This discrepancy has been observed on numerous occasions during my work as a physiotherapist coach. Patients often feel that their therapists do not fully meet their needs or understand them. From my point of view as a physiotherapist coach, it goes beyond "learning": on the one hand, it is about getting to know the patient's everyday strategies, for example, and being able to pass them on to other patients. In my opinion, there is also another potential in "learning": How can the necessary form of therapy (education, therapy, behavioral therapy, etc.) be ideally adapted to the patient's life, suffering, and needs? While this individuality makes the patient feel recognized in their uniqueness, the form of therapy used is implemented more effectively. To a certain extent, the patient becomes the therapist and is thus able to reflect critically on his or her suffering and the therapy applied.

As a coach, I have often talked about the division of roles and awareness of the area of responsibility between patients and therapists. This was often the greatest need for discussion or help for HPs:

Box 1 The Greatest Needs for Discussion or Help for HPs from a Patient Representative, Patient, and Coach

- Starting point: enabling the patient to understand the information available and to categorize it for themselves or their situation. This is a decisive step towards self-empowerment.
- To define for the patient the possibilities and meaningfulness of the therapy and thus also the therapist's role concerning the patient. This results in a shared understanding of the distribution of roles and responsibilities.
- The relationship between therapist (HP) and patient, the distribution of roles, and the awareness of the area of responsibility of each is decisive in leading the patient to self-empowerment.

Depending on the patient's character and expectations, this led to a sense of resignation or even complaints. In most cases, this could have been prevented if the therapist had addressed the patient's needs at the outset. Therapeutic collaboration necessitates a shared understanding of the therapeutic process, the formulation of mutually agreed-upon goals, and the joint pursuit of these goals.

Practical experience in healthcare settings shows that both learners and HPs in EDP benefit from coaching and training in self-reflection. The ability of active reflection cannot be taken for granted. It requires an introduction, guidance, and training in one's ability to reflect.

> The type of complaint and diagnoses are often not entirely clear or difficult to classify. The HPs are "seekers" in their work. Constant reflection on the effects of therapy, preferably together with the patient, is therefore very valuable. It can show whether the course of therapy is meeting expectations and thus invites you to rethink or adapt your method and idea of the symptoms if necessary. (Personal Statement by Frank Clasemann made in 2024)

Examples of guidance for reflection can be described as follows:

> In the training as a coach in the physiotherapy practice, I often slipped into the role of a patient to allow the employees to practice applying the newly trained knowledge. I deliberately tried to portray different characters to show how multifaceted the same clinical picture can be. This was always very much appreciated. (Personal Statement by Frank Clasemann made in 2024)

Snapshot of Practical Insights into Learning Experiences Based on Patient Voices

The following section will provide a snapshot of practical experiences on the reflection of patient voices. The authors want to provide a list of questions to facilitate reflection of HPs as learners or experienced HPs in EDP (see Table 1). These questions are based on first teaching experiences with HPs at the bachelor level in an interprofessional elective module on patient perspective, which can also be applied in EDP settings. This module was based on reading, discussing, and reflecting orally and in writing on different experiences of people with disabilities, using authentic patient narratives accessible via the Internet and with two patients that provide HPs with important information for care, treatment, and goal setting. In 2022/2023, the elective module "Experiencing Patient Perspectives" was offered twice with 20 and 25 LiHPs from each of the five bachelor programs Nursing, Midwifery, Physiotherapy, Occupational Therapy, and Health Promotion and Prevention. The module aims to focus learners' attention on the inclusion and importance of patient voices. This is done by asking the key question: "How do patient experiences change the view of LiHPs on the care situation concerning the prerequisites, framework conditions, responsibilities, professional convictions, etc.?"

The reflection of real recorded narratives from the described sources and databases was extended by live connections with affected persons in an online-supported format, where patients could ask questions about their experiences, discuss them, and reflect together with the students in live sessions. The reflection was initially facilitated by mentors to gain initial experience of what is meant by reflection, for example, how shared reflection works and what it aims to achieve. The reflection then moved to a peer-to-peer setting so that learners could share and reflect on their views of the

Table 1 Dimensions and questions for reflection (own presentation) as a guide for implementation into practice

Dimension of reflection	Guiding questions for reflection (examples)
Perception and description	How do you find the description of the experiences, e.g., using the following? Content Motifs Focal points Manner of description
Personal considerations and effects of implications	How does the narrative affect me? What did I hear apart from what was said, the emotions, concerns, or motivations? What remains unclear to me about the patient's or family member's statements or action strategies, and why?
(Inter)professional considerations and effects or implications	What is important to this person? Can I meet this request or not? What do I take from the descriptions that are relevant to my work as an occupational therapist, physiotherapist, nurse, midwife, health promotion worker, etc.? What aspects of the descriptions are important for us as a team for interprofessional care? Where do I see a need for coordination with my team? What is the patient's or affected person's priorities for treatment?
Learning gain	What new aspects do I take away from the descriptions? What other questions and assumptions arise from this process (reflection and sharing with the group)?

narratives from both a professional perspective and in an interprofessional exchange. Learners were tasked with combining content from selected literature and theoretical input in the form of blended learning with self-directed learning units and combining this with reflection and dialogue in learning groups. Learners kept a reflection journal in their learning groups in a shared, protected digital learning environment. The focus of learning was on reflection on authentic narratives during the units, which took place on different levels with and without guiding questions (see, e.g., Table 1). Experiences from the DIPEx project, live calls with patient representatives, experts from the field from EX-IN, or participation in the Storytelling Café (see description in the appendix) are suitable for such kinds of settings to train skills on active reflection based on questions and common exchange on reflected aspects and how to use and integrate into individual treatment aims, interventions, motivating goals, shared decisions, and further person-centered aspects.

The LiHPs gained a total of 8 weeks of reflective experience in the module, peer-to-peer exchange was part of the reflection, followed by discussions with facilitators in small group sessions. This culminated in a two-stage performance assessment with a formative group assessment (pass/fail). This consisted of (a) an oral presentation by the small group to the whole group and (b) a written reflection report. The LiHPs received written feedback on the small-group performances from the responsible teacher.

Discussion and Conclusion

The discussion refers to central derivations of the outlined procedure of patient voices in different presentation formats from examples of best practice examples integrated into the vice versa process of reflection as LIPHs in an interprofessional learning setting, but also as experienced HPs in EDP. The focus is on small-group reflection as a methodological approach. This is introduced, guided, and actively accompanied by teachers to reflect on issues and cases in an interprofessional and professional manner to identify and share differences and similarities.

The preliminary results of an RCT study using patient stories from the DIPEx database show that students benefit from real patient stories. They are more competent in their communication skills than students in the comparison group, who were taught content by experts [50]. Findings from interprofessional learning settings (physiotherapy and social work) support this initial evidence [43]. People's narratives provide a valuable addition and access to their experiences.

They open the perspective of person-centeredness about the inner experience of illness, treatment outcomes, coping with illness, or experiences with the care system [6]. Charon [12] and Shao-Yin et al. [49] highlight active listening as a crucial factor in strengthening the practitioner–patient relationship, fostering appreciation, respect, and empathy. Strengthening this ability in (future) HPs and developing it as a subcomponent of narrative competence can be supported by video, audio, or text contributions of patient narratives. Additionally, patient narratives are now being used to design case vignettes and prepare simulated persons in medical and health professions training settings for staging to achieve a higher degree of credibility, persuasiveness, and identification with the role to be conveyed [26].

The following aspects of interprofessional lifelong learning can be summarized based on the examples given for the inclusion of patients' and relatives' voices and can be integrated as didactic elements using reflection.

(a) The examples given (EX-IN; DIPEx, authentic experiences by the patient representative, and his involvement) show that there are already several initiatives and movements, and how to implement persons' voices into healthcare. This gives affected persons the opportunity to have a say. Interprofessional learning settings and in-practice settings show that the inclusion of patients' and relatives' voices is possible at a low threshold.

(b) The case descriptions are not constructed or synthetically generated, but "real" persons, patients, and, or family members are integrated life or via media into the learning situation and report closely and authentically about their experiences, according to the motto: "Practice comes to the classroom and reports first-hand."

(c) The examples shown based on the real experiences of patients/relatives serve as a bridge to practice and enable an introduction to the first patient contact. The reflective moment that often follows can be seen as an advantage because the learner can let the situation sink in without immediate time and action pressure, unlike direct contact in practice.

(d) The spectrum of questions, needs, goals, and concerns for therapy that can be reflected on from the patient's perspective is expanded, as well as from the perspective of the concerns of the HPs. Possible mismatches in the perspectives become conscious and recognized.
(e) As already mentioned by patient representatives, a person-centered perspective is associated with an attitude that needs to be sensitized and theoretically underpinned. Patients/relatives are included as equal partners in the interprofessional team and are respected as such. Targeted and respectful communication plays a key role in person-centeredness and collaboration.
(f) Active involvement as stakeholders in the sense of serious shared decision-making empowers patients and has a positive impact on the satisfaction of HPs. Involving and listening to affected persons, as well as collaborating and promoting adherence, are important aspects [15]. Decision-making is highly relevant for goal setting in treatment situations and outcome definition. Without person-centered strategies and a clear negotiation, person-relevant goal setting will remain difficult or will not catch the most reachable motivation of the person possible.
(g) Diseases progress differently and are associated with fluctuations. A sensitive approach is advantageous for the active involvement of patients, as the course of an illness can be associated with instability and vulnerability and therefore needs to be reassessed and reflected upon daily. Questions such as "How are you feeling today?" should be used as serious questions and not as empty phrases.
(h) Reflection functions as a didactic element and cannot always be assumed as a competence of the learner. As a method, reflection should, at best, be specifically linked to a learning object. Especially in the beginning, it is recommended that reflection is actively accompanied and guided by teachers (facilitators) so that learners and or HPs in EDP can benefit from it. Reflection can be topic- or case-related, interprofessional, and profession-specific, to become aware of differences and similarities, share them, and integrate them into the care process in the sense of reflective professional action.
(i) Different levels of education, e.g., at bachelor's or master's level, or in training and continuing education contexts, influence the expected depth of reflection and one's knowledge gain. This must be considered in the methodological design of the respective lifelong teaching/learning situations.

In summary, the authors suggest that:

- Patients' accounts of their individual experiences in dealing with illness and health are an essential approach to understanding, supporting, and comprehending care-related goals, motivations, attitudes, participation, or even decisions. Person-centered care draws on and is enriched by these experiences.
- The active inclusion of the voices of those affected in learning arrangements as a methodological and didactic approach, and interprofessional reflection on them, promotes the ability to change perspectives and the understanding of being

authentic and close to the lifeworld of other people. Learners can thus prepare for practice without being under direct time and action pressure.

- The four person-centered examples of incorporating the perspectives of patients and family members were used to show learners how their views and needs can change professional thinking, action, the goal-setting process, and care management as a health profession. The module example shows that learning from real experiences in the learners' environment can be a helpful preparation if the learners are not yet able to gain their own experience in the practice environment. In this way, "part of the real practice situation comes into the classroom."
- The patient experiences described are real and reach learners through their vividness and authenticity.
- Reflection does not run itself but needs guidance, sharing, and feedback.
- Group reflection provides a "safe space" for learners. It gives learners time to think about questions, ambiguities in understanding and action, and further considerations for which there is often not enough time in practice or opportunity to discuss openly.

Box 2 Good to Know and to Remember Regarding Basics in Patient Voices for EDP and Lifelong Learning

The authors of this chapter would like to encourage and promote the idea that the inclusion of patients/relatives as experts from experience expands the circle of trained experts. The different subjective perspectives and experiences of those affected can broaden professional expertise and enrich the entire spectrum of observation, without being understood as a devaluation of professional expertise. Evidence-based knowledge and skills are vital elements and do not lose their significance when narrative-based experiential knowledge is integrated into interprofessional collaboration and takes its rightful place as the basis for shared decision-making.

The involvement of experienced persons, as in the context of EX-In, DIPEx, or as a patient representative, has proven to be a reliable, methodologically sound approach regarding the credibility of the content of the statements, which are based on real statements by patients/relatives [29, 30, 51] (DIPEx International, https://dipexinternational.org.).

In the context of the Internet and artificial intelligence, it is important to consider the implications of the vast amount of patient information that is freely available or can be generated without attribution or to be transparent to cite sources. The diverse intentions of stakeholders for the use of such data can be used as a critical basis for reflection. The real-life experiences mentioned in this article provide valuable insights into learning situations. It is essential to distinguish between these testimonials and the script templates created for stakeholders. It is often not immediately apparent what motivations, interests, or even unclear or commercial intentions may be behind such contributions. The inclusion of authentic patient/family voices in the educational or care context rarely requires a complete change of approach or mindset. Their sources are disclosed, traceable, and genuine. It is often necessary to be attentive and vigilant to incorporate this perspective at appropriate points. For instance, by expressing an assessment or outcome in a manner that is appropriate, understandable, and comprehensible to the patient, and by ensuring that it has been understood. Investing in a brief period of translation work in terms of comprehensibility initially fosters trust. They are also effective for further relationship work in the therapy and care processes and serve as a basis for interprofessional healthcare.

Finally, regarding the critical reflection on the inclusion of patient/family voices in training and practice units, it should be noted that the inclusion of patient/family voices is subject to a possible implicit bias. This is because these are the voices of people who are motivated and trained to speak openly about their life situations and to go public. This fact must be critically reflected upon in preparation and follow-up. In implementing this approach, it is essential to recognize that it necessitates an individualized approach and negotiation with the individuals involved. It is crucial to identify and agree upon an appropriate level of involvement for the person, which may also be subject to fluctuations.

From the perspective of the patient representative, a crucial element to be considered is as follows:

> One disadvantage of the teaching method with, for example, DIPEx-supported statements, is that the interaction between patient and therapist can only be simulated. However, it is possible to examine the variety of statements from patients with different attitudes toward a topic. The impact of verbal and nonverbal expressions on one another can be profound; however, this cannot be fully appreciated from preserved answers. Such statements are frequently the source of challenging interactions or communication or the cause of misunderstanding. The result can be a misinterpretation, which can lead to a loss of trust. Therefore, training in communication techniques and awareness of the interactions mentioned is fundamental. Based on my experience as a physiotherapist, coach, and patient representative, I believe that a patient (who has been trained to teach) is the most effective didactic tool.

Finally, regarding the critical reflection on the inclusion of patient/family voices in interprofessional education and collaborative practice, it should be noted that the inclusion of patient/family voices is subject to a possible implicit bias, as those who engage in public discourse are often trained and motivated to do so. This fact must be critically reflected upon in preparation and follow-up. In implementing this approach, it is essential to recognize that it necessitates an individualized approach and negotiation with the individuals involved. It is crucial to identify and agree upon an appropriate level of involvement for the person, which may also be subject to fluctuations.

We recommend consciously integrating patient perspectives into IPE and collaborative practice, as this not only transforms how learners and healthcare professionals view care situations, but also deepens their understanding of the needs, experiences, and expectations of those receiving care. Through narrative experiences and interprofessional reflection, LiHPs can develop patient-centered competencies that transcend disciplinary boundaries. Person-centered approaches enhance communication, build stronger relationships, and support meaningful shared decision-making. At the same time, it becomes evident that effective IPC requires the active involvement of patients as partners in the care process. Therefore, we call for continued and systematic efforts to embed patient voices across all levels of IPE and IPC.

Reflective Questions

Questions for reflection are suggested that relate to the content raised in the chapter and can serve as support in different learning and practice contexts. A distinction is made between the three perspectives of learners in education and training (learners), educational staff in higher education and practice (educational staff), practicing HPs in EDP (practitioners), and patients and family members (affected persons).

- How is the inclusion of patient/family voice organized in your place of learning (i.e., IPE) or work (i.e., IPC)?
- In your opinion, how important have patient/family voices been so far in interprofessional education and training or daily interprofessional practice?
- Do you notice differences in the inclusion of the patient/family perspective depending on the specialty, diagnosis, or context?
- How are person-centered needs, goals, and experiences currently reflected in the interprofessional team at your place of study/learning or work?
- In your opinion, what procedures are helpful for the beneficial inclusion of the patient/family perspective in the interprofessional care process?
- In your opinion, which methods and framework conditions are helpful for a profitable reflection process regarding interprofessional collaboration?
- How familiar were you with the practical examples in this chapter? What approaches could you use in your future learning (i.e., IPE) or working (IPC) environment?
- Can you think of other ways to integrate the patient/family perspective into interprofessional education and collaborative practice in your learning and working environment?

References

1. Achberger C. EX-IN Kurse – Teilhabe in der Sozialpsychiatrie. In: Eberle A, Kaminsky U, Behringer L, Unterkofler U, editors. Menschenrechte und Soziale Arbeit im Schatten des Nationalsozialismus. Springer VS; 2019. p. 245–55. https://doi.org/10.1007/978-3-658-19517-5_13.
2. Anderson ES, Ford J, Thorpe L. Perspectives on patients and carers in leading teaching roles in interprofessional education. J Interprof Care. 2019;33:216–25.
3. Bennett-Weston A, Gray S, Anderson ES. A theoretical systematic review of patient involvement in health and social care education. Adv Health Sci Educ. 2022;28(1):279–304. https://doi.org/10.1007/s10459-022-10137-3.

4. Berchtold P, Gedamke S, Schmitz C. Quality through patients' eyes. 2020. https://www.spo.ch/wp-content/uploads/2021/02/Bericht-Quality-through-patients-eyes-final.pdf.
5. Bräuer G. Das Portfolio als Reflexionsmedium für Lehrende und Studierende. Opladen [u.a.]; 2014.
6. Breuning M, Lucius-Hoene G, Burbaum C, Himmel W, Bengel J. Subjektive Krankheitserfahrungen und Patientenorientierung. Das Website-Projekt DIPEx Germany. Bundesgesundheitsblatt Gesundheitsforschung Gesundheitsschutz. 2018;60(4):453–61. https://doi.org/10.1007/s00103-017-2524-y.
7. Brewer M. Interprofessional capability framework. 2011. https://www.healthprecinct.org.nz/wp-content/uploads/2018/12/Brewer-interprofessional-capability-booklet.pdf.
8. Bulman C, Schutz S. Reflective practice in nursing. Wiley; 2013.
9. Bundesamt für Gesundheit (BAG). Schweiz Selbsthilfe. 2024. https://www.bag.admin.ch/bag/de/home/strategie-und-politik/nationale-gesundheitsstrategien/strategie-nicht-uebertragbare-krankheiten/praevention-in-der-gesundheitsversorgung/selbstmanagement-foerderung-chronische-krankheiten-und-sucht/angebote-selbstmanagementfoerderung/selbsthilfe-schweiz.html.
10. Canadian Interprofessional Health Collaborative (CIHC). A national interprofessional competency framework. 2010. https://practiceedportal.health.ubc.ca/wp-content/uploads/2017/01/NationalInterprofessionalCompetencyFramework.pdf.
11. Charité – Universitätsmedizin Berlin (Hrsg.). Mustercurriculum Patientensicherheit der Weltgesundheitsorganisation. Multiprofessionelle Ausgabe. Berlin: Charité – Universitätsmedizin Berlin; 2018. https://cdn.who.int/media/docs/default-source/patient-safety/9783000606267-ger9b27b60a-ce75-43a0-a53d-c45b52ed9aac.pdf.
12. Charon R. What to do with stories. The sciences of narrative medicine. Can Fam Physician. 2007;53(8):1265–7.
13. Charon R. Narrative medicine: a model for empathy, reflection, profession, and trust. JAMA. 2001;286:1897–902. https://doi.org/10.1001/jama.286.15.189.
14. Charon R. Narrative medicine. Honoring the stories of illness. Oxford University Press; 2006.
15. Chung MK, Fagerlin A, Wang PJ, Ajayi TB, Allen LA, Baykaner T, et al. Shared decision making in cardiac electrophysiology procedures and arrhythmia management. Arrhythmia Electrophysiol. 2021;14(12):e007958. https://doi.org/10.1161/CIRCEP.121.007958.
16. Coulter A. Patient engagement – what works? J Ambul Care Manag. 2012;35(2):80–9. https://doi.org/10.1097/JAC.0b013e318249e0fd.
17. Dehnbostel P, Fürstenau B, Klusmeyer J, Rebmann K. Kontextbedingungen beruflichen Lernens: Lernen in der Schule und im Prozess der Arbeit. In: Nickolaus R, Pätzold G, Reinisch H, Tramm T, editors. Handbuch Berufs- und Wirtschaftspädagogik. Klinkhardt; 2010.
18. Deutsche Gesellschaft für Psychiatrie und Psychotherapie, Psychosomatik und Nervenheilkunde (DGPPN). S3-Leitlinie Psychosoziale Therapien bei schweren psychischen Erkrankungen. S3-Praxisleitlinien in Psychiatrie und Psychotherapie. 2nd ed. Springer; 2018.
19. Dingley C, Daugherty K, Derieg MK, Persing R. Improving patient safety through provider communication strategy enhancements. In: Henriksen K, Battles JB, Keyes MA, Grady ML, editors. Advances in patient safety: new directions and alternative approaches (Vol. 3: performance and tools). Agency for Healthcare Research and Quality (US); 2008.
20. Drewniak D, Glässel A, Hodel M, Biller-Andorno N. Risks and benefits of web-based patient narratives: systematic review. J Med Internet Res. 2020;22(3):e15772.
21. Epstein RM, Street RL Jr. The values and value of patient-centered care. Ann Family Med. 2011;9(2):100–3.
22. EX-IN. EX-IN Experten durch Erfahrung in der Psychiatrie. EX-IN in Deutschland e.V. 2024. https://ex-in.de/.
23. Frenk J, Chen L, Bhutta ZA, Cohen J, Crisp N, Evans T, et al. Health professionals for a new century: transforming education to strengthen health systems in an interdependent world. Lancet. 2010;376(9756):1923–58. https://doi.org/10.1016/S0140-6736(10)61854-5.
24. Frommelt P. Salutogenese in der Pflege. Springer; 2010.

25. Gagné JP, Jennings MB. Incorporating a client-centered approach to audiologic rehabilitation. Asha Lead. 2011;16:10–3. https://doi.org/10.1044/leader.FTR1.16082011.10.
26. Glässel A, Zumstein P, Scherer T, Feusi E, Biller-Andorno N. Case vignettes for simulated patients based on real patient experiences in the context of OSCE examinations: workshop experiences from interprofessional education. GMS J Med Educ. 2021;38(5):Doc91. https://doi.org/10.3205/zma001487.
27. Haun M, Bilmayer S, Heuer I, Mahlke C, Puschner B, Wagner M, et al. UPSIDES Erfahrungen in Deutschland aus der Sicht von Peer-Begleiter*innen und -Trainer*innen. Sozialpsychiatrische Inform. 2021:15–8. https://doi.org/10.1486/SI-2021-03_15.
28. Häcker T. Reflexive Professionalisierung. Anmerkungen zu dem ambitionierten Anspruch, die Reflexions-kompetenz angehender Lehrkräfte umfassend zu fördern. In: Degeling M, Franken N, Freund S, Greiten S, Neuhaus D, Schellenbach-Zell J, editors. Herausforderung Kohärenz: Praxisphasen in der universitären Lehrer-bildung. Bildungswissenschaftliche und fachdidaktische Perspektiven. Klinkhardt; 2019. p. 81–96.
29. Health Experience Research Group Researcher's Handbook (HERG). Healthtalkonline modules. Version 42 (unpublished manuscript). 2023.
30. Herxheimer A, McPherson A, Miller R, Shepperd S, Yaphe J, Ziebland S. Database of patients' experiences (DIPEx): a multi-media approach to sharing experiences and information. Lancet. 2000;355(9214):1540–3.
31. Hojat M, Louis DZ, Markham FW, Wender R, Rabinowitz C, Gonnella JS. Physicians' empathy and clinical outcomes for diabetic patients. Acad Med. 2011;86(3):359–64. https://doi.org/10.1097/ACM.0b013e3182086fe1.
32. Kaap-Fröhlich S, Ulrich G, Wershofen B, Ahles J, Behrend R, Handgraaf M, et al. Positionspapier GMA-Ausschuss Interprofessionelle Ausbildung in den Gesundheitsberufen – aktueller Stand und Zukunftsperspektiven. GMS J Med Educ. 2022;39(2):15–28. https://doi.org/10.3205/zma001538.
33. Kunze K. Interprofessionelles Lernen als Grundlage für interprofessionelle Zusammenarbeit in den Gesundheitsberufen – eine Mixed-Methods-Studie zur Relevanz der interprofessionellen Sozialisation im Studium in den Beruf. Dissertation. Universität Osnabrück; 2023. https://doi.org/10.48693/428.
34. Légaré F, Stacey D, Turcotte S, Cossi MJ, Kryworuchko J, Graham ID, et al. Interventions for improving the adoption of shared decision making by healthcare professionals. Cochrane Database Syst Rev. 2014;15(9):CD006732. https://doi.org/10.1002/14651858.CD006732.pub3.
35. Mahlke C, Krämer U, Kilian R, Becker T. Bedeutung und Wirksamkeit von Peer-Arbeit in der psychiatrischen Versorgung. Übersicht des internationalen Forschungsstandes. Nervenheilkunde. 2015;34:235–9.
36. Mead N, Bower P. Patient-centredness: a conceptual framework and review of the empirical literature. Soc Sci Med. 2000;51(7):1087–110.
37. Megatrend Map. 2024. https://content.zukunftsinstitut.de/hubfs/Megatrends/Megatrend-Map%20EN%20Megatrend-Dokumentation%202021.pdf?
38. Mezirow J. Transformative Erwachsenenbildung. Schneider-Verl. Hohengehren; 1997.
39. Moran M, Bickford J, Barradell S, Scholten I. Embedding the international classification of functioning, disability and health in health professions curricula to enable interprofessional education and collaborative practice. J Med Educat Curri Develop. 2020;7:2382120520933855. https://doi.org/10.1177/2382120520933855.
40. Oluoch D, Molyneux S, Boga M, Maluni J, Murila F, Jones C, et al. Not just surveys and indicators: narratives capture what really matters for health system strengthening. Lancet Glob Health. 2023;11(9):e1459–63.
41. Peng Y, Wu T, Chen Z, Deng Z. Value cocreation in health care: systematic review. J Med Internet Res. 2022;24(3):e33061. https://doi.org/10.2196/33061.
42. Pott C. Teilhabeorientierte interprofessionelle ambulante Schlaganfallnachsorge durch Bezugstherapeuten – Etablierung eines innovativen Projekts. Neuroreha. 2020;12:30–4. https://doi.org/10.1055/a-0976-1082.

43. Powell S, Scott J, Scott L, Jones D. An online narrative archive of patient experiences to support the education of physiotherapy and social work students in North East England: an evaluation study. Educ Health. 2013;26(1):25–31.
44. Reichel K, Herinek D. Interprofessionelles Lehren und Lernen – Klärung und Orientierung. In: Ewers M, Reichel K, editors. Kooperativ Lehren, Lernen und Arbeiten in den Gesundheitsprofessionen: das Projekt interTUT. Working Paper No. 17-01 der Unit Gesundheitswissenschaften und ihre Didaktik. Berlin: Charité – Universitätsmedizin Berlin; 2017. p. 9–25.
45. Scholl I, Zill JM, Härter M, Dirmaier J. How do health services researchers understand the concept of patient-centeredness? Results from an expert survey. Patient Prefer Adherence. 2014;8:1153–60. https://doi.org/10.2147/PPA.S64051.
46. Schön DA. The reflective practitioner. Temple Smith; 1983.
47. Schweizerische Akademie der Medizinischen Wissenschaften (SAMW). Charta 2.0 – Interprofessionelle Zusammenarbeit im Gesundheitswesen. 2020. https://doi.org/10.5281/zenodo.3865147.
48. Scura N. Reflexion als didaktische Methode zur Ausbildung und als Schlüsselkompetenz professionellen Handelns. In: Heyse V, Giger M, editors. Erfolgreich in die Zukunft: Schlüsselkompetenzen in Gesundheitsberufen. medhochzwei; 2015. p. 343–64.
49. Shao-Yin C, Chin-Chen W, Chi-Wei L. A qualitative study of clinical narrative competence of medical personnel. BMC Med Educ. 2020;20:415. https://doi.org/10.1186/s12909-020-02336-6.
50. Snow R, Crocker J, Talbot K, Moore J, Salisbury H. Does hearing the patient patient's perspective improve consultation skills in examinations? An exploratory randomized controlled trial in medical undergraduate education. Med Teach. 2016;38(12):1229–35. https://doi.org/10.1080/0142159X.2016.1210109.
51. Spitale G, Glässel A, Tyebally-Fang M, Mouton Dorey C, Biller-Andorno N. Patient narratives – a still undervalued resource for healthcare improvement. Swiss Med Wkly. 2023;153(1):40022. https://doi.org/10.57187/smw.2023.40022.
52. Street RL Jr, Makoul G, Arora N, Epstein RM. How does communication heal? Pathways linking clinician–patient communication to health outcomes. Patient Educ Couns. 2008;92(3):286–91. https://doi.org/10.1016/j.pec.2008.11.015.
53. Towle A, Bainbridge L, Godolphin W, Katz A, Kline C, Lown B, Madularu I, Solomon P, Thistlethwaite J. Active patient involvement in the education of health professionals. Med Educ. 2010;44(1):64–74. https://doi.org/10.1111/j.1365-2923.2009.03530.x.
54. Utschakowski J. EX-IN Ausbildungen: Experienced Involvement – Pro & Kontra. Psychiatr Prax. 2012;39:202–3.
55. Utschakowski J, Sielaff G, Bock T, Winter A. Experten aus Erfahrung. Peerarbeit in der Psychiatrie. Psychiatrie Verlag; 2016.
56. Wilberforce M, Challis D, Davies L, Kelly MP, Roberts C, Loynes N. Person-centredness in the care of older adults: a systematic review of questionnaire-based scales and their measurement properties. BMC Geriatr. 2016;16:63. https://doi.org/10.1186/s12877-016-0229-y.
57. Wissenschaftsrat. Perspektiven für die Weiterentwicklung der Gesundheitsfachberufe: Wissenschaftliche Potenziale für die Gesundheitsversorgung erkennen und nutzen. Köln. 2023. https://www.wissenschaftsrat.de/download/2023/1548-23.pdf?__blob=publicationFile&v=12.
58. World Health Organization (WHO). International classification of functioning, disability and health: ICF. 2001. https://www.who.int/standards/classifications/international-classification-of-functioning-disability-and-health.
59. World Health Organization (WHO). Framework for action on interprofessional education & collaborative practice. Geneva: World Health Organization; 2010.
60. World Health Organization (WHO). Patient safety curriculum guide: multi-professional edition. 2011. https://www.who.int/publications/i/item/9789241501958.

61. World Health Organization (WHO). The European health report 2018: more than numbers – evidence for all. 2018. https://iris.who.int/bitstream/handle/10665/279878/9789289053440-eng.pdf?sequence=1, https://www.who.int/europe/publications/i/item/9789289053440.
62. World Health Organization (WHO). WHO health workforce support and safeguards list 2023. Geneva: World Health Organization; 2023. https://www.who.int/publications/i/item/9789240069787.
63. Ziebland S, Herxheimer A. How patients' experiences contribute to decision making: illustrations from DIPEx (personal experiences of health and illness). J Nurs Manag. 2008;16(4):433–9.
64. Ziebland S, Herxheimer A, Coulter A. What do patients want to know about their medicines, and what do doctors want to tell them? A comparative study. Health Expect. 2004;7(2):109–16.

Further Links & Websites

Deutsche Rheuma-Liga: https://www.rheuma-liga.de.
DIPEx Schweiz: https://DIPEx.ch.
DIPEx Germany: www.krankheitserfahrungen.de.
DIPEx Charity – Healthtalk: www.healthtalk.org.
DIPEx International – Internationaler Dachverband: https://dipexinternational.org.
Health Experiences International (HEXI): https://healthexperiencesinternational.org/.
Health Experiences Insights United Kingdom: https://hexi.ox.ac.uk/.
Health Experience Research Network (HERN): www.healthexperiencesusa.org.
EX-IN Schweiz: Experten durch Erfahrungen in der Psychiatrie: https://www.ex-in-schweiz.ch/.
EX-IN Deutschland: Experten durch Erfahrung in der Psychiatrie: https://ex-in.de/.
Schweizerische Patientenorganisation (SPO): www.SPO.ch.
Schweizerische Rheumaliga: https://www.rheumaliga.ch.
European Patient Forum (EPF): https://www.eu-patient.eu.

Andrea Glässel is a physiotherapist with 10 years of practical experience in neurorehabilitation and a health scientist with a master's degree in neurorehabilitation, public health, and applied ethics. She received her doctorate in rehabilitation sciences from LMU Munich. At the University of Zurich, she is a research associate for patient perspectives and the national representative of Switzerland in the DIPEx, newly renamed "HEXI" Health Experiences International network. Since 2004, she has been teaching students in health professions in interprofessional learning environments. Since 2017, Andrea has been a professor of Interprofessionality and Public Ethics at the ZHAW School of Health Sciences in Winterthur, co-leading the Digital Health Design Living Lab (DHDLL) of the Swiss universities UZH, ZHAW, and Zurich University of Arts (ZHdK).

Katrin Kunze works as a research assistant in Germany. She is an occupational therapist with worked for some years with a focus on psychosocial treatment methods. She completed a master's degree in vocational education for health professions. Since 2015, she has worked on various projects at different universities, focusing on education for health professions. She was a member of the Graduate School for "Interprofessional Teaching in the Health Professions (ILEGRA)." She completed her doctorate in 2023 with a mixed-method study on the relevance of interprofessional socialization during training at the Osnabrück University. In her current project, she is working on user-centered healthcare through the integration of socio-technical systems.

Frank Clasemann has been practicing physiotherapy in Germany since 2003 and in Switzerland since 2009. In 2010, he completed the Master of Advanced Studies in Manual Therapy at the SOMT (University of Physiotherapy in Amersfoort, NL) in Lucerne. In 2016, he obtained a Master of Science (MPT Science) from the universities of Winterthur and Bern. Frank is a physiotherapy coach and honorary lecturer at the University of Basel and the Zurich University of Applied Sciences (ZHAW). Since 2011, Frank has served as a patient representative, delivering lectures as an author, and has been a patient member of the Ethics Committee of the University Hospital Zurich. He is also a co-researcher at the Clinical Trials Center (CTC) and Advisory Board Member of the University of Zurich, and at the Digital Health Design Living Lab of the Swiss universities UZH, ZHAW, and Zurich University of Arts (ZHdK).

Student Voices

Lucas Büsser, Isabella van Setten, and Corina Zweifel

Introduction

This chapter lends a voice to the people most affected by interprofessional (IP) learning activities and the generation expected to succeed in IP collaboration (IPC) directly following graduation: today's healthcare students. They are at the forefront of all efforts regarding IP education (IPE) and experience first-hand how IPE programs (do not) work in practice. Listening to the ones who are affected the most will hopefully help us all to reach a future where IPE can be more effective and more joyful for everyone involved, leading not only to more pleasant experiences for students and facilitators, but ultimately to a more enjoyable working atmosphere and better patient care.

L. Büsser (✉)
SHAPED – Swiss Health Alliance for Interprofessional Education, Bern, Switzerland
e-mail: office@shaped-ip.ch

I. van Setten
Department of Health, Medicine and Caring Sciences, Linköping University, Linköping, Sweden

C. Zweifel
SHAPED – Swiss Health Alliance for Interprofessional Education, Bern, Switzerland

School of Health Professions, University of Applied Sciences, Bern, Switzerland
e-mail: office@shaped-ip.ch; corina.zweifel@students.bfh.ch

A. Xyrichis et al. (eds.), *Building Bridges: A European Perspective on Interprofessional Education, Practice, Policy and Research*,
https://doi.org/10.1007/978-3-032-23222-9_7

Background

Interprofessional education is seen by the World Health Organization (WHO) as a key factor in achieving successful interprofessional collaboration [27]. However, to the authors' knowledge, comprehensive surveys regarding the attitude towards and experience with IPE of European students are lacking. The same is the case with a continental mapping of IPE opportunities for healthcare students, making it difficult to accurately assess the current state of IPE in Europe from any perspective—including the students' perspective. There has recently been a systematic review regarding undergraduate Interprofessional Education in the European Higher Education area (EHEA). However, by definition this was limited to parts of Europe and undergraduate training—and it highlighted the need for further European IPE research [6].

Students' Attitudes and Perceptions of IPE

In general, studies have shown that healthcare students across fields of study and across different countries [2, 4, 16, 18] have a very positive attitude towards IPE.

Furthermore, it is encouraging to see that students explicitly call for IPE and IPC [10, 20]. In 2020, the International Federation of Medical Students' Associations (IFMSA) and the European Regional Office of the International Pharmaceutical Students' Federation (IPSF) started a *"CALL FOR ACTION on Interprofessional Collaboration and Education"* [11]. Their collaboration not only set an example of students working interprofessionally on a project, but also highlighted that a sustainable health workforce will require IPE and IPC in the future more than ever. The endorsement of this call for action by the International (*IADS*) as well as the European Dental Students' Association (*EDSA*), the European Pharmaceutical Student Association (*EPSA*), the European Medical Students' Association (*EMSA*), and the European Federation of Psychology Students' Association (*efpsa*), highlights the importance today's healthcare students—regardless of professional background—place on interprofessional education and collaborative practice (IPECP).

In their call for action, the students call on governments to, among other, *"promote curricular reforms from the standard profession-based education to a longitudinal integrated health professions education that fosters principles of interprofessional collaborations"* [11, p. 4].

Furthermore, healthcare institutions and universities are called upon to *"ensure adequate allocation and institutional support to faculty development and organisation for the implementation of IPE from undergraduate to postgraduate studies"* [11, p. 4].

Similarly, a recent IFMSA policy paper calls on medical schools and universities to *"Initiate curriculum reform to create an educational culture that integrates interprofessional collaboration in everyday working, teaching and learning environments among staff and students"* [10, p. 2].

When surveyed, recent graduates from pharmacy, medicine and nursing reflected in general positively on their IPE activities, putting most value on *"experiences that involved genuine engagement and opportunities to interact with students in other professions working on a relevant problem"* [7, p. 1]. Regardless, the *"overriding message was that a great deal of room for improvement exists"* [7, p. 6]. The existing lack of IPE, as reported around the globe, including in the European region [13], thus can not be attributed to a lack of interest from students.

European IPE Activities

Not all European countries offer the same IP learning opportunities for students [6, 12]. As an example: while in northern European countries, interprofessional training wards (IPTWs) have been implemented for decades [26], in southern Europe they are rarely found [23].

As explored in other chapters of this book, IPE opportunities for students differ vastly: on one hand, between countries, but on the other hand, nationally, between professions, and even between different educational institutions. The issue of substantial program variations across countries as well as fields of studies has been reported on a more global scale as well [9, 13].

Since IPC is essential to face and solve the healthcare challenges of the twenty-first century that Europe (and the world) is already dealing with [27], efforts are needed to ensure equal and sufficient IPE opportunities for all European healthcare students—regardless of their home country or professional background. This becomes even more relevant given the shortage of skilled healthcare workers and increasing costs of healthcare in many countries, as there is evidence that IP interventions improve provider satisfaction and workplace quality [19].

In places where IPE activities exist, more often than not their development and planning seem to lack a theoretical foundation and they are heterogeneous in terms of content [6, 9]. Furthermore, in most cases only few professions are reported to be included in these activities [6, 9].

Students' Integration in the Development of (Future) IPE Activities

While many efforts are aimed at implementing IPE activities more widely, their development seldom includes the people most affected by these activities: the healthcare students. Published data is scarce, but a literature review in 2012 found only 2.4% of investigated IPE activities developed by faculty *and* students, with another 10.8% where students may have been included and 12% where the developers were unclear [1]. This leaves at least ¾ of all IPE activities that were developed without the input and inclusion of students.

Likewise, literature aimed at providing a guide for developing IPE often fails to take the students' view into account [8, 21, 24].

Capturing Students' Voices

In order to (a) establish past and present experiences with IPE as well as concerns for the future of IPE, (b) map IPE opportunities all over Europe, and (c) share best-practice models from a students' perspective, written interviews as well as a group discussion with healthcare students were conducted as follows.

Students from different European countries were approached through fellow authors of this book, via university teachers, and healthcare institutions. Inclusion criteria were: (i) being an enrolled student, (ii) at a European educational institution, (iii) studying any field of healthcare. These criteria were deliberately set quite wide to enable a variety of students to participate, thus capturing a more diverse and inclusive picture. No special interest in IPECP was required, no more than two students per country were allowed, and the aim was to include between 10 and 15 students in total.

The three questions posed to participating students were focused on their own experiences with IPE and IPC. They aimed at highlighting challenges as well as best practice models students had encountered as part of their program/studies. Last but not least, students were asked to provide recommendations to the involved stakeholders regarding the future of IPE and IPC.

A total of eleven students studying in six professional fields (medicine, pharmacy, nursing, speech and language therapy, physiotherapy, and paramedic) in seven countries (Cyprus (CY), Germany (DE), Italy (IT), Netherlands (NL), United Kingdom (UK), Sweden (SW), and Switzerland (CH)) answered the three questions posed by the chapter's authors (Fig. 1).

A consensus towards these answers was discussed between participants during a two-hour online meeting. This section will showcase exemplary snippets of the participants' answers before summing up the group's consensus to each question.

How do you experience interprofessional education and practice in your daily life as a healthcare student in your country?

☒Limited amount of IPE in the curriculum
☒Little to no interaction with students from other professions
☒Few IPE opportunities in the early stages of the curriculum
☒Misalignment of schedules between healthcare professions
☑More elaborate IPE activities seem to have many benefits
☑Internships show great potential to showcase IPC and improve IPE
☑Obvious benefits from working hands-on *and* cross-professions on a project/workshop

Different experiences of IPE and IPC have been reported by the interviewed students. In some places, IPE has become a fixed part of the curriculum: "*During my studies, as a pharmacy student, I have a chance to join an IPE workshop every*

Noel
3. Semester
Paramedic
Switzerland

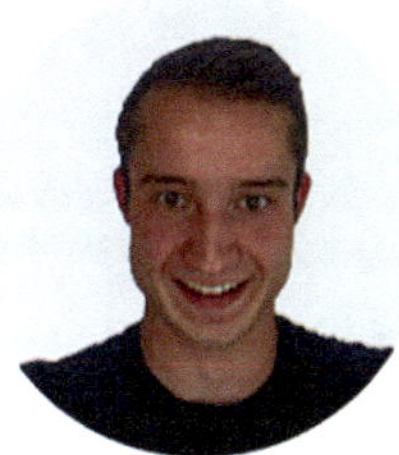

"[...] there are a lot of people who have ambitions to continue their education even after completing their training and it's annoying if they can't continue their education."

"It is inevitable that interprofessional collaborations are the cornerstone of future innovation."

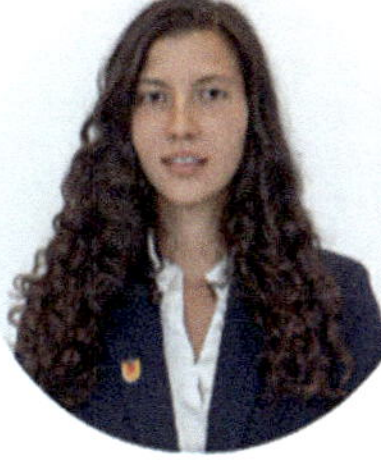

Christiana
4. Semester
Medicine
Netherlands

Clara
6. Semester
Pharmacy
United Kingdom

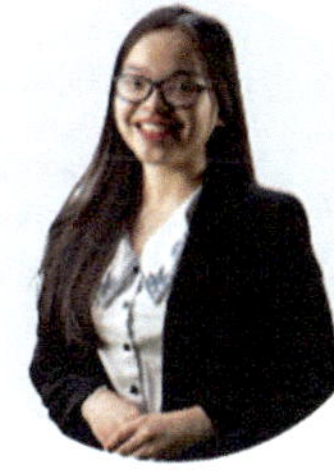

"[...] each university should have a student committee for interprofessional learning and practice so that they could represent the student voices on a larger scale."

"Interprofessional learning and the teaching of non-technical teamwork skills should be an integral part of the curriculum - not just an option for students who are already interested in the subject."

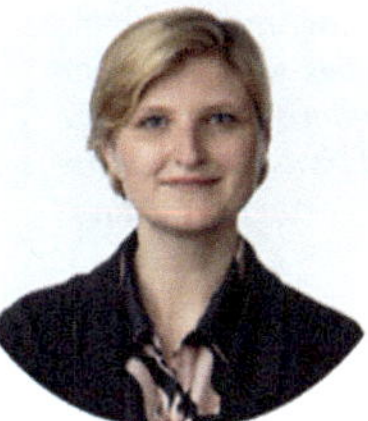

Lina
11. Semester
Medicine
Germany

Antriani
6. Semester
Nursing
Cyprus

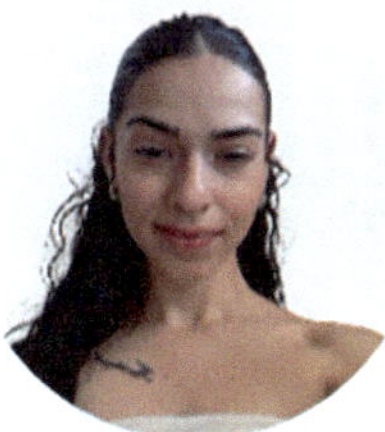

"[...] the stakeholders need to create an appropriate environment to keep students motivated and make them enjoy their IP education."

"[...] it's crucial to allocate the necessary resources. This means providing ample funding for staffing, facilities, and technology to create an environment that actively encourages collaboration between healthcare professionals and students"

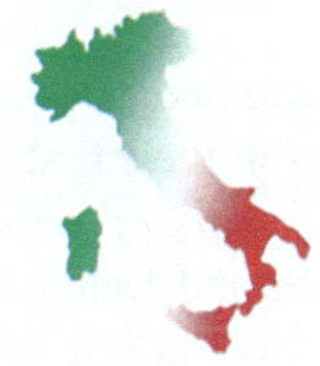

Lorenzo
9. Semester
Medicine
Italy

Fig. 1 Participating European healthcare students and their recommendations for the future of interprofessional education and collaborative practice

Laith
10. Semester
Medicine
Cyprus

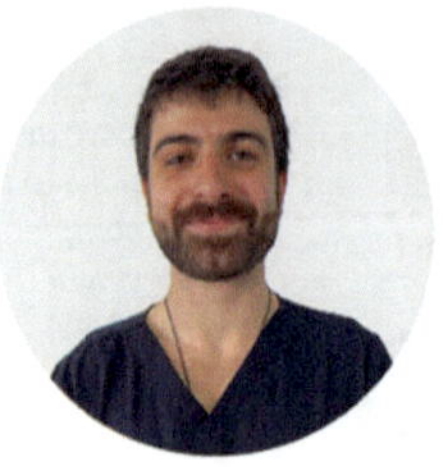

"Use models or simulations based on real clinical scenarios and let students collaborate."

"I see a lot of potential in the placements. During these times it could be a great benefit to get the students together in their daily work life and to exchange at the workplace."

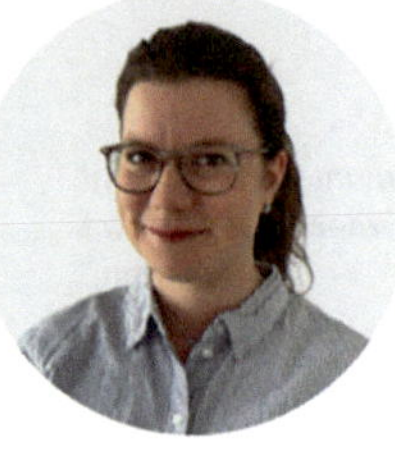

Lina
10. Semester
Physiotherapy
Switzerland

Britt
6. Semester
Speech and Language Therapy
Netherlands

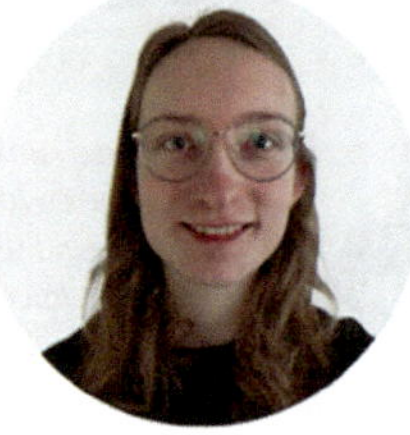

"I think it is really important to get more IP education and have more classes together with other disciplines, to get to know about each others work and how you can assist each other later in life at work"

"[...] it would be good to have more teaching methods such as case studies, workshops and simulations early in the education to engage students more and contribute to better understanding."

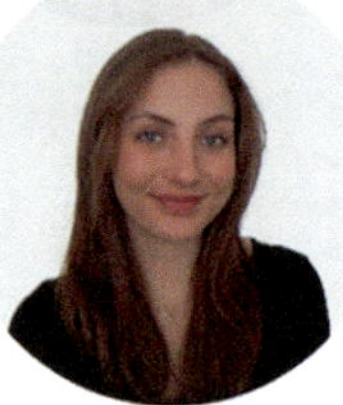

Eleni
4. Semester
Nursing
Sweden

Amanda
9. Semester
Medicine
Sweden

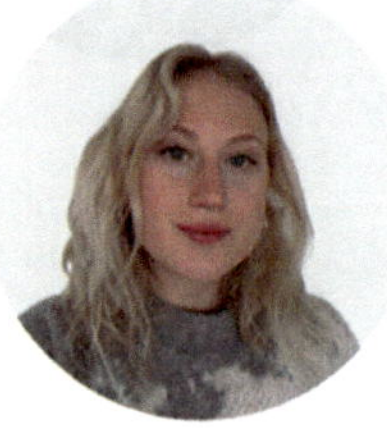

"[...] it would be a great idea to integrate IP education more in the clinic and less in a theoretical way."

Fig. 1 (continued)

year with other medical and health sciences students" (Pharmacy, UK). However, especially among students in their first years of study, IPE can be practically non-existing: *"In the first two years of my study I haven't really had any interprofessional education"* (Speech and Language Therapy, NL). Even later on, IPE was mostly reported to take place on rare occasions only and not to be integrated into everyday study life: *"The fact that KUA [the interprofessional training ward] is a clinical rotation that only lasts for two weeks makes me realize that I really don't experience IP education in daily life as a health care student. I rarely meet students from other disciplines"* (Medicine, SW).

Moreover, what is on offer does not always seem to be of great use and can sometimes fail to connect with reality: *"During the first IPL [Interprofessional Learning] in semester one, we got an overview of the different professions, but I don't feel that it gave much information about what the interprofessional work looks like in practice"* (Nursing, SW). Students recognize that in many places IPE programs are still at a developing stage: *"There seems to be an ongoing search for a way to meaningfully bring nursing and medicine education together for focused sessions"* (Medicine, CY).

Also, the transition from theory to practice poses difficulties in the eyes of students, and the methods taught do not seem to find their way into classrooms: *"The education about how IP should be was pretty precise but the implementation during class not really"* (Physiotherapy, CH). Therefore it sometimes falls to student associations to take the initiative: "*Together with nursing and fellow medical students I engaged in workshops, followed lectures and took part in conferences*" (Medicine, NL).

Internships, on the other hand, seem to foster many IP learning opportunities: *"In my opinion, the mandatory three-month nursing internship was the only real interprofessional education possibility, as we could support nurses in their daily ward routine together with other nursing students. This internship was a very valuable learning experience"* (Medicine, DE). This is supported by statements from other students: *"Our university offers a comprehensive program that includes extensive internship opportunities, which means I have the chance to work directly with professionals from various healthcare disciplines. This has significantly improved my understanding of teamwork dynamics and allowed me to see how different skills integrate to provide comprehensive patient care"* (Medicine, IT). Especially aspiring healthcare professionals who conduct their internships at various professional fields seem to benefit greatly from a better understanding of roles and responsibilities and enhance their (teamwork) skills: *"We complete 8 internships during the 3 years of training (nursing 3 weeks, home care 2 weeks, psychiatry 2 weeks, emergency 2–3 weeks, ICU [Intensive Care Unit] 2–3 weeks, anesthesia 2–3 weeks, elective internship 3 weeks, emergency call center 3 days). Thanks to the insights that we are able to gain through the training, I find that this extremely promotes IP between the different professional groups and that both sides can benefit from each other (both professionally and on a personal level)"* (Paramedic, CH).

During the group discussion, the participating students concluded that while improvements have been made over the past years, there is still insufficient time for IPE in today's healthcare curricula. Additionally, due to a lack of structure, compatibility between the curricula of different professions hinders IPE greatly, calling for more alignment. Where there are IPE activities today, they are often theoretical, while the chances to experience IPC in real-life scenarios are kept to a minimum and are often insufficiently facilitated. Furthermore, it was found that a lack of knowledge about roles and responsibilities of other members of the IP care team in combination with a lack of resources—such as healthcare staff, time, and financial incentives—makes it difficult to actually practice IPECP. Despite these difficulties, the students saw great potential in IPECP, not only in terms of improved patient care, but also in creating a more welcoming and inclusive climate inside the healthcare system.

Where have you experienced challenges when it comes to interprofessional education and practice in the past and what ways did or do you see to overcome them?

Challenges

- ► Not enough emphasis on IPECP in an already packed curriculum
- ► Lack of understanding regarding roles & responsibilities (of other professions)
- ► Lack of common language (profession-specific terminologies make teamwork and communication difficult)
- ► Question of responsibility: Who is responsible for decisions taken by the IP team?

Solutions

- ► Integrate IPE activities in a longitudinal way from the outset to the end of studies
- ► Implement an "IP Health Campus" that would let students learn with, about, and from each other
- ► Reduce the jargon and agree on a common terminology
- ► Introduce sub-responsibilities and define concrete checkpoints to evaluate care

Students reflected vividly on their own experiences with IPECP, trying to come up with answers to both sides of this question. One key issue seems to be a lack of understanding of each other's professions, roles and responsibilities: "*When I started my minor, a lot of people didn't know much about it. Especially about my discipline (Speech and Language therapy) there were a lot of false statements*" (Speech and Language Therapy, NL). This lack of understanding seems to be fuelled by insufficient IPE opportunities and may have grave consequences for collaborative practice: "*Another major challenge is that medical students aren't aware of what nursing students learn. We aren't given any information on what they specialise in, therefore we wouldn't be able to know how to synergise our skills with theirs until we see how it's done in the clinical environment we eventually find ourselves placed in*" (Medicine, CY).

To that point, there is also a more practical side to common (miss-)understanding, which might be rooted more deeply within healthcare professions: "*One challenge has been communication between team members from different healthcare disciplines. I think different professions have a tradition of communicating differently"* (Medicine, SW).

However, students did not only highlight challenges but also the possibilities they saw in overcoming them. This can be exemplified by the lack of understanding and difficulties in communicating: *"Regarding education at university, I found the use of different specific professional terminologies challenging. My team overcame this by reducing the number of jargon, showing visual aids whenever possible, and trying to give relevant examples for explanation"* (Pharmacy, UK).

Students face practical issues when trying to connect with their peers from other healthcare professions: *"I also had the feeling that during studies, every profession has their own timetable and things to learn and with these terms it was harder to connect with a student of another profession"* (Physiotherapy, SW). They envision structural changes that could bring different healthcare students closer together and facilitate better IP exchange: *"An interprofessional health campus would shorten the distances, enable exchange during the lunch break"* (Medicine, DE).

When it comes to IPC, different challenges have been observed by students, such as the decision-making process, which *"might be prolonged due to lengthy deliberations among various professionals"* (Pharmacy, UK). However, there appear to be ways around that, which are already in place in some cases: *"From my experience at hospitals, they overcame this with more effective communication and leadership skills"* (Pharmacy UK).

With increased IPC, students also recognized the question of shared responsibilities as an emerging concern: *"Both or neither parties wanting to take the responsibility upon them"* (Medicine, NL). They offered solutions and did not shy away from evaluating them critically: *"Deciding sub-responsibilities and choosing concrete check and evaluation points. Also, agreeing upon scenarios during which the responsibility shifts may be beneficial (this statement should be taken with a grain of salt because it is not widely applicable)"* (Medicine, NL).

During the group discussion, the participating students concluded that there is a gap between theory and practice in every field of clinical practice, which also includs IPECP. To overcome this, today's healthcare professionals should lead by example and foster better IPC by showing the aspiring generation how it is done well. Additionally, as theoretical explanations do not seem as beneficial as the actual exchange with other healthcare professionals, more emphasis should be put on fostering exchange between students early on during education. This could, for instance, be done by sharing the same campus and having faculty from different professional backgrounds. As there may arise the challenge of students bringing various levels of knowledge to IPE activities, depending on their study progression, IPE could combine students across different semesters for certain topics and let these be collaboratively explored. Furthermore, IPE activities should not be an "add-on" to the curriculum of healthcare students, but rather integrated in a longitudinal way from the outset to the end of their studies and beyond.

Finally, the group agreed that while internships are a great IPE opportunity, there can easily be a lack of motivation for students when they do not feel apprcciated by more experienced members of the healthcare team. To overcome this, internships need to be facilitated by IPECP-experienced educators that can provide guidance and concrete examples for the students to witness the impact of successful IPC.

What advice would you give stakeholders (e.g. policy makers, educational institutions, researchers,...) for them to enable more successful interprofessional education and practice in the future?

- ► Implementing IPE early and continuously throughout the curriculum
- ► Offering more diverse and advanced teaching methods such as simulations and reality-based teaching
- ► Bringing students across fields together
- ► Offering IPE for post-graduates
- ► Providing ample funding and resources for IPE and IPC
- ► Increasing the understanding of roles and responsibilities to ensure functioning IPC
- ► Using placements/internships to experience IPC and to enhance IP understanding and collaboration

The last question focused on the students' recommendation towards different stakeholders with the aim to improve IPECP. In general, there still do not seem to be enough IPE opportunities for students, which they viewed as an integral part to enable them to work collaboratively in the future: *"I think it is really important to get more IP education and have more classes together with other disciplines, to get to know about each other's work and how you can assist each other later in life at work"* (Speech and Language Therapy, NL). The students widely agreed on the fact that IPE should be integrated early on: *"Therefore it would be good to have more teaching methods such as case studies, workshops and simulations early in the education to engage students more and contribute to better understanding"* (Nursing, SW). After early implementation, however, students emphasized that it would be crucial to tailor IPE activities for every step in the curriculum: *"Secondly, integration of IP education is key. It should be seamlessly woven into the curricula of various healthcare professions from the very beginning. This way, students can understand and appreciate the importance of working together as a cohesive team"* (Medicine, IT).

Furthermore, from the students' perspective, IPE should transition from theoretical to more practical approaches: *"I think that it would be a great idea to integrate IP education more in the clinic and less in a theoretical way"* (Medicine, SW). In their view, IPE should be as hands-on and reality-based as possible to enable fruitful collaborations between healthcare students: *"Use models or simulations based on real clinical scenarios and let students collaborate"* (Medicine, CY). They called for modern teaching methods, including learning competitions, to be implemented: *"There should be interactive activities such as workshops or learning competitions at least once every year"* (Pharmacy, UK).

As far as successful IPC goes, students allocated potential in their internships, where a direct translation from IPE and IPC is possible: *"I see a lot of potential in the placements. During these times it could be a great benefit to get the students together in their daily work life and to exchange at the workplace. Then it will lose the theoretical background and profits from the daily need of knowledge and organisation from another profession. For the future it will also create more efficient work within the IP world"* (Physiotherapy, CH).

Furthermore, the participating students agreed on the fact that IPE should not stop with graduation and that for successful IPC post-graduate training opportunities need to exist as well: "*there are a lot of people who have ambitions to continue their education even after completing their training and it's annoying if they can't continue their education*" (Paramedic, CH). However, students acknowledged that there are some challenges in turning these recommendations into reality and urged stakeholders to allocate the necessary resources: *"This means providing ample funding for staffing, facilities, and technology to create an environment that actively encourages collaboration between healthcare professionals and students"* (Medicine, IT).

During the group discussion, the participating students agreed that IPECP should be a natural part of everyday life for a European healthcare student in the twenty-first century. By sharing campuses, lecture halls, and resources—and maybe even attending university-organized social events—students are much more likely to make interprofessional friendships out-of-hospital, which would come in very handy when trying to improve collaborations inside the hospitals (this is also true for the out-patient/primary care sector, of course). From a structural point of view, IPE can only be beneficial if the different study programs are better aligned, IPE is properly integrated into the curricula, enough resources are provided, and teachers have been educated in the field of IPECP. To this point, curriculum-developers should ideally consist of an interprofessional team as well and students (and their feedback) should be included early on. From an educational standpoint, new learning formats such as workshops, competitions, masterclasses, Q&As, simulations, and training wards should be included to ensure sustainable learning experiences for participating students.

Discussion

Participating students—despite studying in a variety of European countries, having diverse professional backgrounds, and being at different stages of their education—could generally agree on the state of IPECP in Europe today.

Their claims of systematic challenges, such as the scarcity of time and space in the curricula of healthcare professionals or the lack of emphasis placed on IPE, are echoed in policy documents of students' associations, and supported by literature since the early 2000s [3, 5].

One vivid example is a literature review from a decade ago, where on a governmental and professional level the *"Lack/limited financial resources"*, on an institutional level the *"Rigid/condensed curriculum"* or the *"Different degree timetables"*, and on an individual level the *"Lack/limited knowledge about other health professions"* have been reported as barriers towards IPE implementation [15, p. 307]. These barriers are almost identical in wording as the concerns voiced by the participating students of this chapter, which aligns with the fact that many of these barriers are still regarded to hinder the successful implementation of IPE today [13].

Many challenges for efficient and effective IPC that have been named by the students, such as the lack of a common language/form of communication, the (miss-)understanding of roles and responsibilities, and the structural deficits with a lack of resources in the workplace have been reported as barriers in a systematic meta-review as well [25]. Consequently, the interviewed students urged stakeholders not to forget about post-graduate students and provide them with ample IPE opportunities—a recommendation that seems widely supported [12, 27].

With regard to the ongoing expansion in the field of IPE—which is welcomed by the students—their wish to be included in the development and evaluation of the mentioned activities should be taken seriously. Not only do international students' associations call for the same [10], but this is also in line with a feedback culture proposed in adult education, as for example in step 6 of the 6-Step-Approach to curriculum development for medical education [22]. Some institutions already implement a student-feedback-culture [26], but as outlined in the introduction and evidenced by the participants' responses, this is still not the current standard of practice. With recent literature such as the AMEE guide Nr. 138 highlighting the value of so-called *"learner involvement in the co-creation of teaching and learning"* [14, p. 924], healthcare faculty have been provided with the necessary evidence and tools. Now it is up to them to include motivated students and make this change a reality.

To answer the question regarding the "right time for IPE", a recent systematic review found evidence that led its authors to advocate for European countries to *"include IPE from the first years of undergraduate education and invest effort into including in IPE a broader representation of professions involved in healthcare settings"* [6, p. 107]. This fits with what interviewed students agreed upon and with what has been done for quite some time in some exemplary parts of Europe [26]; IPE should be started early on in training.

As for how to implement IPE, it is not only the students that call for the implementation of new educational formats when it comes to IPE. Similar recommendations have been made by IPE researchers [12], some explicitly highlighting the differences between uni- and interprofessional student group learning [24] and others recommending to focus on experiential learning [8].

The fact that students call for better education of their teachers on IPE goes in line with a recommendation of the 2022 Position paper of the GMA Committee Interprofessional Education in the Health Professions [12], as well as with the Framework on Action on Interprofessional Education and Collaborative Practice by the WHO [27]. As a matter of fact, the issue of faculty development was already highlighted over a decade ago [17]. However, a global report from 2022 found that only about half of the participating institutions provided *"specific training on how to teach and facilitate interprofessional education to their faculty and academic staff*" [13, p. 31], supporting what European students encounter on a day-to-day basis.

In conclusion, students' views on the challenges of IPECP and their recommendations to overcome them aligned fairly well with what has been reported in literature before. It falls now upon educational institutions, policy makers and other stakeholders to take these recommendations seriously and ensure high-quality IPE for all (European) healthcare students.

Limitations

The obvious limitations of this chapter stem from the small number of interviewees and the use of convenience sampling. The latter opens the door for a selection bias, with results not accurately reflecting the entire population of students. However, the fact that the interviewed students' opinions were mostly in line with what international healthcare students' associations call for with regards to IPECP [11], strengthens their position as representative examples of today's European healthcare students. The rather small sample size was chosen to ensure feasibility of an online discussion with participants, where they could share their experiences with each other and reach a consensus regarding the posed questions.

The objective of this chapter was not to provide a statistically representative account of all European healthcare students on the topic of IPECP. On the contrary, the authors aimed at emphasizing the lived experiences and personal voices of representatives of those affected most directly by IPE, thereby enabling readers to engage with the real individuals behind the often neglected and generalized category of "students".

Recommendations for Policy Makers and Educators

- ► Ensuring pan-European implementation of IPE activities for healthcare students from all professional backgrounds
- ► Integrating IPE early on and continuously throughout the curriculum
- ► Including students (as the primary target group) in the reviewing process of current and the development of new IPE-activities
- ► Offering IPE to post-graduate students and health professionals and helping them become IPC role models for the next generation

Bridging the Gap

Deriving from the answers to *Question 2* it becomes clear that students are generally motivated when it comes to IPE activities and see many benefits in IPC. Challenges for effective IPE, among others, remain the misalignment of curricula of healthcare students, the lack of time and resources allocated to this field, and the often theoretical instead of practice-based approach towards IPE.

As seen in the discussion, the challenges students face when it comes to IPECP are already widely known in literature. However, whilst many IP programs have been piloted during the past decades, there remains a gap between what today's healthcare students need in terms of IPE and what they are offered. As we saw in this chapter, students are ready to tackle the hurdles and improve IPE because they see many benefits of IPECP—not only for patients, but for the healthcare system as a whole. They not only point out challenges but envision solutions as well. Listening to the students and engaging them actively in the development of new IPE activities will likely help us to bridge this gap.

Reflective Questions

- ► Are (your) students from all healthcare professions and over the entire span of their education provided with equal IPE opportunities?
- ► Have (your) students, as the primary target group, been included in the development and reviewing process of IPE activities?
- ► Are you as a healthcare professional and potential IPE educator leading by example in terms of successful IPC?

References

1. Abu-Rish E, Kim S, Choe L, Varpio L, Malik E, White AA, Craddick K, et al. Current trends in interprofessional education of health sciences students: a literature review. J Interprof Care. 2012;26(6):444–51. https://doi.org/10.3109/13561820.2012.715604.
2. Algahtani H, Shirah B, Bukhari H, Alkhamisi H, Ibrahim B, Subahi A, Aldarmahi A. Perceptions and attitudes of different healthcare professionals and students toward interprofessional education in Saudi Arabia: a cross-sectional survey. J Interprof Care. 2021;35(3):476–81. https://doi.org/10.1080/13561820.2020.1758642.
3. Barr H, Koppel I, Reeves S, Hammick M, Freeth D. Effective interprofessional education: argument, assumption and evidence. 1st ed. Wiley; 2005. https://doi.org/10.1002/9780470776445.
4. Berger-Estilita J, Chiang H, Stricker D, Fuchs A, Greif R, McAleer S. Attitudes of medical students towards interprofessional education: a mixed-methods study. Edited by Elisa J. F. Houwink. PLoS One. 2020;15(10):e0240835. https://doi.org/10.1371/journal.pone.0240835.
5. Carlisle C, Cooper H, Watkins C. 'Do none of you talk to each other?': the challenges facing the implementation of interprofessional education. Med Teach. 2004;26(6):545–52. https://doi.org/10.1080/61421590410001711616.
6. Colonnello V, Kinoshita Y, Yoshida N, Villalobos IB. Undergraduate interprofessional education in the European higher education area: a systematic review. Int Med Educ. 2023;2(2):100–12. https://doi.org/10.3390/ime2020010.
7. Gilligan C, Outram S, Levett-Jones T. Recommendations from recent graduates in medicine, nursing and pharmacy on improving interprofessional education in university programs: a qualitative study. BMC Med Educ. 2014;14(1):52. https://doi.org/10.1186/1472-6920-14-52.

8. Hall LW, Zierler BK. Interprofessional education and practice guide no. 1: developing faculty to effectively facilitate interprofessional education. J Interprof Care. 2015;29(1):3–7. https://doi.org/10.3109/13561820.2014.937483.
9. Herath C, Zhou Y, Gan Y, Nakandawire N, Gong Y, Zuxun L. A comparative study of interprofessional education in global health care: a systematic review. Medicine. 2017;96(38):e7336. https://doi.org/10.1097/MD.0000000000007336.
10. International Federation of Medical Students' Associations (IFMSA). IFMSA policy document: interprofessional education and collaborative practice. International Federation of Medical Students' Associations (IFMSA); 2023. https://ifmsa.org/wp-content/uploads/2023/05/IFMSA-Policy-Document-on-Interprofessional-Education-and-Collaborative-Practice.docx.pdf
11. International Federation of Medical Students' Associations (IFMSA), and European Regional Office International Pharmaceutical Students' Federation (IPSF). CALL FOR ACTION on interprofessional collaboration and education. International Federation of Medical Students' Associations (IFMSA) and the European Regional Office of the International Pharmaceutical Students' Federation (IPSF); 2020. https://drive.google.com/file/d/1nJNqN5EjcwBMh3qSwg7YeH-5DXO4L9Dl/view?usp=sharing
12. Kaap-Fröhlich S, Ulrich G, Wershofen B, Ahles J, Behrend R, Handgraaf M, Herinek D, et al. Position paper of the GMA committee interprofessional education in the health professions – current status and outlook. GMS J Med Educ. 2022;39(2)
13. Khalili H, Lackie K, Langlois S, Wetzlmair LC, Working Group. Global IPE situational analysis result final report. Interprofessional Research. Global Publication; 2022. www.interprofessionalresearch.global
14. Könings KD, Mordang S, Smeenk F, Stassen L, Ramani S. Learner involvement in the co-creation of teaching and learning: AMEE Guide No. 138. Med Teach. 2021;43(8):924–36. https://doi.org/10.1080/0142159X.2020.1838464.
15. Lawlis TR, Anson J, Greenfield D. Barriers and enablers that influence sustainable interprofessional education: a literature review. J Interprof Care. 2014;28(4):305–10. https://doi.org/10.3109/13561820.2014.895977.
16. Mohammed CA, Narsipur S, Vasthare R, Singla N, Ran ALY, Suryanarayana JP. Attitude towards shared learning activities and interprofessional education among dental students in South India. Eur J Dent Educ. 2021;25(1):159–67. https://doi.org/10.1111/eje.12586.
17. Reeves S, Tassone M, Parker K, Wagner SJ, Simmons B. Interprofessional education: an overview of key developments in the past three decades. Work. 2012;41(3):233–45. https://doi.org/10.3233/WOR-2012-1298.
18. Rodrigues Da Silva Noll Gonçalves J, Gonçalves RN, Da Rosa SV, Orsi JSR, Moysés SJ, Werneck RI. Impact of interprofessional education on the teaching and learning of higher education students: a systematic review. Nurse Educ Pract. 2021;56(October):103212. https://doi.org/10.1016/j.nepr.2021.103212.
19. Suter E, Deutschlander S, Mickelson G, Nurani Z, Lait J, Harrison L, Jarvis-Selinger S, et al. Can interprofessional collaboration provide health human resources solutions? A knowledge synthesis. J Interprof Care. 2012;26(4):261–8. https://doi.org/10.3109/13561820.2012.663014
20. Swiss Youth Health Alliance (SYHA). Position paper regarding interprofessionality in the education and training of healthcare professions. Swiss Youth Health Alliance (SYHA); 2020. https://files.designer.hoststar.ch/4a/17/4a17c245-e89f-437a-9fac-b26b25805dbd.pdf
21. Teodorczuk A, Khoo TK, Morrissey S, Rogers G. Developing interprofessional education: putting theory into practice. Clin Teach. 2016;13(1):7–12. https://doi.org/10.1111/tct.12508.
22. Thomas PA, Kern DE, Hughes MT, Tachettt SA, Chen BY. Curriculum development for medical education – a six-step approach. 4th ed. Johns Hopkins University Press; 2022.
23. Ulrich G, Hermann A, Glardon O, Kaap-Fröhlich S. Interprofessionelle Ausbildung im Schweizer Gesundheitssystem: Situationsanalyse, Perspektiven und Roadmap. Careum Working Paper 9. Careum Working Paper. Pestalozzistrasse, 3 CH-8032. Zürich: Careum Stiftung; 2020.

24. Van Diggele C, Roberts C, Burgess A, Mellis C. Interprofessional education: tips for design and implementation. BMC Med Educ. 2020;20(S2):455. https://doi.org/10.1186/s12909-020-02286-z.
25. Wei H, Horns P, Sears SF, Huang K, Smith CM, Wei TL. A systematic meta-review of systematic reviews about interprofessional collaboration: facilitators, barriers, and outcomes. J Interprof Care. 2022;36(5):735–49. https://doi.org/10.1080/13561820.2021.1973975.
26. Wilhelmsson M, Pelling S, Ludvigsson J, Hammar M, Dahlgren L-O, Faresjö T. Twenty years experiences of interprofessional education in Linköping – ground-breaking and sustainable. J Interprof Care. 2009;23(2):121–33. https://doi.org/10.1080/13561820902728984.
27. World Health Organization. Framework for action on interprofessional education & collaborative practice. WHO; 2010.

Lucas Büsser MD, is co-founder and current president of the Swiss Health Alliance for Interprofessional Education (SHAPED, www.shaped-ip.ch), a student- and early-career-led organization dedicated to advancing interprofessional education and collaboration in Switzerland. He has led the development, implementation, and evaluation of multiple interprofessional learning initiatives for undergraduate and postgraduate health professions learners.

Isabella van Setten MD, is a trained physician from Linköping University Hospital, where she early during her career initiated an educational focus, such as tutor and mentoring junior medical students and is involved in several educational and patient perspective improvements. She has also served as a member of the "Committee for Interprofessional Learning", contributing to the development and enhancement of interprofessional education and collaboration within the medical faculty.

Corina Zweifel BSc, is a physiotherapist specializing in neurology and a master's student in Bern. She serves as an executive board member of the Swiss Health Alliance for Interprofessional Education (SHAPED, www.shaped-ip.ch), where she advocates for interprofessional education and collaboration in Switzerland. She leads the Interprofessional Case Discussions project team, where students from different healthcare professions join forces to solve a clinical case in a "murder mystery" format.

Interprofessionalism in Action—Building a Bridge Between Person-Centered Practice and Education

Sandra Jorna-Lakke, Anita Kidritsch, Ingrid Aerts, Jaana Paltamaa, Ursula Hemetek, Joost Hurkmans, and INPRO Consortium

The European Commission's support for the production of this publication does not constitute an endorsement of the contents, which reflect the views only of the authors, and the Commission cannot be held responsible for any use which may be made of the information contained therein.

Co-funded by the Erasmus+ Programme of the European Union

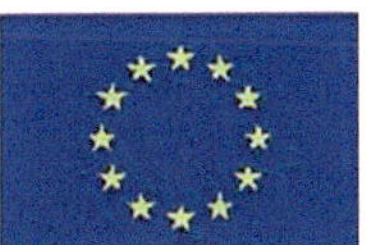

INPRO Consortium

S. Jorna-Lakke (✉)
Research Group Healthy Ageing, Allied Health Care and Nursing, Centre of Expertise Healthy Ageing, Hanze University of Applied Sciences, Groningen, The Netherlands
e-mail: a.e.jorna-lakke@pl.hanze.nl

A. Kidritsch
Institute of Health Sciences, USTP – University of Applied Sciences St. Pölten, St. Pölten, Austria
e-mail: Anita.Kidritsch@fhstp.ac.at

I. Aerts
Department of Health and Sciences, Nutrition and Dietetics Program, AP University of Applied Sciences and Arts, Antwerp, Belgium
e-mail: ingrid.aerts@ap.be

J. Paltamaa
School of Health and Social Studies, Jamk University of Applied Sciences, Jyväskylä, Finland
e-mail: jaana.paltamaa@jamk.fi

U. Hemetek
Department of Health Sciences, University of Applied Sciences, St. Pölten, Austria

J. Hurkmans
Rehabilitation Centre "Revalidatie Friesland", Beetsterzwaag, The Netherlands

A. Xyrichis et al. (eds.), *Building Bridges: A European Perspective on Interprofessional Education, Practice, Policy and Research*,
https://doi.org/10.1007/978-3-032-23222-9_8

Abbreviations

ICF	International Classification of Functioning, Disability and Health
INPRO	Interprofessionalism in Action
INPRO CF	INPRO Competency Framework
IPECP	Interprofessional Education and Collaborative Practice
SR-IPLW	Student-Run Interprofessional Learning Ward

Introduction and Background

Interprofessionalism in Action (INPRO) was an Erasmus+ funded project from 2021 to 2023. It established a "knowledge alliance" involving lecturers, students, managers, and professionals from tertiary education (formally called Higher Education Institutions, here mentioned as education) and Rehabilitation Centers in Austria, Belgium, Finland, and the Netherlands.

The grant proposal for the project was initiated in 2018, reacting to the shift toward more holistic, person-centered healthcare systems. It aimed to integrate Interprofessional Education and Collaborative Practice (IPECP) by creating a robust consortium of diverse professionals from various countries and settings.

The project was initiated as all partners identified the need to adopt a person-centered and practical approach to interprofessionalism. The primary goal of INPRO was to bridge the gap between the competency levels of future professionals and the levels required in rehabilitation practice.

To achieve this, the project team developed various learning materials, tools, and guides that facilitate the transfer from university education to practical IPECP in rehabilitation. Rehabilitation settings are particularly well-suited for IPECP due to the complex and holistic nature of care in these environments.

In this chapter, we share the key INPRO materials, tools, and guides based on the *International Classification of Functioning, Disability and Health (ICF)* as a common language, and the newly created INPRO interprofessional competency framework (INPRO CF). These resources, which are summarized in Tables 1 and 2, were designed to bridge the gap between students' competency levels in IPECP and the levels required in rehabilitation practice. We describe the lessons learned within INPRO and their practical applications to supporting lifelong learning for both students and professionals.

Table 1 A summary of themes ($n = 4$) and ICF-based tools and practices actions ($n = 18$)

Themes	Title	Language	URL
ICF training in the work field ($n = 8$)	ICF and goal-setting workshops	E	https://edu.nl/d7c39
	ICF specialist hours "get to know each other"	E+F	https://edu.nl/gy7ft
	ICF training to all rehabilitation professionals	E	https://edu.nl/jet3e
	Workshop "Setting a Main Goal"	E+D	https://edu.nl/kxjkm
	Training for all the disciplines to explain how ICF is integrated into an electronic device for *persons with disabilities*	E+D	https://edu.nl/fqp4w
	Blackboard course ICF interprofessional: A tool to help the interns make the translation from ICF in education to ICF in practice	E	https://edu.nl/cb49u
	A diary of someone in practice who applies ICF in very small steps	E	https://edu.nl/7k6b8
	Development of a digital escape room	E	https://edu.nl/qxy8p
ICF videos ($n = 4$)	Video between a rehabilitation professional and a *person with disability*	E	https://edu.nl/9c4er
	A series of (short) separate videos that are linked to each other	E	https://edu.nl/wmdqc
	A video on the basic explanation of the ICF	D	https://edu.nl/qw438
ICF-based tools ($n = 4$)	Pilot of ICF-based tools and practices to occupational therapists	E+F	https://edu.nl/9f9ph
	Pilot of ICF-based tools and practices to speech therapists	E+F	https://edu.nl/rnr7p
	Pilot of ICF-based tools and practices to physiotherapists	E+F	https://edu.nl/u9vfj
	Use the "Discussion-tool" for filling in the ICF form	E+D	https://edu.nl/qde9v
ICF documentation ($n = 2$)	Implementation of the ICF documentation system for dietitians—step-by-step guideline	E	https://edu.nl/3ttgc
	Development of an ICF table in an electronic device for *persons with disabilities*	E	https://edu.nl/rjfyj

E English, *D* Dutch, *F* Finnish

Table 2 A summary of the INPRO materials with links as an addition to the ICF-based tools and practices listed in Table 1

Title	URL	
INPRO Competency Framework: User's Guide	https://edu.nl/y4g3f	Aerts et al. [1]
INPRO Competency Framework: Competency Book	https://edu.nl/db9y7	Aerts et al. [2]
INPRO Competentie Raamwerk (in Dutch)	https://edu.nl/y6d7r	Aerts et al. [3]
INPRO Kompetenz Rahmenmodell (in German)	https://edu.nl/dwp37	Aerts et al. [4]
INPRO Competency Framework (in Finnish)	https://edu.nl/vrm7e	Aerts et al. [5]
INPRO Competency Framework (only ICF-related Competencies)	https://edu.nl/vwnkx	Aerts et al. [6]
INPRO CF "INPRO Pilot IPE Intervention"	https://edu.nl/8kbvh	Hemetek et al. [20]
INPRO CF Project "Rehabilitation center"	https://edu.nl/abgb6	Kidritsch et al. [26]
INPRO CF "Jamk Pilots"	https://edu.nl/dgege	Ritsilä et al. [39]
INPRO CF "Coronaria"	https://edu.nl/3vnvy	Enqvist et al. [16]
INPRO CF "Hanze"	https://edu.nl/k8w7f	Lakke et al. [29]
INPRO CF "Revalidatie Friesland"	https://edu.nl/v9gtu	Atsma et al. [9]
INPRO CF Project "Hospital in Belgium"	https://edu.nl/6va4p	De Weerdt and Aerts [12]
INPRO CF "MOHA project"	https://edu.nl/u6r74	Schulner-Weiß et al. [41]
ICF-based tools and practices to promote the use of ICF—a summary on the development actions (a report)	https://edu.nl/umr3m	Paltamaa et al. [36]
ICF education continuum: from basic knowledge to practical ICF implementation material	https://edu.nl/ag44j	Paltamaa and Myllyharju-Puikkonen [34]
ICF in person-centered rehabilitation: Material to support the interprofessional implementation	https://edu.nl/f3vt9	Paltamaa and Myllyharju-Puikkonen [35]
INPRO International Online Learning	https://edu.nl/abvct	Hemetek et al. [21]
INPRO Renewed-interprofessional Skills Day	https://edu.nl/jxfbw	Dielemans et al. [15]
Practice in rehabilitation	https://edu.nl/p8r36	Zimmel et al. [49]
Practice in prevention, with children	https://edu.nl/qca63	Zimmel et al. [50]
Self-esteem meeting	https://edu.nl/jkbqd	Lathi and INPRO Consortium [28]
Role of the coach	https://edu.nl/uy39r	Atsma et al. [9]
Annual employee conversation	https://edu.nl/hthgr	Haumer and Schulner-Weiß [18]
Open Exchange Forum	https://edu.nl/vrh97	[30])

(continued)

Table 2 (continued)

Title	URL	
Design thinking workshops	https://edu.nl/cpg9n	Freisleben-Teutscher et al. [17]
Family group conference	https://edu.nl/hqtqf	Delorette and INPRO consortium [14])
Process guide HEI	https://edu.nl/jgwe9	Hemetek et al. [21]
Student journey	https://www.youtube.com/watch?v=XMuPeKctuZM	De Smedt et al. [11]
Person with disability in IPECP	https://h5p.org/node/1216428	Kidritsch et al. [25]
Business case SR-IPL	https://edu.nl/jbdh9	Tammeling et al. [42]
Guideline SR-IPLW	https://edu.nl/p83u6	Hurkmans et al. [22]
Roadmap SR-IPLW; perspective of management	https://edu.nl/nhwkp	Hurkmans et al. [23]

ICF as a Unifying Language for Interprofessional Collaboration

The importance of the ability to function irrespective of physical and mental health status is increasingly acknowledged. The ICF [47] is a framework designed to describe human functioning and is grounded in a person-centered care approach. The ICF provides both a biomedical and biopsychosocial framework that seamlessly complements this shift toward person-centered care [7].

The ICF conceptualizes an individual's functioning as a dynamic interaction between a person's health condition, environmental factors, and personal factors. This framework situates assessment within a personal context by offering guidance in selecting relevant aspects of functioning and disability for treatment. The ICF, thereby, emphasizes the importance of involving the person as an individual in the assessment process for both validity and ethical reasons [48].

A common language is important to support interprofessional collaborative practice [24, 37]. Using consistent ICF language and concepts facilitates comparisons, complementary information, and knowledge building both between the persons in question and professionals involved and between different professionals [48]. Therefore, in INPRO, the ICF played a central role. The ICF is already widely used in the rehabilitation setting worldwide. INPRO faced a need for well-developed knowledge, values, and attitudes to apply the ICF framework in person-centered social and health services. Overall, the learning materials [34], tools, and guides [35] developed by INPRO promoted the application of the ICF in both education and rehabilitation practice. This allowed us to overcome differences in professional language use and the different languages used according to the various models within different professions, environments, sectors, and countries. ICF-based interprofessional collaboration, communication, and documentation provide insight into the context of available structures and resources in practice. This allows us to deepen our understanding of the needs of a person with disability as an essential foundation for person-centered care.

Each partner was aware of the importance of the ICF before the INPRO project started. At first, we assumed that all partners had relatively similar knowledge bases. However, during the project, differences in perceptions and knowledge levels became apparent. This underlined the importance of the ICF training and ICF-based tools and guides both in education and rehabilitation centers. During the project, we learned that, in IPECP, various stakeholders have their own roles, tasks, and responsibilities. In the following, we will discuss this from different perspectives.

Key Stakeholder Perspectives in INPRO

Persons With disabilities

In INPRO, person-centered rehabilitation occurred at so-called Student-Run Interprofessional Learning Wards (SR-IPLWs; [22]). SR-IPLWs are communities of practice in an inpatient rehabilitation clinic or at outpatient facilities where persons with disabilities, students, healthcare professionals, and lecturers from education work and learn from, with, and about each other in patient care. Equality between all stakeholders at the SR-IPLW is an important value. This means that patients are regarded as equal learners at the SR-IPLW and seen as *persons* with a health question together with their families, instead of patients with an illness or disease. At the SR-IPLW, the "Activities" and "Participation" components of the ICF framework take a central role. After all, persons with disabilities return to daily life, where they try to function in their various social roles as much as possible. Regarding the environmental factors of the ICF, the following questions arise: "Does the person with disability want to return to work?"; "How is the situation at home?"; "Does the person with disability have a partner, children, grandparents?"; "Are hobbies important for functioning in daily life?"; and so on.

The needs and wishes of the person with disability and their family play a central role and are directly related to the environmental factors of the ICF. We wanted to explore how persons perceived their own influence on their needs and wishes during the rehabilitation process at the SR-IPLWs. To answer this question, we interviewed seven persons with disabilities who received rehabilitation treatment at three different SR-IPLWs in three different European countries, namely, at Rehabilitation Center "Revalidatie Friesland" (the Netherlands), Coronaria Rehabilitation and Therapy Services (Finland), and Moorheilbad Harbach Gesundheits- & Rehabilitationszentrum (Austria). We used a common interview guide covering various topics. Our questions encouraged them to outline their journey. Additionally, persons with disabilities were asked to share their experiences with healthcare professionals and their experience of interprofessional collaboration between professionals and students at the SR-IPLW [10].

The results of the Dutch interviews described effective rehabilitation strategies and challenges faced during recovery. All persons with disabilities emphasized the importance of empathic care and individualized therapy during rehabilitation. However, one person encountered limitations in self-regulation during his rehabilitation and highlighted the need for more flexibility and comprehensive explanations of decisions made during treatment. Finnish persons with disabilities described lifelong struggles with multiple health conditions, challenging the goals of the treatment at the activity and participation level of the ICF. Another Finnish person with disability emphasized that a fragmented healthcare system underscored the importance of a holistic, interprofessional care system. The Austrian journeys of persons with disabilities showcased successful rehabilitation after knee surgery, highlighting the critical role of personalized care and the necessity of addressing psychological barriers for complete recovery. Another Austrian person with disability also reported a positive experience, emphasizing the importance of individualized treatment, overcoming movement fears, and incorporating psychological support in the interprofessional collaborative practice of the rehabilitation care [10].

All the interviewees underlined essential qualities of professionals and students at the SR-IPLW, such as empathy, supportiveness, compassion, and a non-judgmental attitude toward persons with disabilities. Additionally, descriptions of persons with disabilities underscored the importance of each person's uniqueness, necessitating personalized care by an interprofessional team. Consequently, the team must communicate adequately to share relevant information within the team. Fragmented care is unacceptable when striving for person-centeredness. Treatment at an SR-IPLW, which emphasizes person-centered care through interprofessional collaboration, seamlessly aligns with the needs and wishes of persons with disabilities as identified in this qualitative study [10].

Professionals and students are prepared for interprofessional learning within a community of practice through well-designed interprofessional education, which may take place both at training institutes and in higher education. Within INPRO, the perspective of the person with disability was included in this design of interprofessional education [17]. This is beneficial not only for the educational process but also for persons with disabilities themselves. According to their statements in INPRO, it helps to identify which people could be asked to get answers on health questions, gain experience-based knowledge, and see their contribution in educating healthcare professionals about their functioning. Including the person with a disability in the IP team makes it easier to formulate their needs and goals, act as equal partners in discussions, weigh different options of healthcare services, and focus on improving their health condition, instead of focusing on deficits [25].

When implementing IPECP, the best way to include persons with disabilities in interprofessional education is, from their perspective, to use plain language and apply the teach-back technique to check a person's understanding. When persons with disabilities pay full attention to their interactions with healthcare professionals or other people, they feel like embracing a "luxury of slowness." This allows them to feel acknowledged in their narrative, individual interests, and environment. They think this can serve as a strong incentive to recognize their own abilities, take action, and develop their resources. In addition, persons with disabilities who participate in IPECP stated in INPRO that they benefit from acknowledging their own and others' intuition and imagination, and their impressions. This can facilitate an open attitude toward an unclear future, which may include potential deviations from their expectations [25].

Professionals

Even though educational institutions offer ICF framework education to students, more needs to be done to enable graduated professionals to implement the ICF in clinical work [37]. Therefore, tools are needed to facilitate competencies in person-centered care that are grounded in ICF as a unifying framework and common language [24]. The ICF-based tools and practices developed (Tables 1 and 2) were intended to improve the person-centered use of the ICF in rehabilitation practice. These tools can be summarized in four themes: ICF training in the work field, ICF-based tools, ICF videos, and ICF documentation (Table 1). Selected examples of tools and practices are explained in the following two subchapters. The whole process is described in a report, "The ICF-based Tools & Practices" [36].

The training and use of ICF-based tools and practices for various professionals and interns were explored in the rehabilitation centers of Finland and the Netherlands. The ICF and goal-setting workshops at Coronaria [33] and Revalidatie Friesland [43, 44] are specific examples of how ICF and person-centered care practices have been developed. The workshops provided an opportunity to reflect upon ICF and goal setting in an interprofessional setting and generated good ideas and further development suggestions. This kind of setting allowed an opportunity to talk more freely about issues around person-centeredness and interprofessionalism. One important message from Coronaria's professionals was "taking the whole person into account." Revalidatie Friesland professionals found that the ICF framework improved goal setting, especially when working across different professions. Using the ICF clarified the main goal and the timeline for achieving this main goal. Additionally, the ICF clearly defined the conditions for discharge, facilitating an earlier discharge.

We observed that interns struggled with the transition from the theoretical understanding of the ICF to applying it to real persons with disabilities in an interprofessional team setting. Therefore, Revalidatie Friesland developed a 5-week course on Blackboard taught by a professional and a lecturer [45]. For each discipline, training was developed to explain how the ICF can be integrated into the electronic data record. A discussion tool was used to complete the ICF form with persons with disabilities.

Professionals received ICF training through practice-based videos. These video materials can also be used to guide students. Overall, four videos were used to facilitate the training of professionals. They included a video of an interaction between a rehabilitation professional and a person with disability, a video on the basic explanation of the ICF, a series of (short) separate videos, and a video of a team meeting ([36], Page 70).

ICF was implemented in the documentation at rehabilitation centers in Austria [19] and the Netherlands [46]. The perception expressed by professionals and lecturers in INPRO was that "Once ICF is properly implemented, it will save time, though it takes time to get started." This underlines the need for long-term commitment to ICF training for professionals and their managers and the importance of educating students in ICF to ensure a smooth transition to internships and professional practice.

Healthcare professionals engaged in learning and working at the previously introduced SR-IPLW act as preceptors. These experienced clinicians function as lecturers and coaches, supervising students during their interprofessional internship and coaching persons with disabilities during their treatment. Their role is to support students and persons with disabilities in translating theoretical learning to real-world clinical practice. To perform this role at the SR-IPLW, preceptors act as so-called "M-shaped" professionals. An M-shaped professional has deepened knowledge of various expertise areas with a holistic view in shared domains. To facilitate planning and assessment of these interprofessional competencies, a competency framework was required and subsequently developed [13].

By utilizing the INPRO CF (Fig. 1), professionals can assess their own skills or those of their team. The framework outlines learning outcomes or behaviors associated with the knowledge and application of interprofessional collaboration, person-centered care, and the ICF. These outcomes are articulated across various levels of complexity within the domains of Interprofessional Practice,

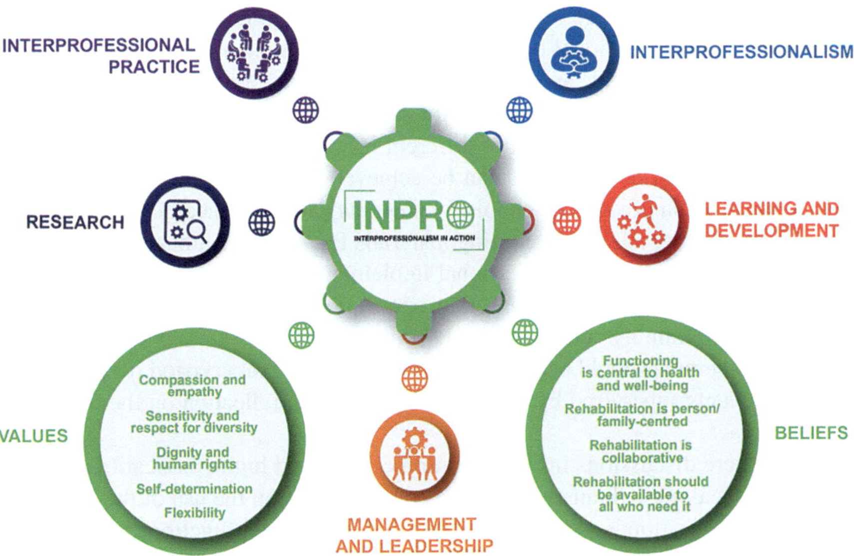

Fig. 1 Overview INPRO CF adapted from WHO-RCF: domains, values, and beliefs [32]

Interprofessionalism, Learning and Development, Management and Leadership, and Research. The framework is available in four languages: English, Dutch, German, and Finnish [2–5]. An overview of only the ICF competencies is also developed [6]. This provides professionals with a solid groundwork for making further developments [1].

Managers

Managers can support professionals in providing person-centered interprofessional care and using the ICF by providing motivation and high-quality training and education for specified learning outcomes. As an example, the INPRO CF and ICF-based tools were used at Moorheilbad Harbach in the annual conversation with employees and their documentation system. Specific training was provided when implementing the tool [18, 41].

Management and Leadership is a domain in the INPRO CF. It delineates interprofessional competencies alongside their associated learning outcomes/behaviors pertaining to teamwork, strategic thinking, management, service development and evaluation, and resource management. This framework serves as a foundational resource for fostering an interprofessional working culture and environment by identifying areas for development and action [1, 12, 29].

The SR-IPLW is based on a strategic agreement between a higher education institution and a rehabilitation center. The SR-IPLW is managed by the Board of Directors of both the rehabilitation centers and the higher education institution, the ward manager, and deans of various academies, and project management. These managers are responsible for achieving the main goal of the SR-IPLW: the implementation of a community of practice where excellent care, high-quality research, innovation, interprofessional education, and collaboration are integrated, designed by students, professionals, and lecturers from various academies [22]. An important success factor of interprofessional education and collaboration is the use of ICF. Therefore, the management at different levels of both organizations needs to facilitate education on ICF. This can be achieved by implementing the ICF basic course in curricula of various schools for students and junior healthcare professionals and introducing advanced learning materials for senior healthcare professionals in order to support the interprofessional implementation of ICF in person-centered care at the SR-IPLW. This means that opportunities for ICF training should be included in the training budget [23, 42]. Additionally, opportunities for interprofessional development should be created, for example, peer supervision for professionals and students supervised by lecturers, during which reflection on the use of ICF can take place.

There were discussions in rehabilitation centers and higher educational institutions about making ICF an everyday practice. To develop the use of the ICF, input from the organization is required. First, the ICF focuses on functional capacity and person-centered clinical reasoning. This can encourage professionals to engage in multi-professional collaboration [8]. However, this requires organizational effort on ICF education in higher educational institutions [40] and ICF training in clinical practice [38]. Second, the professionals and lecturers in INPRO described introducing ICF as follows: "Once ICF is properly implemented, there will be a gain of time, but it takes time to get started." This underlines the need for and long-term commitment to ICF training for professionals and their organizations and the importance of educating students in ICF to ensure a smooth transition to internships and working life. Third, both professionals and lecturers emphasized the importance of management taking an active role when it comes to using ICF. It is, therefore, of the utmost importance that organizational management is fully committed to implementing and teaching ICF before its launch in an organization. The more understanding the managers have of the positive impact of ICF-based practices on their staff members, the better they are at developing implementation strategies for the ICF framework.

The content of this chapter points out that interprofessional use of ICF needs to be initiated and trained. The organizational planning for IPECP (e.g., timelines, financial agreements, and mixing and matching large numbers of learners to equal distributions in interprofessional groups) is challenging for managers as well as administrators [21].

Trainers and Lecturers

At training institutes and in higher education, trainers and lecturers are professionals who influence students and colleagues. They implement interprofessional competencies and ICF-based tools when planning and facilitating educational actions toward interprofessional, shared decision-making. The INPRO project taught us the importance of basic ICF knowledge levels. Different levels of ICF knowledge between professions may hinder progress. During the INPRO project, we became aware of other professionals' paradigms and levels. Therefore, we took more time than expected to address the fact that we needed ICF education within the consortium. For building bridges, we would like to share the insight that your individual needs may not align with those of others at this point.

Trainers and lecturers can achieve individualized learning by using the previously introduced INPRO CF. This framework serves as a fundamental basis for trainers and lecturers to develop assignments and assessment tools. These assignments and assessment tools are designed to align with learning outcomes, which shall be demonstrated in the learners' behaviors, thereby providing a structured foundation for educational initiatives. Selecting suitable learning outcomes was perceived as the most challenging aspect of the process.

Trainers and lecturers can use the INPRO CF to assess their own skills or those of their learners. Because of the INPRO CF, they have a solid foundation to structure and plan further actions. In continuing training and higher education, trainers and lecturers found it beneficial to focus on a smaller set of learning outcomes and realized the importance of avoiding feeling overwhelmed by the multitude of possibilities [9, 16, 41].

As an example from INPRO, interprofessional education was designed for an international online setting. Challenges were the different professional accreditation requirements and inflexible curricula. From each profession and institution, coordinating lecturers had organizing roles. Bridges had to be built between different professional and teaching cultures when lecturers had to take a coaching role [21]. Nevertheless, trainers and lecturers learned when to act or not and created open minds and trust through the additional perspectives they experienced ([21], Page 6). As a consequence, they benefited from the exchange with colleagues and students both on a local and a European level. Next to enhancing their professional competencies, the participants of the international online setting could hone their foreign language skills with English as the main language of communication. This example raises another key stakeholder perspective in INPRO, which will be elaborated on in the following subchapter in more detail.

Students

In INPRO, students participated in the design and implementation of various activities. By using the INPRO CF, students found greater structure and simplicity in reflecting on their progress and setting personal learning outcomes. They discovered the value of concentrating on a limited number of learning outcomes and of giving feedback to their peers from small interprofessional learning groups [1, 15, 20, 26, 39].

In the previously described interprofessional online learning intervention, students achieved the learning outcomes chosen from the INPRO CF [20] by collaborating interprofessionally on the case of a person with disability. By encouraging respect and understanding, they fostered an environment where diverse perspectives were seen as enriching. They honed their professional image and communication skills and learned to ask insightful questions, thereby developing core competencies. Self-confident performance was another benefit:

- "I think that the main learning for me is, that we all can talk English if we want to and that it is possible to have contact and a real conversation about our professions in a multicultural group. Which is really nice, and it boosted my self-confidence" [11].

Learnings of the students were evaluated according to the Kirkpatrick framework [27]:

- Reactions: The students were surprised by the good interprofessional collaboration (communication at eye level, searching together for the best solution) and the precise target definition (very precise goals in terms of body function and structure). They were inspired by the good team atmosphere, in which spirit and coherence were noticeable [49].

- Learnings: In every learning activity, that was evaluated with the use of the Extended Professional Identity Scale, the students' scores improved compared to baseline. The students' learnings were summarized as follows [49]:
  - Taking other professionals on board as a matter of course (accept others' help)
  - Teamwork (learn from the diversity of knowledge of various professional groups)
  - Goal-oriented communication (listening actively, value other opinions)
  - Focus on the person with disability (empathize with their situation, consult a family council if necessary)
- Behavior: Showing the targeted learning outcomes behavior (using the INPRO CF). Students paid attention to the atmosphere of the conversation, applied online counseling/getting to know each other, co-learned, worked in an interprofessional team, got insight into the other's work, saw the perspectives of, and also dealt with reserved/less communicative persons with disabilities. They identified common topics of conversation and noticed what the persons with disabilities could already do or where they could possibly catch up [50].
- Results: The students learned how to network with other professional groups and how to communicate clearly and appreciatively. They realized how important it is to look at the person with disability holistically and to support each other [49].

Lessons Learned by the Researchers of the INPRO Consortium

In the European INPRO project, we collaborated within a large network. Each consortium member was affiliated with their own institute, each with unique strategic goals and stakeholders, including persons with disabilities, researchers, lecturers, managers, students, and financial supporters. Each member of this large network contributed significantly to the success of the INPRO project. We extend our gratitude to them.

Initially, our main focus was on practical tasks: creating materials for the ICF and the INPRO CF, developing SR-IPLWs, and creating and piloting learning materials. However, as we worked on these tasks within our institutes and across different countries, it became clear that effective communication and resource management were crucial for the successful implementation of the INPRO materials. It was also challenging to allocate and use resources such as time, budget, and personnel efficiently. These experiences highlighted the importance of understanding the strategic and tactical aspects in addition to the operational work.

Facilitating and Hindering Factors During the INPRO Project

Throughout the INPRO project, we encountered more factors that either facilitated or hindered our progress in both process and content development. Recognizing these factors was crucial for navigating challenges and leveraging opportunities for success.

Facilitating Factors

- One of the primary facilitating factors was the "Open Exchange Forums" [30]. These forums were organized to foster dialogue and knowledge sharing among project participants. Through these open discussions, we became aware of similarities in the types of facilitating and hindering factors experienced at different levels within our institutes and surrounding networks. Listening to each other's solutions enabled us to address and overcome our own hindering factors more effectively.
- Using the same terminology based on the ICF was a huge facilitating factor that helped us to overcome the language barriers between diverse professions and cultural contexts.
- We also highly valued the shared-decision meetings within the INPRO project [14]. These meetings enabled us to foster competency-oriented communication between the person with disability and the interprofessional team based on the ICF in order to better achieve our goal of person-centered care [28].
- Another significant facilitator was the adoption of a process-oriented approach, which was grounded in design-based research [31]. Involving all stakeholders allowed us to develop and pilot learning materials rapidly. By embracing the concept of learning by doing, we observed firsthand the power of practical, iterative development. This hands-on approach not only accelerated our progress but also ensured that the materials we created were robust and well-suited to real-world applications.
- Additionally, we leveraged existing learning materials, adapting them for interprofessional education. Developing new courses from scratch can be time-consuming for lecturers. We argued that re-using and customizing materials that had already proven effective and received positive feedback from students was a practical and efficient strategy. This approach allowed us to build on established resources, saving time and ensuring quality.

Hindering Factors

While these facilitating factors significantly contributed to our progress, we also faced several hindering factors. These challenges included:

- Diverse organizational cultures: Differences in organizational cultures across the various institutes involved in the project sometimes led to misunderstandings and misalignments in objectives and expectations.
- Resource constraints: Limited resources, in terms of both time and budget, occasionally hindered our ability to execute plans as swiftly or comprehensively as desired.
- Coordination issues: Coordinating efforts among multiple stakeholders and across different geographical locations posed logistical challenges, impacting the smooth execution of activities.
- Cultural competences: Professionals need to be culturally competent to effectively apply ICF principles. This involves understanding and respecting cultural differences, which can be complex and require ongoing education and adaptation.

Overcoming Hindering Factors

By acknowledging and addressing these hindering factors, we implemented several strategies to mitigate their impact:

- Enhanced communication: Regular and structured communication channels were established to ensure clarity and alignment among all participants.
- Resource optimization: We prioritized activities and allocated resources strategically to maximize efficiency and effectiveness.
- Collaborative online tools: Utilization of collaborative tools and technologies facilitated better coordination and interaction among geographically dispersed team members.

Summary of Lessons Learned

The INPRO project demonstrates the critical importance of establishing a common language and framework, in this case, the ICF, to facilitate interprofessional collaboration and person-centered care in rehabilitation. The development and implementation of ICF-based tools and practices across education and clinical settings highlights how such a unifying approach can bridge gaps between theory and practice.

Importantly, the chapter underscores the need to engage all stakeholders—persons with disabilities, professionals, managers, and educators—in adopting and applying the ICF. By highlighting the diverse perspectives and experiences of these groups, the findings illustrate how IPECP requires a multilevel, collaborative effort to be successful and sustainable.

The INPRO project highlighted the importance of understanding both facilitating and hindering factors in a complex, multilevel network organization. Open forum exchanges and the learning by doing principle proved to be powerful facilitators, especially for the implementation of the ICF and the INPRO CF. Challenges that required strategic intervention were, for example, the diverse organizational cultures and resource constraints. By learning from these experiences, we were able to navigate the project more effectively and achieve our goals.

These lessons are particularly relevant for rehabilitation settings across Europe, where consistent use of the ICF can enable more holistic, person-centered care. Furthermore, the INPRO CF provides a valuable resource for aligning educational and professional development with the competencies required for effective IPECP.

Understanding these dynamics is crucial for future projects, particularly those involving interprofessional education and collaboration. Being aware of the different network levels at which communication and interaction occur, and aligning efforts accordingly, can significantly enhance the quality and impact of collaborative endeavors.

Practical next steps for educators who facilitate the transition from education to practice would be to engage persons with disabilities as equal partners in the design and delivery of IPECP, to integrate the INPRO CF into curriculum planning and student assessment, and to adopt ICF-based training and tools for students and professionals.

Policymakers should mandate the use of the ICF as a unifying framework in rehabilitation settings and provide resources to support the adoption and application of the ICF. For more collaborative, person-centered care, bridges between education and rehabilitation institutes are needed.

Researchers could explore strategies for overcoming organizational and cultural barriers and evaluate the impact of ICF-based IPECP interventions on outcomes and experiences of persons with disabilities. In addition, factors that contribute to the long-term sustainability of IPECP should be investigated.

Reflective Questions

- What strategies can be used to ensure the meaningful involvement of persons with disabilities and their families in the design and delivery of interprofessional education and practice?
- What are the long-term impacts of using ICF as a foundation for interprofessional education?
- How can the INPRO CF and ICF-based tools be adapted and applied in other healthcare contexts beyond rehabilitation to promote interprofessional competencies?
- What additional tools, resources, or support do professionals and managers need to effectively implement the ICF and person-centered, interprofessional practices in rehabilitation settings?

References

1. Aerts I, De Weerdt C, INPRO Consortium. INPRO competency framework: user's guide; 2023a. https://doi.org/10.48544/f417fb2f-7323-4941-861e-26c21a1c94c3.
2. Aerts I, De Weerdt C, INPRO Consortium. INPRO competency framework: competency book; 2023b. https://doi.org/10.48544/55b4f885-e839-4bf4-a0d0-7d0fa46dcfdb.
3. Aerts I, De Weerdt C, INPRO Consortium. INPRO competentie raamwerk; 2023c. https://doi.org/10.48544/12f77ff3-154c-4e73-ad77-3d43c2c4cb8f.
4. Aerts I, De Weerdt C, INPRO Consortium. INPRO Kompetenz Rahmenmodell; 2023d. https://doi.org/10.48544/b215aa9e-1491-4acd-9fa6-e7c2d5dc30bf.
5. Aerts I, De Weerdt C, INPRO Consortium. INPRO competency framework (in Finnish); 2023e. https://doi.org/10.48544/8ea6014a-5704-4bcb-b8dc-f99064a50f74.
6. Aerts I, De Weerdt C, INPRO Consortium. INPRO competency framework (only ICF); 2023f. https://doi.org/10.48544/6856cbbb-d3d5-40b8-a306-374a1a493bba.
7. Alford VM, Ewen S, Webb GR, McGinley J, Brookes A, Remedios LJ. The use of the International Classification of Functioning, Disability and Health to understand the health and functioning experiences of people with chronic conditions from the person perspective: a systematic review. Disabil Rehabil. 2015;37(8):655–66. https://doi.org/10.3109/09638288.2014.935875.
8. Allan CM, Campbell WN, Guptill CA, Stephenson FF, Campbell KE. A conceptual model for interprofessional education: the international classification of functioning, disability and health (ICF). J Interprof Care. 2006;20(3):235–45. https://doi.org/10.1080/13561820600718139.

9. Atsma L, Van der Velde IR, Petiet L, Aerts I, De Weerdt C. INPRO CF Revalidatie Friesland; 2023. https://doi.org/10.48544/56ef59a1-f062-4484-96db-cc5b8da9ed0b.
10. Colman KSF, Hurkmans J, van Lingen E, Mutanen L, Haumer C, INPRO Consortium. Patient Journeys, A path with challenges that you do not need to walk alone! INPRO; 2023. 7.4.e Patient Journey; report – INPRO
11. De Smedt C, Hemetek U, Freisleben-Teutscher CF, Szuszkiewicz P, Kidritsch A. INPRO Journey of the Student. [Video]. YouTube; 2022. https://www.youtube.com/watch?v=XMuPeKctuZM&t=264s
12. De Weerdt C, Aerts I. INPRO CF project hospital in Belgium; 2022. https://doi.org/10.48544/bc7d10ce-0273-4c84-8b68-33ea2390541d.
13. De Weerdt C, Aerts I, Lakke S, Paltamaa J, Reinders JJ. Proposing an interprofessional competency framework for personcentered care connecting interprofessional education and collaborative practice. Health Interprof Pract Educ. 2024;6(5):1–14. https://doi.org/10.61406/hipe.315.
14. Delorette M, INPRO Consortium. Family group conference. INPRO; 2023. https://doi.org/10.48544/c0556534-511f-4915-87ef-69f547a360e1.
15. Dielemans R, Lakke S, Reinders J. INPRO renewed-interprofessional skills day; 2023. https://doi.org/10.48544/72a4c747-bbad-4250-9152-b381d09b594b.
16. Enqvist M, Lahti L, Aerts I, De Weerdt C. INPRO CF "Coronaria"; 2023. https://doi.org/10.48544/47365505-9547-48ca-a825-28017789bec8.
17. Freisleben-Teutscher CF, Kidritsch A, INPRO Consortium. Design thinking workshops. INPRO; 2023. https://doi.org/10.48544/3028fd2d-46e2-4c0c-a3fd-2657cff43886.
18. Haumer C, Schulner-Weiß S. Annual employee conversations. INPRO; 2023. https://doi.org/10.48544/ae25288a-d516-42ee-94f5-ca7211dfcc3e.
19. Haumer C, Schulner-Weiß S, INPRO Consortium. Implementation of ICF documentation system for dietitians – step-by-step guideline. INPRO; 2023. https://doi.org/10.48544/33b444f6-aa4d-4892-8db8-eff0f71b2d56.
20. Hemetek U, Kidritsch A, Myllyharju-Puikkonen A, Aerts I, De Weerdt C, Lakke S. INPRO CF "INPRO Pilot IPE intervention"; 2022. https://doi.org/10.48544/9923bd2f-4258-483a-a215-ad552cfdb232.
21. Hemetek U, Kidritsch A, Aerts I, Jorna-Lakke S, Kolm A, Ritsilä J, Freisleben-Teutscher CF, INPRO Consortium. INPRO process guide for lecturers in higher education institutions. INPRO; 2023. https://www.inproproject.eu/material/6-2-c-process-guide-hei
22. Hurkmans J, Colman KSF, Atsma LT, van Lingen E, Tammeling P. INPRO ConsortiumINPRO student-run interprofessional learning ward, guideline. INPRO; 2023a. https://doi.org/10.48544/0a918421-166b-48da-bab1-c6978a8d89ba.
23. Hurkmans J, Colman KSF, Atsma LT, van Lingen E, Tammeling P. INPRO ConsortiumINPRO student-run interprofessional learning ward, roadmap. INPRO; 2023b. https://doi.org/10.48544/91b3e9ea-b7f5-406f-918f-b61c7dd16ec9.
24. Johansen T, Kvaal AM, Konráðsdóttir ÁD. Developing and implementing ICFbased tools for occupational rehabilitation supporting the communication and return to work process between sickness absentees, clinical team and jobcentre contacts. Front Rehabil Sci. 2022;15(3):830067. https://doi.org/10.3389/fresc.2022.830067.
25. Kidritsch A, Freisleben-Teutscher CF, Hemetek U, INPRO Consortium. INPRO journey of the person in interprofessional education [Interactive Slides]. H5P; 2021. https://h5p.org/node/1216428
26. Kidritsch A, Freisleben-Teutscher C, Hemetek U, Glösmann J, Haumer C, Zimmel C, Hackl V, Schulner-Weiss S, Aerts I, De Weerdt C. INPRO CF project "Rehabilitation center"; 2022. https://doi.org/10.48544/9923bd2f-4258-483a-a215-ad552cfdb232.
27. Kirkpatrick JD, Kirkpatrick WK. Kirkpatrick's four levels of training evaluation. Association for Talent Development; 2016.
28. Lahti L, INPRO Consortium. Self-esteem meeting. INPRO; 2023. https://doi.org/10.48544/7998e46e-be6c-4539-b213-b366ad22b92a.
29. Lakke S, Aerts I, De Weerdt C. INPRO CF Hanze; 2023. https://doi.org/10.48544/48a43021-ef93-490e-b8c7-ffaa32414329.

30. Lang C, Kidritsch A. Open Exchange Forum; 2023. https://doi.org/10.48544/d77443fe-fd38-40d7-9c63-6559af9abdb8.
31. McKenney S, Reeves TC. Conducting educational design research. Routledge; 2019. https://doi.org/10.4324/9781315105642.
32. Mills J, Cieza A, Short S. Development and validation of the WHO rehabilitation competency framework: a mixed methods study. Arch Phys Med Rehabil. 2021;102(6):113–1123. https://doi.org/10.1016/j.apmr.2020.10.129.
33. Mutanen L, Kuohuva-Jokinen E, Metsalu P, INPRO Consortium. ICF and goal setting workshops. INPRO; 2023. https://doi.org/10.48544/574f93f8-82d1-4a92-98bd-d54520f075d4.
34. Paltamaa J, Myllyharju-Puikkonen A. ICF education continuum: from basic knowledge to practical ICF implementation material. INPRO; 2023a. https://doi.org/10.48544/0abcde0c-2bfe-4b9f-9d5a-aa4f3ac22bd2.
35. Paltamaa J, Myllyharju-Puikkonen A. ICF in person-centred rehabilitation: material to support the interprofessional implementation. INPRO; 2023b. https://doi.org/10.48544/91b0f1e7-8352-4365-bf45-7e55b7f04856.
36. Paltamaa J, Mutanen L, van Lingen E, Haumer C, Schulner-Weiß S, Kidritsch A, Aerts I, INPRO Consortium. ICF-based tools and practices to promote the use of ICF – a summary on the development actions (a report). INPRO; 2023. https://doi.org/10.48544/2b741b92-7153-49cb-ab0c-7b2c0ef3848d.
37. Paltamaa J, van Lingen E, Haumer C, Kidritsch A, Aerts I, Mutanen L. Specific ICF training is needed in clinical practice: ICF framework education is not enough. Front Rehabil Sci. 2024;5 https://doi.org/10.3389/fresc.2024.1351564.
38. Reed GM, Dilfer K, Bufka LF, Scherer MJ, Kotzé P, Tshivhase M, Stark SL. Three model curricula for teaching clinicians to use the ICF. Disabil Rehabil. 2008;30(12–13):927–41. https://doi.org/10.1080/09638280701800301.
39. Ritsilä J, Myllyharju-Puikkonen A, Paltamaa J, Aerts I, De Weerdt C. INPRO CF "Jamk Pilots"; 2023. https://doi.org/10.48544/2ab508c8-ae05-4301-bed1-cfcaa95f6b0d.
40. Scholten I, Barradell S, Bickford J, Moran M. Twelve tips for teaching the International Classification of Functioning, Disability and Health with a view to enhancing a biopsychosocial approach to care. Med Teach. 2021;43(3):293–9. https://doi.org/10.1080/0142159X.2020.1789082.
41. Schulner-Weiß S, Zimmel C, Haumer C, Aerts I, De Weerdt C. INPRO CF at MOHA project; 2022. https://doi.org/10.48544/a20c28a8-544d-4dc0-900d-101e58125b40.
42. Tammeling P, Hurkmans J, INPRO Consortium. INPRO student-run interprofessional learning ward, social business case. INPRO; 2023. https://doi.org/10.48544/d792c0b3-f53e-4e7a-90fa-bab7e8dbf9e4.
43. Van Lingen E, INPRO Consortium. ICF table in electronic patient device. INPRO; 2023a. https://doi.org/10.48544/38c631ec-3701-4f42-b331-b58dbd807050.
44. Van Lingen E, INPRO Consortium. Training for all the disciplines to explain how ICF is integrated in our EPD. 2023b. https://www.inproproject.eu/wp-content/uploads/2023/12/5.5.b13-Blackboard-course-ICF-interprofessional.pdf
45. Van Lingen E, Jager I, Atsma L, Knol M, INPRO Consortium. Workshop setting a main goal. INPRO; 2023a. doi.10.48544/9e052e9e-20b8-4b2a-ad5e-07dbabe1ef60 https://doi.org/10.48544/51c1754b-636a-42fa-bc46-e3701704c5a7.
46. Van Lingen E, Vloet J, Leurink L, INPRO Consortium. Blackboard course ICF interprofessional. INPRO; 2023b. https://doi.org/10.48544/9e052e9e-20b8-4b2a-ad5e-07dbabe1ef60.
47. World Health Organization. International classification of functioning, disability and health: ICF. World Health Organization; 2001. https://apps.who.int/iris/handle/10665/42407
48. World Health Organization. How to use the ICF: a practical manual for using the International Classification of Functioning, Disability and Health (ICF). Exposure draft for comment. WHO; 2013. https://www.who.int/docs/default-source/classification/icf/drafticfpracticalmanual2.pdf?sfvrsn=8a214b01_4

49. Zimmel C, Schulner-Weiß S, Hackl S, Grünstäudl I, Preißinger S, Wagner-Jakisic J, Delorette M, Freisleben-Teutscher CF, Kidritsch A, INPRO Consortium. Practice in rehabilitation. INPRO; 2023a. https://doi.org/10.48544/5332d3e5-5dbe-4796-ab27-b17c0607f736.
50. Zimmel C, Kidritsch A, Hemetek U, Fux W-D, Neubauer M, Freisleben-Teutscher CF, INPRO Consortium. Practice in prevention, with children. INPRO; 2023b. https://doi.org/10.48544/2a597d52-9e42-4670-8a8a-848efb77fd45.

Sandra Jorna-Lakke, P.hD., is a physical therapist who has worked in several clinical environments. Sandra is now a healthcare scientist and lecturer at the Hanze University of Applied Sciences, Groningen (the Netherlands). At the Interprofessionalism in Action (INPRO) project, Sandra acted as an overall coordinator and worked on several work packages. Sandra is motivated to improve interprofessional healthcare through facilitating interaction between therapists, students, lecturers, and researchers.

Anita Kidritsch, M.Sc., is a trained physiotherapist and works as a senior researcher at at the University of Applied Sciences St. Pölten (USTP, Austria). Within the INPRO project, she was the coordinator of USTP's contributions and was involved in developing and implementing interprofessional education. She is a Ph.D. student at the University of West Attica, Department of Public and Community Health, working on the topic of "Digitised Interprofessional Collaboration of Health Teams in Education."

Ingrid Aerts, M.Sc., is a lecturer and researcher at the Nutrition and Dietetics program at AP University of Applied Sciences, Antwerp (Belgium). She graduated as a dietitian, specialized in sports nutrition. She also has a master's degree in Training and Education Sciences. Since 2008, she has been involved in IPCIHC (InterProfessional Collaboration in Healthcare). Within the INPRO project, she was responsible for the work package that elaborated on interprofessional competencies and their assessment.

Jaana Paltamaa, Ph.D., is a senior researcher at JAMK UAS (Finland). She led the International Classification of Functioning, Disability and Health (ICF) and dissemination work package of the INPRO project. As a physiotherapist, Ph.D., and an associate professor, she has a long experience in applied research and development with partners from the working life. She has a special interest in functioning and is familiar with the training and implementation of the WHO ICF classification. Since 2013, she has been a collaborator of the family of international classifications network WHO-FIC (Family of International Classifications Network) FDRG (Functioning and Disability Reference Group).

Dr. Ursula Hemetek, MPH, is a trained dietitian and works as a lecturer in the study program of Dietetics at the University of Applied Sciences St. Pölten (USTP, Austria). Within the INPRO project, she was involved in developing and implementing (international) interprofessional education in study programs for health professionals.

Joost Hurkmans, (J.J.S.), Ph.D., is a senior researcher in rehabilitation medicine at the rehabilitation center "Revalidatie Friesland" in the Netherlands. He worked for 20 years as a speech and language pathologist and clinical linguist in a rehabilitation clinic. Now, he uses his expertise in the research on neurological speech and language disorders and interprofessional education and collaboration. He is the project manager of the Student-Run Interprofessional Learning Ward, a work package under his lead within the INPRO project.

Integrating and Implementing IPE in Health and Social Curricula—A Practical Emphasis

Anita Iversen and Annika Lindh Falk

Introduction

European Union (EU) directives, in line with World Health Organization [44–46] policies, lend support to interprofessional education (IPE) to enhance health outcomes by standardizing professional qualifications across Member States and incorporating interprofessional learning into higher education frameworks. The adoption of IPE in Europe's health and social care curricula is driven by the need for collaborative practice to address complex healthcare demands, reduce clinical errors, and improve safety [31]. Furthermore, a critical shortage of healthcare personnel and recommendations from various professional bodies highlight the necessity for innovative educational approaches [9, 38, 47].

Regional interprofessional Networks in Europe are enhancing IPE visibility and integration through conferences, projects, and best practice exchanges. Despite these efforts, the implementation of IPE varies significantly across countries and institutions, and many IPE programs are not fully documented and described [1, 11, 33]. Addressing challenges and improving collaborative practices remain essential for advancing IPE in European health professions education. Language barriers and cultural differences pose additional challenges in documenting and sharing IPE

Authors Anita Iversen and Annika Lindh Falk have contributed equally to this chapter.

A. Iversen (✉)
Faculty of Health Sciences, Centre for Faculty Development, UiT The Arctic University of Norway, Tromsø, Norway
e-mail: anita.iversen@uit.no

A. Lindh Falk
Faculty of Medicine and Health Sciences, Linköping University, Linköping, Sweden
e-mail: annika.lindh.falk@liu.se

A. Xyrichis et al. (eds.), *Building Bridges: A European Perspective on Interprofessional Education, Practice, Policy and Research*,
https://doi.org/10.1007/978-3-032-23222-9_9

designs. This chapter will provide insights into the design and implementation of IPE, introduce a four-dimensional (4-D) model for curriculum development, and discuss the enablers and barriers to integrating IPE into higher education, with specific examples from Sweden and Norway.

Design and Implementation of IPE in Curricula

Integrating IPE into mainstream education is a complex, global endeavor, facing numerous barriers and challenges that necessitate a clear strategy for successful and sustainable implementation [4, 12, 19]. Maddock et al. [22] describe a collaborative approach to curriculum design that considers the evolving landscape of healthcare practice and education. This involves maintaining continuous dialogue between academic institutions and healthcare education stakeholders [38].

A common framework for IPE curriculum design in undergraduate education includes learning objectives (knowledge, skills, attitudes), intended learning outcomes (for assessment), and the competencies to be developed [37]. Recommendations from a scoping review by Shakhovskoy et al. (2020) suggest considering participant attributes, including educational level, stage of progression, the disciplines they represent, and the size and composition of interprofessional groups. The recommendations also explore learning constructs, encompassing foundational theories, educational frameworks, and specific learning objectives. Diverse learning approaches such as exchange, observation, simulation, and direct clinical application are also discussed in their review.

Academic institutions aim to establish IPE programs that engage students from various health professions, with learning activities designed to enable students to interpret their experiences and achieve IPE objectives. These activities range from structured assignments to impromptu interactions in clinical settings [41], promoting the application of diverse professional knowledge and skills for optimal patient-centered care [23].

The timing for integrating IPE into healthcare education is debated. Early introduction during undergraduate studies can counteract negative professional socialization [10, 18], while others argue for its integration post-qualification for a more profound impact [31]. Regardless of timing, creating a learning environment that ensures students' psychological safety is crucial [23], supporting the principle of lifelong learning where IPE starts at the undergraduate level and continues throughout a professional's career.

To address the varying documentation of IPE designs and strategies, we employ the 4-D framework [20] to critically analyze and reflect on examples from Linköping University (Sweden) and UiT The Arctic University of Norway (Norway). This approach aims to enhance practical aspects of incorporating IPE into health and social care curricula.

The 4-D Model of Curriculum Development

The 4-D model, introduced by Lee et al. [20], provides a theoretical framework for developing new curricula and reviewing existing curricula in health and social care professions education (Table 1). This model highlights the importance of considering four interrelated dimensions when designing an IPE curriculum, as shown in Fig. 1. Moran et al. [30] further demonstrate the model's applicability in both the creation and refinement of IPE curricula.

Table 1 The 4-D curriculum development framework [20]

Dimension	Description
D1. Identifying future healthcare practice needs	*This dimension seeks to connect health professionals' practice needs to new and changing workplace demands in all health sectors. Curriculum considerations take into account global health and educational reforms; how these link to the development of knowledge, competencies, capabilities, and practices; as well as local institutional delivery conditions*
D2. Defining and understanding capabilities	*This dimension describes the knowledge, capabilities, and attributes health professionals require. This component addresses how changing health services impact expertise, identities, and practice, which ultimately impacts the training and preparation of future health professionals*
D3. Teaching, learning, and assessment	*This dimension pertains to the development of appropriate learning, teaching, and assessment experiences, all of which have been guided by the messages inherent within D1 and D2*
D4. Supporting institutional delivery	*This dimension focuses on the impact of local university structure and culture in the shaping of curriculum design and delivery, such as timetabling, logistics, and entry requirements*

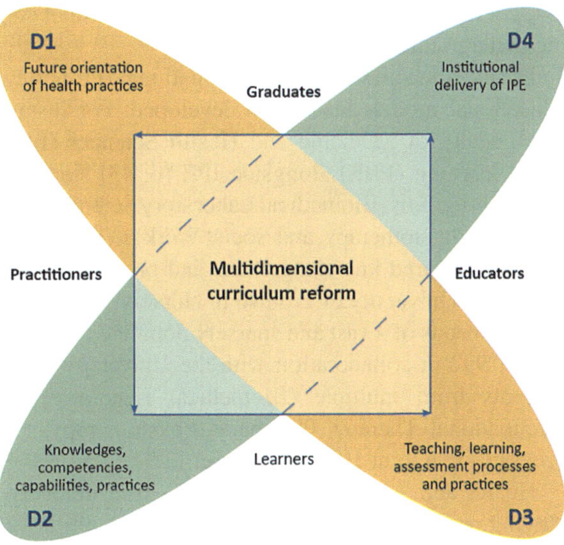

Fig. 1 The 4-D model of curriculum development [20]

The 4-D framework (Table 1) facilitates the design and conceptualization processes crucial for curriculum development. It aids educators in structuring curricula that effectively prepare students for the complexities of future healthcare roles. It emphasizes the interconnectedness and mutual dependency of the four dimensions, essential for capturing the "whole picture" of educational practice, health policies, professional practices, and healthcare complexities (Fig. 1).

A Retrospective Lens on IPE Designs in Sweden and Norway

Dimension 1: Identifying Future Healthcare Practice Needs—The Why?

This dimension explores the global and local challenges in future health and social services, focusing on Norway and Sweden. Both countries, known for their "Scandinavian model" of welfare [42], have a strong governmental influence in shaping health policies and implementing public sector initiatives. Despite their similarities, each country has distinct approaches to healthcare and education, governed by separate ministries but intertwined historically.

In Sweden, the Ministry of Health and Social Affairs has been proactive in reorganizing healthcare to enhance patient care since 2016 [35], emphasizing primary care and interprofessional collaborative practice [36]. Norway's significant policy, The Coordination Reform [27], aimed to enhance healthcare efficiency and patient orientation, continuously evolving through political guidelines.

Both countries have integrated IPE into their health and social care education systems, focusing on team-based care. In Sweden, the Higher Education Ordinance [34] mandates that health profession education programs include IPE to foster teamwork competencies. Similarly, Norway's educational policies and legislation [24, 25, 26] emphasize acquiring interprofessional collaborative competencies during undergraduate studies.

Despite the absence of a unified national IPE policy in both countries, innovative educational models have been developed. For instance, at Linköping University, The Faculty of Medicine and Health Sciences (FMHS) has embraced problem-based learning (PBL) alongside IPE [6, 43] since 1986, involving students from various programs (Biomedical Laboratory Science, Medicine, Nursing, Occupational Therapy, Physiotherapy, and Social Work) in a mandatory, 10-week course designed to build a shared knowledge base and prevent stereotypical views of professional roles. The University of Tromsø in Norway, established in 1968 to address the educational needs of a vast and sparsely populated area, introduced a similar IPE initiative in1992 in collaboration with the University College of Tromsø [8], engaging students from multiple (Biomedical Laboratory Science, Medicine, Nursing, Occupational Therapy, Pharmacy, Physiotherapy, Psychology, and Radiography) programs in a joint 10-week course.

Health and social care continue to face unresolved challenges globally, with varying patient outcomes despite similar conditions worldwide. Universities strive to enhance students' collaborative skills, but growing student numbers and logistical issues, such as arranging clinical placements, complicate these efforts. For instance, Linköping University has developed a collaboration with several regional healthcare providers and other universities to ensure IPE for all students.

In Sweden, recent initiatives focus on addressing people's needs through enhanced collaboration across health and social care sectors. In Norway, particularly in the north, a shortage of healthcare personnel and large geographical distances between institutions pose risks to patient outcomes. Technological solutions are limited by economic constraints, professional shortages, and skill gaps. In response, Norway's Ministry of Health and Care Services has assessed and initiated plans for sustainable health services and workforce competencies [28, 29]. A 2015 structural policy by the Ministry of Education and Research aimed to consolidate resources into fewer, stronger institutions, exemplified by the creation of UiT The Arctic University of Norway, which faces its own challenges due to its current size and diversity.

Despite being pioneers in integrating IPE, institutions such as Linköping University and UiT The Arctic University of Norway must continually adapt their educational strategies to meet evolving demands and ensure effective professional and IPE.

Dimension 2: Defining and Understanding Capabilities—The What?

This dimension focuses on the current and future essential knowledge and capabilities required by healthcare professionals. Although Nordic countries lack a specific competency framework for interprofessional collaboration and such skills are not directly linked to accreditation in health and social care, various interprofessional competency frameworks are available. These frameworks aim to pinpoint crucial competencies for effective interprofessional collaborative practice to enhance health outcomes. Despite regional and contextual variations in healthcare, these frameworks typically include core competencies across domains such as interprofessional communication, patient-centered care, role clarification, team functioning, collaborative leadership, conflict resolution, and ethics and values [39]. These competencies provide a foundation for interprofessional learning activities, helping students develop the necessary skills for effective teamwork in their future professional roles.

Since 1999, the Bologna process has aimed to enhance coherence in higher education across Europe by introducing new strategies that impact teaching and learning. This initiative introduced a shift from a teaching-oriented to a learning-oriented approach, emphasizing the definition of learning outcomes, and uses active verbs to describe competencies in three strands: knowing and understanding, knowing how to act, and knowing how to be [7]. National qualifications frameworks in Sweden [34] and Norway [32] support this shift. In the context of IPE, this means focusing on clearly defined learning outcomes. Sweden and Norway, while similar, show subtle differences in their IPE learning outcomes, as illustrated in examples from

Linköping University and UiT The Arctic University of Norway (referenced in Table 2). These examples specifically pertain to IPE for first-year undergraduate students.

The latest IPE model at Linköping University, based on Interprofessional Education Collaborative (IPEC) [13] guidelines, was introduced in 2016 and encompasses undergraduate programs in Biomedical Laboratory Science, Medicine, Nursing, Occupational Therapy, Physiotherapy, and Speech and Language Pathology. This model includes three mandatory modules [5, 21] and is currently under systematic evaluation for implementation and sustainability [16]. The FMHS has also established a local learning outcome for all programs, emphasizing that students should attain interprofessional competence for effective teamwork across professional groups.

In Norway, the development of collaborative skills follows a spiral curriculum model, also informed by IPEC [13], which progressively exposes students to interprofessional learning from understanding health and social systems to engage in simulations and with patients in clinical placements [15]. Both Swedish and Norwegian models aim to guide learning levels of IPEC competencies [13] and foster interprofessional identity through socialization [17]. However, several challenges, such as the COVID-19 pandemic, economic constraints in healthcare, changes in educational regulations [26], and leadership, have hindered the full implementation of the planned IPE curriculum at UiT The Arctic University of Norway.

Dimension 3: Teaching, Learning, and Assessment—The How?

Dimension 3 focuses on the development of effective teaching, learning, and assessment activities within IPE, guided by foundational dimensions D1 and D2. Learning theories play a crucial role in shaping these activities, promoting interprofessional learning where students from various professions engage collaboratively to understand each other's perspectives, expand competencies, and establish a foundation for joint action [6]. At Linköping University, PBL is employed across the FMHS to facilitate IPE. This involves students working in small tutorial groups on real-life scenarios to enhance their understanding of different professional viewpoints and patient needs. The curriculum progresses from initial scenario-based learning with dedicated supervisors to more complex real-case scenarios focused on quality improvement and culminates in clinical placements where students work in teams under the guidance of both team and profession-specific supervisors (Table 3). These supervisors are pivotal in fostering effective interprofessional interactions, requiring a deep understanding of interactive learning, group dynamics, and a commitment to IPE and collaboration.

At UiT The Arctic University of Norway, unlike the Swedish model with PBL, there is no uniform pedagogical framework guiding all teaching and learning activities. Instead, the IPE curricula within the Faculty of Health Sciences are informed by social constructivism, critical reflection, relational pedagogy, and

Table 2 Definitions of learning outcomes: examples from IPE curricula in Sweden and Norway at the first-year IPE module

Strands [7]	Strands Sweden	Examples of descriptions from FMHS[a], Sweden[b]	Strands Norway	Examples of descriptions from Norway[c]
Knowing and understanding	Knowledge and understanding	Describe the assignments and responsibilities of healthcare and social services in Sweden Explain the basics of evidence-based practice	Knowledge	Describe how the Norwegian health and welfare system is organized, including the general distribution of tasks Explain the significance that interprofessional collaboration can have for users of health and welfare services Account for basic ethical theories and concepts and describe key aspects of communication in interactions between individuals within the health and welfare system Provide examples of innovation, creativity, and flexibility in the health and welfare system Describe how inclusion, equality, non-discrimination, and the right to equitable services are important for all groups in society Are aware of the Sami peoples' rights to equitable health and welfare services and have knowledge of and understanding of the Sami's status as an indigenous people
Knowing how to act	Skills and abilities	Identify communication patterns within a group and explain how these influence group processes	Skills	Reflect on the types of common competencies required by professional practitioners in the health and welfare system Discuss one's own relational and communication skills and the various roles involved in interprofessional collaboration Contribute with one's own and recognize others' knowledge and expertise in solving collaborative projects in groups Apply ethical theories and concepts to concrete issues

(continued)

Table 2 (continued)

Strands [7]	Strands Sweden	Examples of descriptions from FMHS[a], Sweden[b]	Strands Norway	Examples of descriptions from Norway[c]
Knowing how to be	Values and attitudes	Motivate the importance of having a holistic view of the person and her health in relation to the future profession Reflect on your own values from a diversity perspective Describe the consequences of ethical standpoints based on ethical principles, laws, and evidence	General competence	Reflect on the types of shared competencies required by professional practitioners in the health and welfare system Reflect on how one's own values, cultural background, and communication style affect interactions with patients, service users, relatives, and other health personnel

[a]*FMHS* Faculty of Medicine and Health Sciences

[b]At Linköping University: The learning outcomes outlined for the first-year IPE module (6 ECTS) that includes students from Biomedical Laboratory Science, Medicine, Nursing, Occupational Therapy, Physiotherapy, and Speech and Language Therapy

[c]At UiT The Arctic University of Norway: The learning outcomes are outlined in a first-year joint course: Hel 0700 (10 ECTS) that includes students from the following programs: Biomedical Laboratory Science, Clinical Nutrition, Dentistry, Dental Hygiene, Medicine, Nursing, Occupational Therapy, Paramedicine, Pharmacy, Physiotherapy, Psychology, Radiography, and Social Education. These learning outcomes are continuously being refined and expanded

Table 3 A simplified model of the overarching study progression in interprofessional collaborative learning

Examples	Early (first year of study)	In the middle	Late (last year of study)
Sweden (FHMHS)	IPE 1, Professionalism in Health Care, 6 ECTS (see Table 2)	IPE, Quality improvement and learning in practice, 3 ECTS	IPE, Professional perspectives in collaboration, 3 ECTS Interprofessional Clinical Placement at a hospital ward/ healthcare center
Norway	10 ECTS joint course (see Table 2)	Varying durations Selected interprofessional learning activities, for example: innovation projects, shadowing, case-based learning, etc. Students from at least two different programs	Interprofessional Simulation in Acute Situations (1 day) Interprofessional Clinical Placement at Hospital Ward/ Healthcare Center/ Municipality Care. Students from at least two different programs (varying durations)

feedback theory, including a student-centered approach with small group learning and supervision. A key component of this approach, however, not yet fully implemented, is the interprofessional clinical placements conducted during the final year of the curriculum. These placements, lasting 1–5 days, are integrated into the students' regular clinical rotations at community nursing homes, health centers, or hospitals. During these placements, interprofessional groups of three to six students from various programs such as medicine, nursing, occupational therapy, physiotherapy, and pharmacy collaborate while providing care to typically older patients with complex health issues. Students are expected to be self-directed and produce a written report detailing care suggestions for each patient. Supervisors provide guidance and facilitate interprofessional reflections at the end of each placement. This model emphasizes practicality and flexibility, allowing interprofessional activities to be initiated by the university or health practitioners, and encourages such collaborations whenever opportunities arise during clinical placements. UiT uses constructive alignment [2] as a design principle for IPE, ensuring that learning outcomes, activities, and assessments are interconnected and clearly communicated to students. At Linköping University, the plan to implement an IPE portfolio for assessment, which would include students' documentation and reflections, has not been fully realized. In Northern Norway, interprofessional collaborative practice with patients is crucial for meeting learning outcomes aligned with IPEC competencies [13]. However, the planned implementation of the Individual Teamwork Observation and Feedback Tool [40] and a model for critical reflection on teamwork of IPE [14] has faced delays, possibly due to a lack of faculty development in IPE, among other reasons. To address these challenges, a joint faculty development course was created between UiT The Arctic University of Norway and Linköping University, offering credits for master's and Ph.D. students to enhance faculty and healthcare personnel's capabilities in developing and sustaining IPE.

Dimension 4: Supporting Institutional Delivery—The Where?

Dimension 4 emphasizes the support for implementing IPE activities by integrating local culture and structural considerations into the curriculum design and delivery. The model by Lee et al. [20] underlines the importance of including various stakeholders' perspectives in the development process. Lawlis et al. [19] identify key success factors for effective IPE implementation, which include adequate financial resources, sustainable organizational structures that facilitate IPE, comprehensive faculty development programs, and consideration of the personal and professional factors that affect IPE faculty.

Since its inception in 1986, IPE funding has been a core component of FMHS's educational system, consistently supported by its leadership and faculty. Despite this, there remains a need for ongoing faculty development in PBL and IPE. The organizational structure has adapted over time, with a notable change being the appointment of an IPE program director to the Board of Education, facilitating regular discussions on IPE-related matters such as scheduling and content. To further integrate IPE across all programs, an IPE committee with a facilitator from each program was established a year ago. Additionally, student involvement in the development, implementation, and evaluation of IPE is prioritized, with students participating in every board and committee to ensure their input shapes the educational framework. At UiT The Arctic University of Norway, leaders and faculty have dedicated funding and time allocation to IPE's success, despite fluctuating organizational commitment due to leadership changes and economic challenges in healthcare. These issues may intermittently affect the IPE curriculum's development and implementation, but are not expected to hinder students' interprofessional collaboration learning significantly. An active steering group representing all programs supports the joint IPE course, and the faculty board has outlined plans for further development, suggesting expected systematic changes and enhancements in IPE implementation.

Discussion

Integrating IPE into healthcare education programs is essential for preparing students to collaborate effectively in the health workforce. This chapter outlines a systematic approach, highlighting key considerations for planning and implementing IPE. The 4-D model [20] serves as a general framework for curriculum development and aligns well with findings from Lawlis et al. [19], which emphasize specific factors critical for successful IPE implementation. These factors, including governance and management, financial conditions, teacher competence, and commitment to developing IPE content, can present both opportunities and challenges. Acknowledging the dual impact of these factors highlights the complexity of implementing IPE.

The WHO has consistently emphasized the importance of adopting a health-promoting and preventive approach across health services. A key focus is on strengthening primary healthcare and fostering integrated healthcare systems, which are common challenges across Europe [47]. In Sweden, and even more so in Norway, the government has established clear strategies for IPE and collaborative practice. However, one could argue that without adequate financial resources, realistic changes might remain theoretical.

Nevertheless, healthcare education must continuously evolve, adapting its content to include crucial elements, such as public health perspectives, cultural competence, sustainable healthcare, and interprofessional skills. Educational approaches should also empower students to navigate ongoing changes, fostering a mindset of lifelong learning and encouraging them to stay informed and responsive to emerging challenges.

These arguments highlight a critical challenge within the education system: maintaining a delicate balance between theory and practice while addressing the concern that an overload of content competes for students' attention in the curriculum. Effective collaboration across educational programs requires a consensus on shared content that aligns with the needs of sustainable healthcare. Faculty members from various programs, in collaboration with healthcare professionals, must identify core concepts, formulate relevant learning outcomes, and coordinate schedules for learning activities at the university and in clinical placements. Simultaneously, they must ensure that the students' workload remains manageable. Addressing this challenge is crucial for the success of IPE. Additionally, the learning outcomes should reflect the depth and breadth of interprofessional competences, formulated through a progressive process.

A notable challenge in developing a course or curriculum is the inconsistency between the intended curriculum (the formal content decided by institutions) and the implemented curriculum (what teachers or supervisors deliver) [3]. To overcome this challenge, it is essential to have teachers and healthcare professionals with strong educational competences, supported by knowledge-informed leadership and robust organizational structures [19]. For teachers and healthcare professionals, it is crucial to understand that engagement in IPE requires a fundamental understanding of IPE and collaborative practice. Additionally, teachers and healthcare professionals need to be aware of the various roles they have, along with the corresponding knowledge and skills required for each role. These roles include being a planner, resource developer, information provider, supervisor and/or facilitator, role model, and examiner.

Having policies and trained teachers and healthcare professionals is essential, but not sufficient, for successfully integrating and implementing IPE in health and social curricula. A major challenge for IPE is the high workload among teachers and healthcare professionals, coupled with staff shortage in healthcare. Additionally, the strain of accommodating numerous students in clinical placements calls for innovative solutions, such as reorganizing students from uniprofessional to interprofessional groups and developing new models for supervision and feedback.

To address the challenging logistics and the need for innovation in organizing IPE, administrative staff must be trained and work collaboratively with teachers and healthcare personnel. Ultimately, the sustainability of IPE may hinge most critically on the vision and support from leaders. Leaders must ensure financial commitment from the university to embed IPE within educational infrastructures. They must also engage in and support the establishment of organizational structures, such as committees, boards, and directors, to ensure arenas where collaboration between programs can sustain high-quality IPE for all healthcare students. Furthermore, systematic evaluation, for instance, using the 4-D model [20], or other models, should be systematically addressed to align with future needs.

Reflective Questions for the Reader

By reflecting on these questions, you can gain a deeper understanding of the context in which IPE operates in your country and at your university, as well as the historical factors that have shaped the interplay between health, social policies, and education.

Culture at Your University

- Investigate whether your university has specific guidelines or frameworks that support IPE.
- Consider how these guidelines influence the curriculum, teaching methods, and learning outcomes.
- Reflect on the extent to which these policies are implemented and their impact on students' preparedness for collaborative practice.
- How are patients as a stakeholder visible in educational practice and documents regulating IPE?
- How do organizational and administrative structures enable and/or hinder integration and implementation of IPE?

Interconnections Between Health and Social Policies and Education

- Look into the historical development of health and social policies in your country and how they have influenced educational practice, IPE in particular.
- Reflect on significant reforms or milestones that have shaped the relationship between healthcare, social welfare, and education.
- How is systematic evaluation of IPE performed and by whom?

Knowledge Base and Theoretical Underpinnings

- Are the interprofessional competency frameworks familiar in your institution? How can you use these frameworks when building a sustainable module for IPE?
- What learning theories and approaches underpin your institution, and how can that enable and/or hinder the development of IPE?

References

1. Anderson E, Smith R, Hammick M. Evaluating an interprofessional education curriculum: a theory-informed approach. Med Teach. 2016;38(4):385–94. https://doi.org/10.3109/0142159X.2015.1047756.
2. Biggs J, Tang C. Teaching for quality learning at university: what the student does. 3rd ed. Maidenhead: McGraw-Hill/Society for Reserach in Higher Education and Open University Press; 2007.
3. Biggs J, Tang C, Kennedy G. Teaching for quality at university. 5th ed. Maidenhead: McGraw-Hill education; 2022.
4. Clark PG. Looking below the surface of interprofessional education uncovering organizational factors and forces. J Allied Health. 2021;50(3):182–9.
5. Dahlberg J, Abrandt Dahlgren M, Ekstedt M, Hammar M, Lindh FA. The Linköping journey. In: Forman D, Jones M, Thistletwaite J, editors. Sustainability and interprofessional collaboration: ensuring leadership resilience in collaborative health care. Springer; 2020.
6. Dahlgren LO. Interprofessional and problem-based learning: a marriage made in heaven? J Interprof Care. 2009;23(5):448–54. https://doi.org/10.1080/13561820903163579.
7. The European higher education area (EHEA) in 2020: Bologna process implementation report, 2020. https://doi.org/10.2797/756192. https://eurydice.eacea.ec.europa.eu/publications/european-higher-education-area-2020-bologna-process-implementation-report
8. Ekeli B-V. Tvetydighet. En studie av samarbeid i helsetjenester og samarbeidslæring i helsepersonellutdanning. [Ambiguity. A study of cooperation in health services and collaborative learning in health personnel education] (Doctoral dissertation). 2014. Retrieved from http://hdl.handle.net/10037/5863
9. Frenk J, Chen L, Bhutta ZA, Cohen J, Crisp N, Evans T, Fineberg H, Garcia P, Ke Y, Kelley P, Kistnasamy B, Meleis A, Naylor D, Pablos-Mendez A, Reddy S, Scrimshaw S, Sepulveda J, Serwadda D, Zurayk H. Health professionals for a new century: transforming education to strengthen health systems in an interdependent world. The Lancet (British Edition), 2010;376(9756):1923–58. https://doi.org/10.1016/S0140-6736(10)61854-5
10. Gilbert JHV. Interprofessional learning and higher education structural barriers. J Interprof Care. 2005;19(suppl 1):87–106. https://doi.org/10.1080/13561820500067132.
11. Grace S. Models of interprofessional education for healthcare students: a scoping review. J Interprof Care. 2021;35(5):771–83. https://doi.org/10.1080/13561820.2020.1767045.
12. Handgraaf M, Wallin J, Groll C, Posenau A. Identification of barriers and facilitators of successful interprofessional education (IPE) – a scoping umbrella review/Identifizierung der Einflussfaktoren für die interprofessionelle Ausbildung (IPE) – ein Umbrella Scoping Review. Int J Health Prof (Warsaw, Poland). 2023;10(1):117–35. https://doi.org/10.2478/ijhp-2023-0009.
13. Interprofessional Education Collaborative (IPEC). Core competencies for interprofessional collaborative practice: 2016 update. Washington, DC: Interprofessional Education Collaborative; 2016.
14. Iversen A, Hauksdottir N. Tverrprofesjonell samhandling og teamarbeid: kjernekompetanse for fremtidens helse- og velferdstjenester (Interprofessional Collaboration and Teamwork: Core Competencies for the Future Health and Welfare Services) (1. utgave.). Gyldendal; 2020.
15. Jensen CB. The patient's role in undergraduate health students' interprofessional clinical placements (Doctoral dissertation). UiT The arctict university of Norway; 2023.
16. Karlsson EA, Kvarnström S, Kvarnström M. Exploring a revised interprofessional learning curriculum in undergraduate health education programs at Linköping University. BMC Med Educ. 2024;24:466. https://doi.org/10.1186/s12909-024-05458-3.
17. Khalili H, Orchard C, Laschinger HKS, Farah R. An interprofessional socialization framework for developing an interprofessional identity among health professions students. J Interprof Care. 2013;27(6):448–53. https://doi.org/10.3109/13561820.2013.804042.

18. Langendyk V, Hegazi I, Cowin L, Johnson M, Wilson I. Acad Med. 2015;2015(90):732–7. https://doi.org/10.1097/ACM.0000000000000714.
19. Lawlis TR, Anson J, Greenfield D. Barriers and enablers that influence sustainable interprofessional education: a literature review. J Interprof Care. 2014;28(4):305–10. https://doi.org/10.3109/13561820.2014.895977.
20. Lee A, Steketee C, Rogers G, Moran M. Towards a theoretical framework for curriculum development in health professional education. Focus Health Prof Educ. 2013;14(3):70–83.
21. Lindh Falk A, Dahlberg J, Ekstedt M, Heslyk A, Whiss P, Abrandt DM. Creating spaces for interprofessional learning: strategic revision of a common IPL curriculum in undergraduate programs. In: Vyt A, Pahor M, Tervaskanto-Maentausta T, editors. Interprofessional education in Europe: policy and practice. Antwerpen: Garant Publishers Limited; 2015. p. 49–66.
22. Maddock B, Kumar A, Kent F. Creating a collaborative care curriculum framework. Clin Teach. 2019;16(2):120–4. https://doi.org/10.1111/tct.12796.
23. Maddock B, Dārziņš P, Kent F. Realist review of interprofessional education for health care students: What works for whom and why. J Interprof Care. 2023;37(2):173–86. https://doi.org/10.1080/13561820.2022.2039105.
24. Ministry of Education and Research. Education for welfare – interaction in practice (Meld. St.13 (2011–2012)). 2012. Retrieved from https://www.regjeringen.no/no/dokumenter/meld-st-13-20112012/id672836/?ch=1
25. Ministry of Education and Research. Quality Culture in Higher Education (Meld. St.16 (2016–2017)). 2017a. Retrieved from https://www.regjeringen.no/no/dokumenter/meld.-st.-16-20162017/id2536007/?ch=1
26. Ministry of Education and Research. National Curriculum Regulations for Norwegian Health and Welfare Education (RETHOS). 2017b. Retrieved from https://lovdata.no/dokument/SF/forskrift/2017-09-06-1353
27. Ministry of Health and Care Services. The Coordination Reform – Proper treatment – at the right place and right time (Meld.St. 47 (2008–2009)). 2009. Retrieved from https://www.regjeringen.no/contentassets/d4f0e16ad32e4bbd8d8ab5c21445a5dc/no/pdfs/stm200820090047000dddpdfs.pdf
28. Ministry of Health and Care Services. NOU 2023:4. Time for action: The personnel in sustainable health and care services. Oslo; 2023. Retrieved from https://www.regjeringen.no/no/dokumenter/nou-2023-4/id2961552/
29. Ministry of Health and Care Services. National Health and Coordination Plan, Our Common Health Service. (Meld.St.9 (2023–2024)). Oslo; 2024. Retrieved from https://www.regjeringen.no/no/dokumenter/meld.-st.-9-20232024/id3027594/
30. Moran MC, Steketee C, Forman D, Dunston R. Using a Research-Informed Interprofessional Curriculum Framework to guide reflection and future planning of interprofessional education in a multi-site context. J Res Interprof Pract Educ. 2015;5(1) https://doi.org/10.22230/jripe.2015v5n1a187.
31. Reeves S, Fletcher S, Barr H, Birch I, Boet S, Davies N, McFadyen A, Rivera J, Kitto S. A BEME systematic review of the effects of interprofessional education: BEME Guide No. 39. Med Teach. 2016;38(7):656–68. https://doi.org/10.3109/0142159X.2016.1173663.
32. Regulation on NQF (Norwegian NKR) and EQF. Regulation on the National Qualifications Framework (NQF) for Lifelong Learning and the Reference to the European Qualifications Framework (EQF) for Lifelong Learning (FOR-2017-11-08-1846). Legal Data; 2017. https://lovdata.no/dokument/LTI/forskrift/2017-11-08-1846
33. Shakhovskoy R, Dodd N, Masters N, New K, Hamilton A, Nash G, Barr N, George K, Pelly F, Reid C, Taylor J, Bogossian F. Recommendations for the design of interprofessional education: findings from a narrative scoping review. Focus Health Prof Educ Multi-Prof J. 2022;23(4):82–117. https://doi.org/10.11157/fohpe.v23i4.608.
34. The Swedish Ministry of Education and Research. Högskoleförordning (English title: University regulation). 1993. Retrieved from https://www.riksdagen.se/sv/dokument-och-lagar/dokument/svensk-forfattningssamling/hogskoleforordning-1993100_sfs-1993-100/

35. The Swedish Ministry of Health and Social Affairs. Effektiv vård (English title: Effective healthcare). 2016. Retrieved from https://www.regeringen.se/contentassets/42b0aef4431c4ebf9410b8ee771830eb/effektiv-vard%2D%2D-slutbetankande-av-en-nationell-samordnare-for-effektivare-resursutnyttjande-inom-halso%2D%2Doch-sjukvarden_sou-2016-2.pdf
36. The Swedish Ministry of Health and Social Affairs. God och nära vård – En primärvårdsreform. (English title: Good and immediate care. A primary care reform). 2018. Retrieved from https://www.regeringen.se/rattsliga-dokument/statens-offentliga-utredningar/2018/06/sou-201839/
37. Thistlethwaite J, McLarnon N. Learning in and about interprofessional teams and wider collaborations. In: Alnaami MY, Alqahtani AA, Alfaris AA, Abdulghani HM, Mohammed CA, editors. Novel health interprofessional education and collaborative practice program: strategy and implementation. 1st ed. Singapore: Springer; 2023. p. 69–92.
38. Thistlethwaite J, Xyrichis A. Forecasting interprofessional education and collaborative practice: towards a dystopian or utopian future? J Interprof Care. 2022;36(2):165–7. https://doi.org/10.1080/13561820.2022.2056696.
39. Thistlethwaite J, Forman D, Matthews LR, Rogers G, Steketee C, Yassine T. Competencies and frameworks in interprofessional education: a comparative analysis. Acad Med. 2014;89(6):869–75. https://doi.org/10.1097/ACM.0000000000000249.
40. Thistlethwaite J, Dallest K, Moran M, Dunston R, Roberts C, Eley D, Fyfe S. Introducing the individual Teamwork Observation and Feedback Tool (iTOFT): development and description of a new interprofessional teamwork measure. J Interprof Care. 2016;30(4):526–8. https://doi.org/10.3109/13561820.2016.1169262.
41. Van Diggele C, Roberts C, Burgess A, Mellis C. Interprofessional education: tips for design and implementation. 2020; https://doi.org/10.1186/s12909-020-02286-z.
42. Vrangbæk K, Iversen A. Health systems of Scandinavia. In: Quah S, editor. International encyclopedia of public health, vol. 6. 3rd ed. Elsevier; 2025. p. 677–82.
43. Wilhelmsson M, Pelling S, Ludvigsson J, Hammar M, Dahlgren LO, Faresjo T. Twenty years experiences of interprofessional education in Linkoping-ground-breaking and sustainable. J Interprof Care. 2009;23(2):121–33.
44. World Health Organization (WHO). Framework for action on interprofessional education and collaborative practice. 2010. Retrieved from: https://www.who.int/publications/i/item/framework-for-action-on-interprofessional-education-collaborative-practice
45. World Health Organization (WHO). Transforming and scaling up health professionals' education and training. 2013. Retrieved from: https://www.who.int/publications/i/item/transforming-and-scaling-up-health-professionals%E2%80%99-education-and-training
46. World Health Organization (WHO). Framework on people-centred health services. 2016. Retrieved from: https://apps.who.int/gb/ebwha/pdf_files/WHA69/A69_39-en.pdf
47. World Health Organization (WHO). Global competency and outcomes framework for universal health coverage. 2022. Retrieved from: https://www.who.int/publications/i/item/9789240034662

Anita Iversen is an Associate Professor, at the Centre for Faculty development (HelPed), the Faculty of Health Sciences, UiT The Arctic University of Norway. She is a distinguished teacher, Ph.D., in Health Sciences with extensive experience in research, teaching, and leadership within medical and health sciences education and professional development for academic staff.

Annika Lindh Falk is a senior lecturer, M.Sc., in occupational therapy and Ph.D. in medical education, and the Program Director for Interprofessional Education. She is involved in higher education and a supervisor for master and doctoral students in medical education. Her research interest is interprofessional learning and collaboration in health and social care.

How to Bridge Interprofessional and Simulation-Based Education? The State of the Art in IP-Sim

Tove Törnqvist, Simon Wiss Tidén, Patricia Picchiottino, and Thomas Fassier

Abbreviations

CRM	Crisis resource management
IPE	Interprofessional education
IP-Sim	Interprofessional simulation
IPECP	Interprofessional education and collaborative practice
RCDP	Rapid Cycle Deliberate Practice
SBE	Simulation-based education
SP	Simulated and standardized persons
WHO	World Health Organization

T. Törnqvist (✉)
Department of Health, Medicine and Caring Sciences, Linköping University, Linköping, Sweden
e-mail: tove.tornqvist@liu.se

S. Wiss Tidén
Clinical Training Centre, Faculty of Medicine and Health Sciences, Linköping University, Linköping, Sweden

P. Picchiottino
Geneva University of Applied Sciences, Geneva, Switzerland

Center for Interprofessional Simulation, Geneva, Switzerland

T. Fassier
Faculty of Medicine, University of Geneva, Geneva, Switzerland

Center for Interprofessional Simulation, Geneva, Switzerland

A. Xyrichis et al. (eds.), *Building Bridges: A European Perspective on Interprofessional Education, Practice, Policy and Research*,
https://doi.org/10.1007/978-3-032-23222-9_10

Introduction

Simulation-based education (SBE) and interprofessional education (IPE) are increasingly recognized globally as important for training healthcare students and professionals. However, the terminology and acronyms used to describe the amalgamation of SBE and IPE differ internationally, causing confusion. To ensure clarity in this chapter, we adopt the following definitions. We define simulation as "a technique—not a technology—to replace or amplify real experiences with guided experiences that evoke or replicate substantial aspects of the real world in a fully interactive manner" [19]. This definition underscores simulation's roots in experiential learning, akin to IPE [4], and encompasses a wide range of simulation methods, including high-fidelity mannequins, role-playing, simulated individuals, and screen-based simulations [19]. Virtual reality, another simulation modality, is explored in another chapter. Concerning IPE, we concur with the World Health Organization's (WHO) definition: "when two or more professions learn about, from and with each other to enable effective collaboration and improve health outcomes" [40].

The concept of simulation-enhanced IPE (Sim-IPE) lies at the intersection of SBE and IPE. The International Nursing Association for Clinical Simulation and Learning (INACSL) defines Sim-IPE as follows: "Simulation-enhanced interprofessional education (Sim-IPE) enables learners from different healthcare professions to engage in a simulation-based experience to achieve linked or shared objectives and outcomes" [34]. Some scholars differentiate between Sim-IPE and interprofessional simulation (IP-Sim), suggesting that Sim-IPE is more focused on achieving IPE outcomes [33]. In this chapter and within the European context, we align with INACSL's definition of Sim-IPE. Additionally, we define "multiprofessional simulation" as situations where trainees collaborate on the same task but do not engage in learning from or about each other.

This chapter bridges the SBE and IPE literature, reflecting on the current state of the art and challenges in education, practice, policy, and research concerning IP-Sim for healthcare students and professionals. Our reflection began with two seminal textbooks in the field [2, 31], incorporating best-evidence guidelines on simulation and IP-Sim [29, 34], and comprehensive literature reviews on these subjects [4, 26, 33]. We enriched the chapter with select studies from European countries and our own experiences integrating simulation into IPE curricula at Linköping University and the Geneva Center for Interprofessional Simulation. The chapter is organized around six interrelated questions (Fig. 1), following Kern's six-step curriculum design framework [36], which serves as a practical guide for health professions educators in systematically designing, evaluating, or updating a curriculum.

The hexagon made of plain arrows illustrates the six-step cyclical process of curriculum development and revision. Internal dotted bidirectional arrows illustrate that all steps are interdependent, with thicker ones indicating more frequent interconnections. The external dotted double arrow illustrates the congruence of learning objectives, educational strategies, assessment, and evaluation.

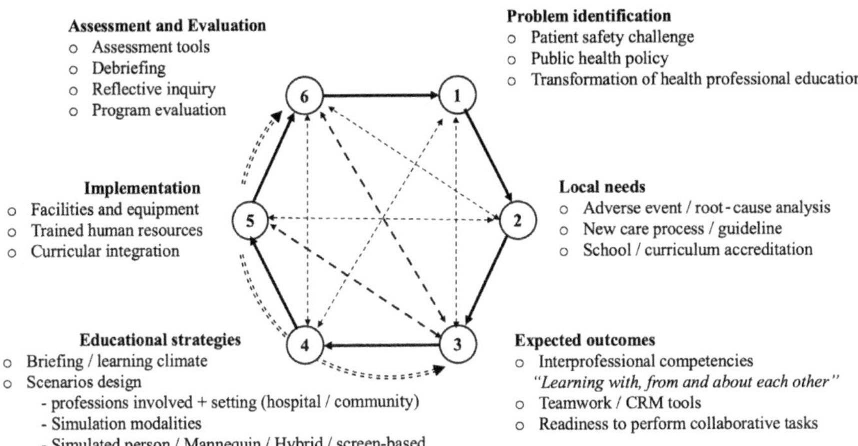

Fig. 1 IP-Sim curriculum design framework, recreated by the authors

IP-Sim to Address Global Challenges

Healthcare systems worldwide face complex challenges, as noted by Frenk et al. [15] and the WHO [40]. IPE and collaborative practice (IPECP) are crucial for effectively addressing these issues, and IP-Sim is a response to three key international challenges: patient safety, public health, and health profession education [15, 16, 40]. Tackling the underlying causes of these challenges and implementing strategic interventions is vital for the future of healthcare delivery and education. The WHO [40] stresses the need for collective action and dedicated discussions from multiple perspectives. Students, especially, require time to contemplate these matters, and IP-Sim's integration into educational and healthcare settings has the potential to support this reflective process.

Patient safety has been a longstanding healthcare concern, highlighted by the report "To Err Is Human" [22]. Errors often stem from poor teamwork and communication, jeopardizing patient safety [29]. Ongoing efforts aim to enhance care quality and patient safety [31]. IP-Sim plays a pivotal role in improving collaborative skills, confidence, interprofessional communication, and, consequently, patient care and safety [5]. In general, SBE also aids in developing human factor skills, such as cognitive and social-behavioral competencies, decision-making, and understanding human psychology interactions, all of which positively influence patient safety [1].

Public health faces issues such as an aging population, the prevalence of noncommunicable diseases, and environmental concerns. IPECP is essential for transitioning to care models that can adapt to the evolving complexities of public health [40]. IP-Sim enables students and healthcare professionals to engage in realistic collaborative scenarios, bolstering their ability to address both current and future intricate public health problems [16]. It provides a contextual learning environment to examine public health challenges and devise appropriate care strategies.

As healthcare systems reorganize in response to the challenges mentioned, health professional education must adapt. Both educational and health systems should foster IPE and collaboration [15, 16, 40]. IP-Sim acts as a tool for learning, allowing students to learn in collaborative environments that reflect their future clinical settings. Education must also anticipate trends like telemedicine and eHealth integration and incorporate them into the curriculum. Engaging in IP-Sim collaborations prepares us not only to form effective teams but also to proactively address potential future healthcare scenarios. This proactive stance equips us to navigate the healthcare landscape of the future more adeptly [16].

Your Local Needs

The successful integration of simulation into existing curricula necessitates the dedication of innovators and early adopters who believe that simulation fulfills the needs of the academic healthcare community [23]. According to Kern's model, Step 2 involves collaboration among policymakers, academics, trainers, students, patients, and relatives to assess local needs using various tools: stakeholder analysis, quantitative surveys, leader interviews, and root-cause analysis of adverse events, among others [36]. Recent examples from European countries demonstrate the application of IP-Sim to address the general needs identified in Kern's first step at a local level.

IP-Sim is extensively utilized in hospitals and acute care medicine to meet patient safety needs. In Geneva, Switzerland, Boloré et al. [6] described an IP-Sim training program focusing on interprofessional and patient safety competencies for hospital teams managing patients with rapid clinical deterioration, such as septic shock. Another example from the university hospital in Geneva used a root-cause analysis of a fatal adverse event that highlighted teamwork dysfunctions. In response, the Geneva Interprofessional Simulation Center developed and implemented a new crisis resource management (CRM) training program for physicians, nurses, and technicians to address this issue.

Experts suggest that patient safety is a topic amenable to developing IPE experiences, not just in hospitals but also in community settings [16]. IP-Sim offers valuable opportunities in this regard. For example, in the United Kingdom, Kayyali et al. [24] trained pharmacy and nursing students to collaborate in simulated environments, including hospital wards and general practice offices, with scenarios covering chronic conditions such as dementia, diabetes, Parkinson's disease, and various patient safety concerns, such as therapy duplication, drug interactions, and treatment modifications post-hospital discharge.

Regarding public health needs, IP-Sim can prepare students and professionals for collaborative work in community settings [28] and address the growing demand for palliative medicine and advanced care planning amid an aging population [18]. For instance, Lunde et al. [28] in Norway explored interprofessional teamwork in primary care scenarios where medical and nursing students worked together to evaluate, diagnose, and create a joint management plan for an elderly patient in a nursing home post-hip surgery.

Although IP-Sim is gaining traction in health professions education, its adoption in Europe appears limited. Currently, there is no comprehensive survey detailing the integration of IP-Sim in health professional schools across Europe. A recent systematic review by Colonnello et al. [13] of IPE within undergraduate medical education programs in 49 European higher education area countries (up to 2022) identified 32 studies from 14 countries. Only eight studies reported the incorporation of IP-Sim into IPE curricula: three from the United Kingdom, two from Sweden, and one each from Italy, Norway, and Turkey. A prior systematic review by Palaganas et al. [33] of 54 studies on prelicensure Sim-IPE (up to 2019) found that only nine originated from Europe: eight from the United Kingdom and one from Norway. These reviews indicate unmet needs in IP-Sim, including more diversity in health professions training together, more community-based scenarios, a deeper understanding of the theoretical frameworks underpinning IP-Sim, and more robust research designs. These needs are consistent with findings from other literature reviews (such as [4, 26]).

Regardless of the local needs identified, they present opportunities to promote IP-Sim, which enhances IPECP at both local and national levels. The rise of IP-Sim in Switzerland exemplifies this complex interplay. The demand for IPE across professions at the University of Applied Sciences in Geneva sparked the initial IP-Sim activities in the early 2010s. Initially, medical student participation was voluntary. The Geneva Faculty of Medicine and the Faculty of Pharmacy incorporated IPE into their curricula in 2013 and 2018, respectively. In 2020, the Federal Office of Public Health issued a policy brief highlighting exemplary local initiatives to encourage IPE at the national level. Presently, all medical schools in Switzerland are required to demonstrate IPE integration for accreditation by the Swiss Agency of Accreditation and Quality Assurance. In Israel, Brezis et al. [7] described a similar experience, where an IP-Sim training program in end-of-life communication skills was initiated in one university hospital and then spread throughout the country and ultimately influenced national end-of-life care policy.

Expected Training Outcomes

In Kern's model, Step 3 is crucial for ensuring educational consistency (Fig. 1): learning goals and objectives translate the identified needs (Step 2) to inform decisions regarding simulation modalities (Step 4), implementation (Step 5), and, to some extent, assessment and program evaluation (Step 6) [36]. Thus, when determining goals and objectives, one should consider the ultimate outcome of any IPE curriculum: a collaborative practice-ready health workforce [40].

To prepare for interprofessional collaboration, healthcare professionals must develop interprofessional competencies in conjunction with their profession-specific skills [15]. However, the relationship between interprofessional and professional competencies is intricate, and the scope of interprofessional competencies remains debated [35]. Revisiting the semantic distinction between interprofessional and multiprofessional simulation aids in developing learning goals and objectives that are explicitly oriented toward IPE. In IP-Sim (akin to IPE-enhanced simulation), trainees cultivate interprofessional competencies by learning about, from, and with other professions. Conversely, in multiprofessional simulation, they develop similar competencies concurrently. Distinguishing between these can be challenging; scrutinizing scenarios for explicit interprofessional learning outcomes is beneficial. For instance, in cardiac life support, IP-Sim would incorporate specific teamwork-related objectives, while multiprofessional simulation would focus primarily on practicing cardiopulmonary resuscitation skills, which are common across all professions.

To effectively align learning goals and objectives with IPE outcomes in IP-Sim programs, adopting an interprofessional competency framework is advisable [34]. Four renowned frameworks are utilized globally, developed in the United Kingdom, Canada, the United States, and Australia [35]. In Geneva, the National Interprofessional Competency Framework by the Canadian Interprofessional Health Collaborative is employed, while in Linköping, the IPE Collaborative Core Competencies for Collaborative Practice are used [35]. A study exploring the diversity of competency frameworks for IPE across European countries has yet to be identified.

To demonstrate interprofessional competencies, health professionals must utilize appropriate teamwork tools and strategies. Grounded in human factors research, CRM tools are increasingly incorporated into IP-Sim training programs [5, 9]. International standards suggest designing IP-Sim based on established competency frameworks or CRM-models [34]. In our experience, they serve different purposes and should be used complementarily. CRM-models are more practical for writing learning objectives and guiding assessment in IP-Sim activities. In the French-speaking part of Switzerland, we implemented TeamSTEPPS® [9] as a CRM tool at both undergraduate and postgraduate levels. Competency frameworks, being more conceptual, provide overarching goals to structure the entire IPE curriculum, integrate IP-Sim with other educational strategies, and ensure constructive alignment (i.e., congruence) with assessments.

Another critical aspect to clarify when formulating learning goals and objectives is the theoretical perspective underpinning IP-Sim [34]. While learning theories are instrumental in informing decisions and maintaining consistency in IPE curriculum design, this element is often underrepresented or absent in IP-Sim programs documented in the literature [4]. In two systematic reviews that reported this information, only 21–50% of the studies articulated the underlying conceptual or theoretical framework [13, 33]. Numerous theories examine the learning mechanisms during IPE, making it challenging to navigate among them [2]. Hean et al. [20] summarized the main trends stemming from behaviorism and constructivism theories, offering guidance for educational practitioners. In this chapter, we emphasize the significance of experiential learning theory in both IPE and SBE, which is congruent with social constructivism [4]. Lunde et al.'s [28] study exemplifies how such a theoretical perspective can inform operational research. We also advocate for the application of instructional design theories, such as the innovative four-component instructional design (4C/ID) model. In 4C/ID, learning goals are directed toward complete, real-life clinical tasks to prevent fragmentation, enhance complex learning, and facilitate the transfer of learning outcomes from simulated settings to the workplace [17]. This task-centered approach holds promise for designing innovative IP-Sim programs that train health professionals to perform tasks collaboratively, share responsibilities, and, at times, shift tasks [15].

Blending IPE and SBE Learning Strategies into IP-Sim

The fourth step in Kern's model builds upon the preceding steps, particularly the third, and concentrates on educational strategies [36]. Given this chapter's focus on IP-Sim, it is natural that the strategies should amalgamate the best of IPE and SBE: "to learn about, from and with each other" [40] and to offer "guided experiences that evoke or replicate substantial aspects of the real world" [19]. We contend that a primary benefit of integrating IPE and SBE is the shared emphasis on fostering collaborative competence among healthcare students and professionals. IPE, with its focus on understanding and valuing diverse roles and responsibilities [15], finds a complementary partner in SBE, which provides a dynamic environment for experiencing interprofessional teamwork in simulated contexts [2, 27, 30]. This integration fosters an atmosphere where individuals not only recognize the importance of their roles but also understand the synergies that arise from collaboration [30].

Guidelines are available to support academics and clinicians in designing SBE to ensure best-standard practice [29, 34]. However, it is essential to acknowledge that IP-Sim is inherently diverse, and there are no absolute rights or wrongs. The blending of IPE and SBE into IP-Sim is more about making intentional choices within the framework of constructive alignment [2] and addressing didactic questions such as who, when, how, and why. In designing an IP-Sim, considerations should be made regarding the scope of the scenario and the modalities used to represent it.

The scenario's scope (identified during Step 3) informs the learning content and guides learners in grasping collaborative competencies such as communication, roles, and responsibilities. Crafting a meticulously considered scenario is thus paramount, and there are various approaches to this [27, 30]. To the best of our knowledge, most IP-Sim activities have centered on specialized care within hospital settings [8, 25]. While simulations in primary care and municipal healthcare contexts are emerging, they remain relatively rare. However, we argue that IP-Sim has the potential to adapt to the swift transitions in care currently underway and can be one of the solutions to this evolving challenge. By crafting scenarios that envisage potential future developments in healthcare, such as more care being given by municipal healthcare, we can acquaint students with novel care models and collaborative methods.

We also propose that IP-Sim presents unique opportunities to depict a more intricate healthcare landscape, surpassing the limitations of isolated scenarios illustrating specific events in a care process. In Linköping, we have developed an IP-Sim scenario that traces a simulated patient and their relative over a 21-day period. This simulation spans an entire day and encompasses four distinct phases of the patient's care trajectory: the acute phase, two intervals in the hospital ward separated by several days, and the concluding scenario in a home setting. By structuring the simulation this way, we equip our diverse student body to not only comprehend a patient's healthcare journey but also to discern when their own and others' competencies are most pertinent to the patient and their family.

SBE can be implemented using various modalities, with mannequins and simulated or standardized patients (SPs) being the most prevalent [19, 29]. High-fidelity mannequins were initially developed for the in-service training of professional teams in acute care settings, such as emergency medicine, anesthesiology, and obstetrics and gynecology [29]. In contrast, human simulation was designed for pre-service training to evaluate and enhance students' clinical competencies with SPs. Each modality has its pros and cons. Literature indicates that SPs afford students higher-level practice in communication and interaction compared to mannequins [11]. Conversely, studies suggest that mannequins help students concentrate better on tasks and bolster teamwork skills [2]. When orchestrating IP-Sim, selecting the modality should, therefore, align with the specific learning objectives.

The conventional method of conducting simulations comprises an introduction, the simulation itself, which is followed up by a debriefing [2]. Nonetheless, alternative proven methods for IP-Sim exist, such as Rapid Cycle Deliberate Practice (RCDP). RCDP offers a different approach to simulation training for interprofessional teams. Unlike the traditional format, RCDP integrates simulation and reflection within the situation. For instance, participants can reflect on events immediately after practicing specific tasks without the simulation being over yet. Moreover, RCDP facilitates effective problem-solving by allowing pauses at critical junctures for reflection on, for example, teamwork, communication, and leadership [12].

Where, How, And With Whom to Implement IP-Sim

In Kern's fifth step, IP-Sim is implemented [36]. A seminal paper in simulation posited Issenberg's three-factor equation, pivotal for grasping effective simulation-based healthcare education: the equation [training resources] × [trained educators] × [curricular integration] [23], lays out a comprehensive blueprint for IP-Sim deployment. Astbury et al. [4] scrutinized 15 literature reviews to distil the finest IPECP practices, pinpointing facilitators and barriers aligning with Issenberg's factors.

Training resources encompass facilities, equipment, simulators, task trainers, and accessories to emulate all targeted healthcare settings, alongside computers and software. They also incorporate educational materials developed or refined in Kern's preceding steps: syllabi, scenarios, debriefing guides, and checklists [23]. The versatility of simulation facilities affords the necessary adaptability for IP-Sim [4]. Our experience suggests that IP-Sim's realism hinges more on emotional authenticity in human interactions than on physical verisimilitude with equipment and mannequins. This paradigm shift bolsters the learning journey. Hence, simulation spaces with a neutral arrangement and essential audio–video tech are preferable for IP-Sim over high-tech hospital-like rooms. Such setups foster scenario diversity for training interprofessional collaborative practice across hospital and community settings, including care transitions. To navigate IP-Sim's inherent scheduling and logistical hurdles, distributing simulations beyond the center—via in-situ and computer-based methods—is sometimes imperative [29].

Maintaining educator availability and proficiency is as critical as securing physical resources for simulation operations [4, 23]. IP-Sim instructors require dual training in IPE and SBE. Overcoming this challenge is formidable. At this juncture, revisiting Kern's second step to reevaluate local faculty development and train-the-trainer initiatives is advisable [36]. An individual might excel in simulation yet lack awareness of the IPE competencies and CRM tools integral to the proposed IP-Sim curriculum. Conversely, an IPE facilitator might lack simulation facilitation and debriefing expertise [29]. In Geneva, our IP-Sim endeavors pair professionals from two disciplines in dyads, each bringing complementary IPE and SBE skills [37]. We also offer structured feedback through direct observation and debriefing to these IP-Sim pairs, utilizing validated instruments [32]. Beyond educators, IP-Sim's human resource needs extend to administrative and technical personnel, key figures for running a simulation program, and SPs. We deliberately expand human simulation's scope in IP-Sim scenarios to include not just simulated patients but also simulated relatives and other professionals. Training and engaging SPs must adhere to best-evidence standards for their safe and proper participation. Furthermore, thoughtful consideration is warranted when integrating SPs as educational allies in IP-Sim to optimize learning effects [11]. Whether actual patients or actors, their involvement in scenario crafting, team training, and debriefing can markedly enhance IP-Sim.

Curricular integration, often overlooked in simulation rollouts, is arguably the most formidable aspect of IP-Sim implementation [4, 13, 26]. Principal obstacles include scheduling clashes, logistical and spatial limitations in simulation venues, and discrepancies in anticipated learning results and evaluation methods among health profession academies [4, 33]. Furthermore, curricular integration necessitates optimal placement of IP-Sim within an IPE educational continuum [4]. Such distribution and sequencing should afford learners ample simulation opportunities over time for deliberate practice and skill mastery. The curriculum must also engage students or trainees in a deliberate learning trajectory [29], incorporating modalities such as e-learning, shadowing, and collaborative clinical practice, pre- and post-IP-Sim. Nonetheless, ideal distribution and sequencing are often constrained by scheduling and logistical challenges [4, 26].

Assess Learning and Evaluate IP-Sim Training

The final step in Kern's model pertains to assessment and evaluation [36]. While it is an integral part of the learning process, determining the appropriate methods for assessing learners and evaluating programs can be challenging. A core principle of simulation is to offer students a risk-free environment where they can hone various skills and procedures without endangering patient safety [26]. This opportunity to err and learn from mistakes is vital, not only for students but also for professionals, as it significantly contributes to enhancing patient safety. Such an environment necessitates psychological safety within the group, fostered through an accepting and non-judgmental atmosphere [29]. However, academic discourses often drive us toward evaluating students and verifying if they have achieved specific learning objectives, such as those outlined by the Bologna process. Balancing these needs is crucial when implementing IP-Sim, as the requirement for a safe learning space and the imperative to measure learning must be carefully managed.

In assessing interprofessional learning, several tools are employed in the field of IPE, including the Interprofessional Collaborative Competency Assessment Scale and the Interprofessional Socialization and Valuing Scale [3, 39]. These instruments can evaluate students' interprofessional learning and competencies. Yet, the literature offers scant examples of tools designed specifically for use within IP-Sim. Instead, emphasis is placed on reflection through debriefing and co-briefing sessions [38]. In simulation pedagogy, reflection is underscored as an essential means of assessing simulated scenarios and assimilating the lessons learned. Merely performing tasks is insufficient for learning; reflection on actions is necessary [14].

Research underscores the significant value of debriefing (reflection), yet it also highlights the challenges associated with conducting effective debriefing sessions, particularly in IP-Sim contexts. Holmes and Mellanby [21] explored how an interprofessional group of students influences debriefing strategies and the challenges associated with the student group being interprofessional. Their findings indicate that facilitators often respond with "It depends" when queried about their debriefing tactics, suggesting the absence of a one-size-fits-all approach. A key takeaway from their study is the importance of tailoring debriefing to the learners' needs and leveraging the diverse perspectives of an interprofessional group of facilitators who can support one another and serve as role models for the students.

IP-Sim typically necessitates multiple facilitators to steer the simulation, so-called co-debriefing. If done effectively, co-debriefing can incorporate various perspectives to enrich the discussion. However, it is crucial to recognize differing viewpoints, shaped by respective disciplines and professions. Steering the reflection toward interprofessional learning objectives and fostering an appreciation for diverse perspectives can propel the reflection process forward. It is easy to default to discipline-specific knowledge, but the true challenge lies in guiding the reflection in an interprofessional direction. Other important considerations include defining roles within a co-debriefing context and being cognizant of hierarchical dynamics [10].

Finally, a significant challenge in evaluating IP-Sim is ensuring the simulation's interprofessional nature, as opposed to a multiprofessional one. Distinguishing between these concepts is not straightforward, and it is all too easy to misconstrue a multiprofessional simulation as interprofessional. Following Palaganas et al. [33] and international guidelines, a simulation program or activity is deemed IP-Sim when its objectives and assessments are explicitly linked to IPE [33, 34]. As an IP-Sim instructor, one's role is to cultivate a learning environment that motivates students to pursue defined learning objectives and assess their progress accordingly. The teaching focus should center on the students' learning needs and how to facilitate this learning, rather than on the instructor's teaching preferences [2]. To maintain an interprofessional emphasis throughout the IP-Sim, it is imperative that all educators and coordinators concur on prioritizing the interprofessional element in all simulation phases. This entails setting clear objectives for the simulation, ensuring that the interprofessional scope informs the introduction, simulation, and reflection stages. Constructive alignment is pivotal, requiring that the IP-Sim be designed with interprofessional learning objectives from the outset, allowing these objectives to be enacted during the simulation and reflected upon subsequently [2].

Conclusion

IP-Sim is an educational approach aimed at enhancing IPE and training of healthcare students and professionals. IP-Sim offers a unique opportunity to unite professionals from various disciplines, featuring scenarios with the potential to support interprofessional learning. IP-Sim also offers an opportunity to adapt to the swift transitions in care currently underway, as well as depict a more intricate healthcare landscape. For the effective design and implementation of IP-Sim, it is recommended that policymakers, researchers, and academics utilize recognized interprofessional competency frameworks, support established CRM models, and apply proven learning theories, instructional design methods, and validated assessment tools. The implementation of IP-Sim accumulates the challenges associated with both simulation and IPE, including securing material and financial resources, training personnel, and integrating activities into a curriculum supported by multiple institutions. Prompt engagement of all stakeholders, centered around clearly defined needs, will enhance the likelihood of successful initiation and ongoing development. In the European context, IP-Sim faces the challenge of fostering a community of practice that spans across nations, with a particular emphasis on development in Eastern Europe.

Reflective Questions for the Reader

- How can IP-Sim be tailored to meet the specific healthcare needs of your local community?
- What are the essential factors to consider when implementing IP-Sim in your educational or clinical setting?
- How can IP-Sim be integrated into the curriculum to ensure constructive alignment with IPE objectives?
- How should learning be assessed in IP-Sim, and what tools or methods would be most effective?

References

1. Abildgren L, Lebahn-Hadidi M, Mogensen CB, Toft P, Nielsen AB, Frandsen TF, Steffensen SV, Hounsgaard L. The effectiveness of improving healthcare teams' human factor skills using simulation-based training: a systematic review. Adv Simul. 2022;7(1):12. https://doi.org/10.1186/s41077-022-00207-2.

2. Abrandt Dahlgren M, Rystedt H, Felländer-Tsai L, Nyström S, editors. Interprofessional simulation in health care: materiality, embodiment, interaction. Springer; 2019.
3. Almoghirah H, Nazar H, Illing J. Assessment tools in pre-licensure interprofessional education: a systematic review, quality appraisal and narrative synthesis. Med Educ. 2021;55(7):795–807. https://doi.org/10.1111/medu.14453.
4. Astbury J, Ferguson J, Silverthorne J, Willis S, Schafheutle E. High-fidelity simulation-based education in pre-registration healthcare programmes: a systematic review of reviews to inform collaborative and interprofessional best practice. J Interprof Care. 2021;35(4):622–32. https://doi.org/10.1080/13561820.2020.1762551.
5. Boet S, Bould MD, Fung L, Qosa H, Perrier L, Tavares W, Reeves S, Tricco AC. Transfer of learning and patient outcome in simulated crisis resource management: a systematic review. Can J Anesth. 2014;61(6):571–82. https://doi.org/10.1007/s12630-014-0143-8.
6. Boloré S, Fassier T, Guirimand N. Effect of an interprofessional simulation program on patient safety competencies of healthcare professionals in Switzerland: a before and after study. J Educ Eval Health Prof. 2023;20:25. https://doi.org/10.3352/jeehp.2023.20.25.
7. Brezis M, Lahat Y, Frankel M, Rubinov A, Bohm D, Cohen MJ, Koslowsky M, Shalomson O, Sprung CL, Perry-Mezare H, Yahalom R, Ziv A. What can we learn from simulation-based training to improve skills for end-of-life care? Insights from a national project in Israel. Isr J Health Policy Res. 2017;6(1):48. https://doi.org/10.1186/s13584-017-0169-9.
8. Buljac-Samardzic M, Doekhie KD, van Wijngaarden JDH. Interventions to improve team effectiveness within health care: a systematic review of the past decade. Hum Resour Health. 2020;18(1):2. https://doi.org/10.1186/s12960-019-0411-3.
9. Chen AS, Yau B, Revere L, Swails J. Implementation, evaluation, and outcome of TeamSTEPPS in interprofessional education: a scoping review. J Interprof Care. 2019;33(6):795–804. https://doi.org/10.1080/13561820.2019.1594729.
10. Cheng A, Palaganas J, Eppich W, Rudolph J, Robinson T, Grant V. Co-debriefing for simulation-based education: a primer for facilitators. Simul Healthc. 2015;10(2):69–75. https://doi.org/10.1097/SIH.0000000000000077.
11. Cleland JA, Abe K, Rethans J-J. The use of simulated patients in medical education: AMEE Guide No 42. Med Teach. 2009;31(6):477–86. https://doi.org/10.1080/01421590903002821.
12. Coleman N, Wiltrakis SM, Holmes S, Hwu R, Iyer S, Goodwin N, Mathai C, Gillespie S, Hebbar KB. A comparison of rapid cycle deliberate practice and traditional reflective debriefing on interprofessional team performance. BMC Med Educ. 2024;24:122. https://doi.org/10.1186/s12909-024-05101-1.
13. Colonnello V, Kinoshita Y, Yoshida N, Bustos Villalobos I. Undergraduate interprofessional education in the European higher education area: a systematic review. Int Med Educ. 2023;2(2):100–12. https://doi.org/10.3390/ime2020010.
14. El-Awaisi A, Jaam M, Wilby KJ, Wilbur K. A systematic review of the use of simulation and reflection as summative assessment tools to evaluate student outcomes following interprofessional education activities. J Interprof Care. 2022;36(6):882–90. https://doi.org/10.1080/13561820.2022.2026899.
15. Frenk J, Chen L, Bhutta ZA, Cohen J, Crisp N, Evans T, Fineberg H, Garcia P, Ke Y, Kelley P, Kistnasamy B, Meleis A, Naylor D, Pablos-Mendez A, Reddy S, Scrimshaw S, Sepulveda J, Serwadda D, Zurayk H. Health professionals for a new century: transforming education to strengthen health systems in an interdependent world. Lancet. 2010;376(9756):1923–58. https://doi.org/10.1016/S0140-6736(10)61854-5.
16. Frenk J, Chen LC, Chandran L, Groff EOH, King R, Meleis A, Fineberg HV. Challenges and opportunities for educating health professionals after the COVID-19 pandemic. Lancet. 2022;400(10362):1539–56. https://doi.org/10.1016/S0140-6736(22)02092-X.
17. Frerejean J, Van Merriënboer JJG, Condron C, Strauch U, Eppich W. Critical design choices in healthcare simulation education: a 4C/ID perspective on design that leads to transfer. Adv Simul. 2023;8(1):5. https://doi.org/10.1186/s41077-023-00242-7.
18. Friedman MI, Attivissimo LA, Kiszko KB, Rimar A, Yezzo PM, Torroella Carney M. The development and piloting of a goals of care conversation education program for an advanced

illness population. Gerontol Geriatr Educ. 2020;41(1):52–62. https://doi.org/10.1080/02701960.2019.1623210.

19. Gaba DM. The future vision of simulation in health care. Qual Saf Health Care. 2004;13(Suppl_1):i2–i10. https://doi.org/10.1136/qshc.2004.009878.
20. Hean S, Craddock D, O'Halloran C. Learning theories and interprofessional education: a user's guide. Learn Health Soc Care. 2009;8(4):250–62. https://doi.org/10.1111/j.1473-6861.2009.00227.x.
21. Holmes C, Mellanby E. Debriefing strategies for interprofessional simulation—a qualitative study. Adv Simul. 2022;7(1):18. https://doi.org/10.1186/s41077-022-00214-3.
22. Institute of Medicine. To err is human: building a safer health system. Washington: The National Academies Press; 2000. https://doi.org/10.17226/9728.
23. Issenberg SB. The scope of simulation-based healthcare education. Simul Healthc. 2006;1(4):203–8. https://doi.org/10.1097/01.SIH.0000246607.36504.5a.
24. Kayyali R, Harrap N, Albayaty A, Savickas V, Hammell J, Hyatt F, Elliott K, Richardson S. Simulation in pharmacy education to enhance interprofessional education. Int J Pharm Pract. 2019;27(3):295–302. https://doi.org/10.1111/ijpp.12499.
25. Kiessling A, Amiri C, Arhammar J, Lundbäck M, Wallingstam C, Wikner J, Svensson R, Henriksson P, Kuhl J. Interprofessional simulation-based team-training and self-efficacy in emergency medicine situations. J Interprof Care. 2022;36(6):873–81. https://doi.org/10.1080/13561820.2022.2038103.
26. Lee CA, Pais K, Kelling S, Anderson OS. A scoping review to understand simulation used in interprofessional education. J Interprof Educ Pract. 2018;13:15–23. https://doi.org/10.1016/j.xjep.2018.08.003.
27. Lunde L, Moen A, Jakobsen RB, Rosvold E, Brænd A. Exploring healthcare students' interprofessional teamwork in primary care simulation scenarios: collaboration to create a shared treatment plan. BMC Med Educ. 2021;21:416. https://doi.org/10.1186/s12909-021-02852-z.
28. Lunde L, Moen A, Jakobsen RB, Møller B, Rosvold EO, Brænd AM. A preliminary simulation-based qualitative study of healthcare students' experiences of interprofessional primary care scenarios. Adv Simul. 2022;7(1):9. https://doi.org/10.1186/s41077-022-00204-5.
29. Motola I, Devine LA, Chung HS, Sullivan JE, Issenberg SB. Simulation in healthcare education: a best evidence practical guide. AMEE Guide No. 82. Med Teach. 2013;35(10):e1511–30. https://doi.org/10.3109/0142159X.2013.818632.
30. Oxelmark L, Nordahl Amorøe T, Carlzon L, Rystedt H. Students' understanding of teamwork and professional roles after interprofessional simulation—a qualitative analysis. Adv Simul. 2017;2:8. https://doi.org/10.1186/s41077-017-0041-6.
31. Paige JT, Sonesh SC, Garbee DD, Bonanno LS, editors. Comprehensive healthcare simulation: interprofessional team training and simulation. Springer; 2020.
32. Paignon A, Wiesner Conti J, Cerutti B, Fassier T. French translation and validation of the interprofessional facilitation scale for simulation. J Interprof Care. 2021;35(5):803–7. https://doi.org/10.1080/13561820.2021.1879750.
33. Palaganas JC, Brunette V, Winslow B. Prelicensure simulation-enhanced interprofessional education: a critical review of the research literature. Simul Healthc. 2016;11(6):404–18. https://doi.org/10.1097/SIH.0000000000000175.
34. Rossler K, Molloy MA, Pastva AM, Brown M, Xavier N. Healthcare simulation standards of best PracticeTM simulation-enhanced interprofessional education. Clin Simul Nurs. 2021;58:49–53. https://doi.org/10.1016/j.ecns.2021.08.015.
35. Thistlethwaite JE, Forman D, Matthews LR, Rogers GD, Steketee C, Yassine T. Competencies and frameworks in interprofessional education: a comparative analysis. Acad Med. 2014;89(6):869–75. https://doi.org/10.1097/ACM.0000000000000249.
36. Thomas PA, Kern DE, Hughes MT, Tackett S, Chen BY, editors. Curriculum development for medical education: a six-step approach. 4th ed. Johns Hopkins University Press; 2022.
37. van Gessel E, Picchiottino P, Doureradjam R, Nendaz M, Mèche P. Interprofessional training: start with the youngest! A program for undergraduate healthcare students in Geneva, Switzerland. Med Teach. 2018;40(6):595–9. https://doi.org/10.1080/0142159X.2018.1445207.

38. Webster KLW, Keebler JR. Best practices for interprofessional education debriefing in medical simulation. In: Paige J, Sonesh S, Garbee D, Bonanno L, editors. Comprehensive healthcare simulation: InterProfessional team training and simulation. Comprehensive healthcare simulation. Cham: Springer; 2020. https://doi.org/10.1007/978-3-030-28845-7_5.
39. Wooding EL, Gale TC, Maynard V. Evaluation of teamwork assessment tools for interprofessional simulation: a systematic literature review. J Interprof Care. 2020;34(2):162–72. https://doi.org/10.1080/13561820.2019.1650730.
40. World Health Organization (WHO). Framework for action on interprofessional education & collaborative practice. 2010. https://www.who.int/publications/i/item/framework-for-action-on-interprofessional-education-collaborative-practice.

Tove Törnqvist (BSc, MSc, PhD) is a registered occupational therapist and an assistant professor at the Department of Health, Medicine and Caring Sciences, Linköping University, Sweden. Tove's research interests are focused on interprofessional collaboration and learning, with an emphasis on students' learning. She is also engaged in education and pedagogical development within the bachelor's program in occupational therapy, the master's program in medical sciences, and specific interprofessional learning activities such as interprofessional simulations at Linköping University.

Simon Wiss Tidén (BSc, MSc) is a nurse anesthetist by profession and currently works as senior coordinator for simulations at the Clinical Training Centre of the Faculty of Medicine and Health Sciences, Linköping University, Sweden. His work involves planning, executing, and evaluating a variety of simulations. Simon has a keen interest in simulation as a pedagogical approach for learning and has been involved in the development and establishment of interprofessional simulations at the faculty.

Patricia Picchiottino (MAS, BSc) is a senior lecturer at the University of Applied Sciences and Arts of Western Switzerland HES-SO, Geneva, Switzerland. Deputy Director of the Center for Interprofessional Simulation, she coordinates the interprofessional education (IPE) curriculum at the Geneva School of Health Sciences HES-SO, Geneva. Midwife by training, she has a special interest in simulation-enhanced IPE (Sim-IPE).

Thomas Fassier (PhD, MD, MHPE, MPH) is a senior lecturer at the University of Geneva and an attending physician at the Geneva University Hospitals. Director of the Center for Interprofessional Simulation, he coordinates the IPE curriculum at the Faculty of Medicine. Physician by training, he has a special interest in Sim-IPE.

Extended Reality in Interprofessional Education Across Europe

Paul Dudley and Monika Bolliger

Introduction

Interprofessional education (IPE) is a critical component of healthcare training, promoting collaboration among professionals to improve patient outcomes [17]. Traditionally, IPE has relied on face-to-face simulations, problem-based learning, and role-playing exercises to foster teamwork and communication [15]. While these methods are well-established, they can be resource-intensive, requiring significant logistical planning, physical space, and faculty involvement [16]. Consequently, there is growing interest in technological innovations that can enhance IPE while reducing associated costs and barriers.

Extended reality (XR), an umbrella term encompassing virtual reality (VR), augmented reality (AR), and mixed reality (MR), has emerged as a promising tool for healthcare education [13]. XR offers immersive and interactive learning environments that can simulate clinical scenarios with high fidelity, providing learners with opportunities to practice skills and engage in collaborative problem-solving without the constraints of traditional in-person training [5]. In IPE, XR technologies facilitate realistic role-playing, communication exercises, and

P. Dudley (✉)
City St George's, University of London, London, UK

Faculty of Life Sciences and Medicine, King's College London (KCL) University, London, UK
e-mail: Paul.dudley@citystgeorges.ac.uk

M. Bolliger
Institute for Public Health, Zurich University of Applied Science, Winterthur, Switzerland

Faculty of Medical Sciences, Private University in the Principality of Liechtenstein (UFL), Triesen, Liechtenstein
e-mail: bolg@zhaw.ch

A. Xyrichis et al. (eds.), *Building Bridges: A European Perspective on Interprofessional Education, Practice, Policy and Research*,
https://doi.org/10.1007/978-3-032-23222-9_11

decision-making processes among healthcare students from different disciplines, even when they are geographically dispersed [14].

The integration of XR into IPE aligns with broader trends in digital learning and simulation-based education. Advances in XR technology have improved accessibility and usability, allowing students to engage with virtual scenarios via standard computers, mobile devices, or VR headsets [12]. These innovations have the potential to address existing challenges in healthcare education, such as limited access to physical training spaces, variability in patient cases, and time constraints for both learners and educators [8]. Furthermore, research suggests that XR-based training can enhance learners' engagement, knowledge retention, and teamwork skills compared to traditional methods [7].

This chapter explores the transformative role of XR in IPE, focusing on case studies from King's College London (KCL) and Zurich University of Applied Sciences. Examining XR applications such as virtual home environments and patient safety simulations highlights the benefits and challenges of integrating XR into healthcare training. Through these examples, the chapter provides practical insights into how XR can be leveraged to enhance interprofessional collaboration, reduce training costs, and create accessible learning experiences for a diverse range of students. Designed for a diverse audience, from XR experts to beginners, it provides an overview of XR applications in healthcare education, dispels common misconceptions, and provides practical guidance for its implementation.

Drawing on a range of sources, including existing literature, case studies, and personal experiences in university healthcare education, the chapter presents a compelling case for the integration of XR in IPE. It showcases how XR can be used to create authentic learning environments that mirror real-world scenarios, enhancing students' understanding and preparing them for their future roles in healthcare.

The chapter demystifies XR, explaining its various forms, the language used in its context, and how it compares to AR, other forms of MR, and VR. It delves into the technology's workings, its limitations, and the advantages it offers over conventional simulation methods of teaching.

The unique contribution of this chapter lies in its practical and technical approach. It not only discusses the theoretical aspects of XR in IPE but also provides practical guidance for creating XR projects. This guide is designed to inspire educators to experiment with XR and adapt it to their specific teaching contexts.

Looking ahead, the chapter also explores the future trends in XR and IPE, highlighting the areas that educators and practitioners need to watch out for, including artificial intelligence (AI). It concludes with a reflection on the challenges and opportunities that lie ahead in this exciting field.

Key Phrases with Definitions to Help You Understand Extended Realities

Understanding these basic XR terms can help healthcare professionals and educators appreciate how immersive technologies might be used for training, patient care, and therapy, offering innovative approaches to traditional challenges in the medical field.

- *XR*: XR is an umbrella term that encompasses various forms of immersive technologies, including VR, AR, and MR.
- *VR*: Think of VR like a computer-created world that you can step into and explore. For healthcare professionals, this could mean walking through a detailed 3D model of the human heart or practicing a surgical procedure in a risk-free, simulated environment.
- *AR*: AR is like having a magic lens that overlays extra information on what you're already seeing in the real world. For instance, a doctor could see a digital overlay of a patient's vein structure on their skin before inserting a needle.
- *MR*: MR blends the real world with digital elements more seamlessly than AR. In a medical training context, this might mean practicing on a mannequin that reacts in real-time to treatment, guided by digital cues seen through special glasses.
- *360-Degree Video/Image*: Imagine being inside a sphere, and the face of that sphere has an image or video projected onto it. You are able to look around in all directions from a single point, as if you are standing in the center of a room and can see every corner by just turning your head. This could be used to immerse health professionals in a clinical scenario, allowing them to understand patient experiences or to visualize complex procedures from multiple angles, or as an introduction to a new space.
- *Presence*: This term is all about feeling like you are truly "there" in the VR environment. It is crucial for learning in healthcare, as feeling present in a simulated medical scenario can enhance learning and retention of skills.
- *Latency*: Latency refers to any delay between your actions and what you see in the VR world. In a healthcare setting, low latency is vital to ensure that when you practice a procedure in VR, the response is immediate and accurate, just like in real life.
- *Field of View (FOV)*: FOV is how wide you can see within the VR environment. A wider FOV can make VR training tools more immersive for healthcare professionals, offering a broad and realistic view of the virtual scene.
- *Tracking*: This is about how the VR system follows your movements. Accurate tracking ensures that when you move or look around in a virtual space, everything responds just like it would in real life, which is crucial for realistic training experiences in healthcare.
- *Three Degrees of Freedom (3DoF)*: Degrees of freedom refer to your ability to move through a virtual environment in a head-mounted display (HMD). 3DoFs

correspond to the user's rotational movement on the *x*, *y*, and *z* axis also known as pitch, yaw, and roll. When viewing a 360-degree image in an HMD, you can look left and right, up and down, and can tilt your head side to side; these are the 3DoFs.

- *Six Degrees of Freedom*: This phrase includes the 3DoFs described above, but also includes three more, which are thought of as the translational movement along the *x*, *y*, and *z* axes. When viewing a computer-generated virtual world, you can move back and forward, side to side, and up and down throughout the world; this is not achievable with a 360-degree image.

Integrating XR in Health Professions Education: Collaborative Experiences from KCL and Zurich University of Applied Sciences, Switzerland

The authors of this chapter have developed and tested XR technologies for IPE at KCL and Zurich University of Applied Sciences, demonstrating their pivotal role in IPE within health professions. The examples from these two institutions illustrate the transformative potential of XR to enhance educational practices, develop critical competencies, and foster teamwork among healthcare students.

XR Development at KCL

At KCL, the integration of XR into health professions education has been exemplified through a detailed, photorealistic 360-degree virtual tour of a patient's home. This project, developed in collaboration with physiotherapist Chloe Apps, was designed to simulate a range of home-based hazards, such as trip hazards, inaccessible necessities, and signs of neglect. Originally intended for immersive use with VR headsets, the application was adapted to a web-based platform hosted on Moodle (a virtual learning environment) during the pandemic, ensuring that training remained accessible to all students, regardless of location and access to an HMD.

This move not only preserved the integrity and continuity of the educational experience but also actively engaged students in assessing and managing potential risks, thus preparing them for practical, real-world clinical scenarios.

Aligned with the principles of IPE as endorsed by the World Health Organization "Interprofessional education occurs when two or more professions learn about, from and with each other to enable effective collaboration and improve health outcomes" [17] and highlighted by Buring et al. [1] "The goal of these efforts is to develop knowledge, skills and attitudes that result in interprofessional team behaviors and competence." The virtual simulated home environment promotes collaborative learning and a deeper understanding of patient care within home settings. Students from various healthcare disciplines were given time to interact with this environment and develop details of a care plan from their profession's perspective. Students then worked together in a mixed profession group to discuss the details of the care plan and to hear from each other about the concerns they found that they felt needed actioning. The project enhances teamwork and improves patient outcomes by preparing students to effectively address complex care scenarios and think about care from other professions.

Details of the patient's recent hospital admission, past medical history, medication history, and social history were shared with the students before they had an opportunity to explore the patient's virtual home.

Students convened in pre-set interprofessional groups to discuss the patient case they observed in the home environment. Their task was to develop a patient-centered management plan using a multi-disciplinary team (MDT) approach. Educational scaffolding, in the form of paperwork, guided their assessment, analysis, and understanding of roles and responsibilities within the clinical team.

After participating in the synchronous team-based activity, students proceeded to engage in independent post-activity work. This allowed for individual reflection on their learning experiences and provided an opportunity to review an exemplary MDT discussion related to the patient case, which had been developed by members of the project team.

XR Innovations at Zurich University of Applied Sciences, Switzerland

Zurich University of Applied Sciences, Switzerland, developed two XR applications specifically for an interprofessional module. These applications immersed approximately 280 B.Sc. students from diverse health fields such as nursing, physiotherapy, midwifery, occupational therapy, and public health in detailed patient safety scenarios. Inspired by the effectiveness of immersive VR training demonstrated in studies by Cieslowski et al. [4] and Choi et al. [3], these applications were designed to create a dynamic learning environment.

Students used these applications—one web-based and the other optimized for VR headsets—to engage with a "Room of Horrors," where they identified and assessed safety risks and potential errors within a healthcare setting. This practical exercise not only utilized the collaborative learning and teamwork benefits of XR technologies, as supported by research from Grassini et al. [6] and Liaw et al. [9], but also encouraged students to engage in interprofessional dialogue and reflection. This reflective practice is essential for deep learning and professional development, significantly enhancing their learning outcomes and clinical readiness. The experiences bridged the gap between theoretical knowledge and practical application, fostering an understanding of different professional perspectives and preparing students for real-world scenarios.

Lessons Learned

XR has a lot of potential to be a powerful teaching tool. There are many types of XR, and understanding the limits, challenges, and costs associated with each type is just as important as understanding the learning outcomes you are trying to achieve. There will be cases where things like 360-cinematography may be cheaper and easier to produce than other forms of XR, but does it meet the needs of your students? Is there an easier and cheaper way of doing it that does not involve XR? What does XR offer your learning needs that other modalities do not?

XR has many places in education, but be mindful of the trap that the allure of XR technology brings. It is a very good hook to get interest and buy-in from others.

Conclusion

The integration of XR technologies at both KCL and Zurich University of Applied Sciences demonstrates novel ways of using this technology to teach interprofessionally. These technologies have been used as complementary training methods in a way that has put limited demands on academics to deliver and oversee. These initiatives show that XR can enhance students' practical skills and underscore how technological innovations can revolutionize educational outcomes in healthcare. Insights from these experiences offer valuable guidance for other institutions considering the adoption of similar technologies in their curricula, highlighting the benefits of XR in improving educational practices in the health sector.

Shaping the Future: XR Empowered by AI

The authors take a look into the future, which has already begun with the combination of XR and AI. XR and AI are on the brink of redefining our physical reality, offering transformative potentials in various domains, particularly in healthcare and medical education. This fusion represents a potentially dynamic interplay between immersive experiences and intelligent algorithms, shaping the future landscape of education and practice.

The integration of AI technology with XR technologies unlocks new opportunities for personalized, adaptive learning experiences. Through dynamic interactions and intelligent feedback mechanisms, AI enhances the XR experience and tailors it to individual needs and preferences. AI imbues XR experiences with intelligence, interactivity, and responsiveness, adapting to users' behavior, preferences, and even emotions. This enhanced interactivity is particularly beneficial for interprofessional learning, where students from various healthcare domains collaborate and role-play complex scenarios. For instance, AI-driven virtual characters can simulate realistic patient encounters, enabling nursing, medical, and other healthcare students to practice teamwork, communication, and decision-making in a safe and controlled environment.

In summary, by harnessing the potentials of XR and AI, we embark on a journey to redefine our physical reality. Through collaborative efforts and ethical considerations, we can leverage the transformative potential of these technologies to shape a future where healthcare education transcends boundaries and empowers learners to thrive in an ever-evolving landscape.

Discussion

The transformative integration of XR and AI into IPE is poised to revolutionize healthcare training. By offering personalized, adaptive learning experiences, these technologies enhance the depth and breadth of healthcare education. Central to this revolution is XR's unique capability to foster communication, teamwork, and a deep understanding across various healthcare disciplines, as evidenced by the work of Mistry et al. [10] and supported by practical healthcare applications. The importance of immersive technologies in creating effective collaborative learning environments is further reinforced by research from Choi et al. [3] and initiatives by the Canadian Interprofessional Health Collaborative [2].

Adding a vital, practical dimension to this discussion are the firsthand experiences of the authors who have embarked on developing XR applications for IPE. These insights show the substantial benefits of XR in simulating complex healthcare scenarios, providing students with immersive, collaborative problem-solving activities that closely mirror real-world patient care. Such practical applications underscore the academic findings and highlight the invaluable role of immersive learning environments in fostering interprofessional collaboration. The authors have demonstrated that once made, tested, and evaluated, XR applications can be scaled up to large numbers of students, crossing professions and schools across universities with relative ease. Once made, you can exponentially expand the number of users with minimal extra work.

The introduction of AI into the XR landscape opens new avenues for innovation, promising to enhance the realism and personalization of learning experiences even further. This synergistic relationship between AI and XR holds the potential to revolutionize healthcare education by providing adaptive, responsive educational environments that cater to the individual needs and learning styles of students.

However, it is essential to address the considerable privacy and ethical challenges that accompany the advancement of XR and AI technologies. The development of systems capable of offering highly personalized experiences through biometric data necessitates rigorous ethical scrutiny and robust data protection measures. Ensuring the responsible use of XR in educational settings is paramount as these technologies evolve, highlighting the need for ongoing research and dialogue within the healthcare and academic communities to navigate these complex issues.

Despite these challenges, the promise of XR and AI in healthcare education remains vast. Addressing issues such as equitable access to technology, the ethical implications of its use, and the development of content that accurately reflects the complexities of interprofessional healthcare delivery is crucial for the successful integration of XR into healthcare education. By combining firsthand development experiences with academic insights, educators and developers can work toward a more integrated, efficient, and empathetic healthcare system, navigating both the opportunities and challenges presented by XR and AI technologies.

This synthesis seeks to encapsulate the excitement and potential of XR and AI in healthcare education, thoughtfully integrating concerns and ethical considerations into a narrative that remains optimistic about the future of interprofessional learning.

Getting Started with XR in IPE: A Beginner's View

Understanding Your Educational Needs

For many educators, the idea of integrating XR into IPE can feel overwhelming. The technology itself—whether VR, AR, or MR—is evolving rapidly, and for those new to this field, the initial steps can seem daunting. However, XR does not have to be an all-or-nothing approach. With careful planning, strategic investment, and a clear understanding of its educational value, even novice educators can begin incorporating immersive technology into their teaching in meaningful ways.

Before adopting XR, the most crucial step is to reflect on your educational needs. What specific learning challenges do your students face, and can XR offer a solution that traditional teaching methods cannot? XR is a powerful tool, but it should never be used simply for the sake of technology. If a simpler and more cost-effective approach—such as traditional role-playing, video-based learning, or standard simulations—can achieve the same objectives, then XR may not be necessary. However, if you aim to provide a risk-free environment for students to practice high-stakes decision-making, expose them to a variety of realistic clinical scenarios, or facilitate collaboration among geographically dispersed learners, then XR could be a valuable addition to your curriculum.

Choosing the Right XR Modality

Understanding the different types of XR available is another critical step. VR offers full immersion, transporting learners into computer-generated environments where they can interact with scenarios that mimic real-life healthcare settings. This is particularly useful for high-risk clinical training, such as emergency response or surgical procedures.

On the other hand, AR overlays digital elements onto the real world, allowing learners to interact with both virtual and physical components simultaneously. This can be highly beneficial for skill-based training, such as guiding students through a complex medical procedure with digital prompts. MR takes this one step further by allowing users to manipulate virtual objects within their real-world environment, offering hands-on learning experiences that are deeply interactive.

For educators who want a more accessible starting point, 360-degree videos can provide an effective, low-cost alternative, offering students the ability to observe and analyze clinical environments without the need for expensive VR headsets. These videos allow learners to explore a scene from all angles, making them particularly useful for observational training or introducing students to complex healthcare environments.

Practical Considerations Before Implementation

Once an educator determines that XR is a suitable addition to their teaching, practical considerations come into play. Accessibility is a key concern. If an XR-based activity requires specialized headsets, will all students have access to the necessary hardware? If not, is there a web-based or mobile alternative? Cost is another major factor. Developing fully interactive VR simulations can be expensive, and funding may be a barrier. In some cases, investing in existing XR applications, rather than creating custom content, may be a more practical solution.

Additionally, technical support is essential. Educators need to ensure that they have access to IT professionals who can troubleshoot hardware and software issues, as well as provide training to faculty members who may be unfamiliar with immersive technologies. Without adequate technical support, even the best-designed XR experiences may fail to deliver their intended learning benefits.

Getting Started with Minimal Investment

For those just starting out, it is advisable to begin with minimal investment and gradually scale up. Rather than committing to a large-scale XR implementation immediately, educators can first explore free or low-cost XR applications that align with their curriculum. Google Arts & Culture offers free access to 360 content. Although this is not designed for healthcare teaching, it offers an insight into how 360 content can be utilized. Alternatively, companies like Oxford Medical Simulation may offer free trials or demonstrations for you to trial before investing.

Universities may already have existing resources, such as simulation labs or media production teams, which can support XR projects. Open-source tools also provide an opportunity to create interactive experiences without the financial burden of commercial software. Taking advantage of these existing resources can make the transition to XR smoother and more cost-effective.

Piloting XR in Your Curriculum

Once an XR approach is selected, piloting the technology within a small student group is a crucial step. A pilot project allows educators to assess usability, engagement, and overall effectiveness before rolling out XR to a larger audience. During this phase, collecting feedback from both students and faculty is essential. Are students finding the XR experience engaging? Does it enhance their understanding of interprofessional collaboration? Are there technical issues that need to be addressed? This iterative approach ensures that any necessary adjustments can be made before full-scale implementation.

Pilots also help educators refine the way they integrate XR into their teaching. They can determine whether students need additional guidance before using the technology, whether certain scenarios need to be adjusted for clarity, and whether the technology itself is enhancing learning in the way it was intended. By making these adjustments early, educators can increase the likelihood of a successful broader rollout.

Overcoming Common Challenges

Like any educational innovation, the integration of XR comes with challenges. Technical barriers, such as software compatibility or hardware malfunctions, can be frustrating, especially for educators with limited experience in digital learning technologies. Ensuring that students are fully engaged is another consideration. While XR can be highly immersive, it requires clear learning objectives and structured activities to ensure that students remain focused on educational outcomes.

Additionally, ethical and privacy concerns should not be overlooked. Some XR applications collect user data, so educators need to be aware of data security policies and ensure compliance with institutional regulations. Understanding what data is being collected and ensuring that student privacy is protected is crucial when integrating new technology into an educational setting.

Long-Term Vision and Scaling XR in IPE

For those who successfully navigate the early stages of XR integration, there is significant potential for long-term growth. Once a small-scale XR project proves effective, educators can consider expanding to larger student groups or even collaborating with other institutions. One of the key advantages of XR is its scalability—once an interactive learning experience is developed, it can be used repeatedly with minimal additional cost or effort.

The future of XR in IPE also extends beyond current technologies, with AI playing an increasingly important role in creating adaptive, personalized learning experiences. AI-driven XR applications can respond dynamically to student actions, providing real-time feedback and adjusting scenarios based on individual learning needs. Staying informed about emerging trends in AI-enhanced XR will help educators prepare for the next wave of innovations in healthcare education.

Summary

In summary, adopting XR as a novice educator does not require an advanced technical background or a massive budget. With thoughtful planning, a clear understanding of learning objectives, and a willingness to experiment, educators can begin incorporating XR into IPE in ways that are both meaningful and sustainable. Starting small—by leveraging existing resources, exploring low-cost applications, and piloting XR experiences—can provide valuable insights and set the stage for more advanced implementations in the future.

By addressing key considerations such as accessibility, cost, technical support, and ethical implications, educators can make informed decisions that ensure XR enhances, rather than complicates, the learning experience. As XR continues to evolve, its potential to transform IPE will only grow, offering innovative new ways to engage students and prepare them for the collaborative demands of modern healthcare.

An Advanced Understanding of VR

For those considering investing in XR and VR, it is important to gain a technical understanding of what VR is and how it works. This section will provide a comprehensive overview of VR, explaining its various forms and the language used in its context.

VR, as defined by the Oxford Dictionary, is a computer-generated simulation of a three-dimensional image or environment [11]. This simulated world can be interacted with in a seemingly tangible manner by an individual using specialized electronic equipment, such as a helmet fitted with a screen or gloves equipped with sensors.

This definition captures the most commonly recognized form of VR, where the user dons an HMD and is virtually transported to a different environment. In this immersive environment, the user might find themselves in a fully computer-generated world, akin to a video game, or they might be presented with a photorealistic environment, a 360-degree image, or a video to explore. As they move their head around, the headset tracks their location and orientation, adjusting the in-screen visuals accordingly, so that their real-world movements are mimicked in the virtual experience.

However, VR is not limited to HMDs. It can also be experienced on a PC, laptop, or mobile smartphone. A well-known example of this is Google Maps' Street View, where users can navigate 360-degree images mapped against GPS locations using a mouse or touchscreen. It is important to remember that this format is an option when producing your own VR experiences, particularly for individuals who might find wearing or using VR headsets challenging, uncomfortable, or even impractical.

Another variant of VR is known as an immersion room. Here, images or computer-generated environments are projected or displayed on the walls. This setup is typically paired with a touch screen interface, allowing users to interact with the projected images. While users can explore the environment in an immersion room, they are less immersed compared to HMDs and can easily discern their location in the real world. Conversely, HMDs offer a more immersive experience, making users feel as if they have been fully transported to the virtual environment.

A 360-degree image provides a panoramic view that captures everything in a seamless circular format. These images are created by stitching together photos or videos captured by a purpose-built 360-degree camera. These cameras have two or more lenses, each facing different directions with overlapping fields of view. An example leading 360-degree camera in the market is the Insta360 Titan (Image 1), which has eight lenses. Each lens captures an image that overlaps with its neighboring image at what is known as "the stitch line." Ideally, the stitch line should be invisible so that the viewer does not notice any discontinuity or distortion in the image. However, this is not always easy to achieve, especially when there are moving objects or complex textures in the scene. The camera has software that uses advanced algorithms and sensors to detect and adjust the stitch line dynamically, ensuring that the final image is as smooth and natural as possible. When filming or capturing images, it is important to consider where the areas are that the viewers are going to be most interested in, trying to get this central in the lens and keep the stitch lines on something plain and away from areas the viewers will be watching.

In 360-cinematography, there are two options: monoscopic and stereoscopic. Monoscopic in VR is where one image is shown to both eyes, creating a flat 360-degree image. Whereas stereoscopic there are two images shown, one for each eye. The two images are shown from slightly different angles, which is how human eyes work and allows your brain to calculate depth. Stereoscopic VR allows you to create a sense of depth in your virtual world (3D), but has limitations. Stereoscopic VR can only be viewed in an HMD, as it is showing two different images and is limited to a lower resolution when filming.

An example of where we have used this is in a home environment that was a small room with furniture and props. The stitch lines struggled to handle this, but shooting in 3D produced an image with cleaner stitch lines than the 2D-360 equivalent. The 3D effect caused props in the scene to pop off the screen more, with some of the props having a 3D effect. There have been no studies or comments on whether 360-3D offers any more benefits than 2D-360, from a user's point of view, with regard to an increased feeling of presence that we can find.

Resolution is part of an important consideration in VR and something that may feel familiar. Resolution refers to the number of pixels in the horizontal and vertical axes of the screen and is familiar to most in commercial TVs. The resolution influences the level of detail perceived by the human eye. The Varjo XR-4 (one of the most powerful HMDs currently on the market) has a resolution of 3840 x 3744 pixels; however, Varjo says, "Resolution is best measured as pixels per degree (or PPD) in a user's field of view." An HMD resolution can be misleading because it does not take into account the size of the display or location of the pixels; a headset with the same number of pixels spread over a larger area will reduce the sharpness and quality of the image displayed or if the pixels are most concentrated around the edges of your FOV the area of interest will appear blurry or pixelated.

The PPD is the number of pixels within 1 degree of vision in front of the eye. To calculate the PPD, you divide the number of pixels in a horizontal display line by the horizontal FOV provided by the lens. For example, if a VR headset has 1280 pixels in a horizontal display line and a horizontal FOV of 90 degrees, it would have a PPD of approximately 14.2 (1280/90). A higher PPD results in a sharper, more realistic image, which is one of the factors that influence immersion and presence in

VR. However, any display above 60 pixels/degree is essentially wasting resolution because the eye cannot pick up any more detail; the human eye can view approximately 60 PPD. This is called retinal resolution, or eye-limiting resolution. PPD takes into account how the optical lenses affect visible pixel density. Therefore, it provides a more honest metric for VR pixel density.

AR works by projecting holographic images in the real world. This is achieved by headsets using a computer connected to glasses; the glasses generate the holographic image, which gives it the illusion of being present in the real world. The experience for the user is different from VR in the sense that the user is still aware of their surroundings; they are not transported to a new virtual environment but stay grounded in reality. This allows for an interesting approach to teaching. AR headsets are expensive; the HoloLens 2 and Apple Vision Pro are relatively new expensive technologies. In the United Kingdom, there are a few HoloLens packages available, like HoloPatient or Lucina (a birthing manikin with an AR training package), but the cost of such applications has limited the usability and buy-in from institutions. Institutions need to decide if it is cheaper or more cost-effective to hire simulated patients or look to alternative options to train students rather than pay an annual subscription to AR training packages.

Creating and Implementing VR

With a strong background in technology-enhanced learning, particularly through working in complex busy simulation centers, we have found 360-cinematography is the simplest and most accessible way to create XR. This may be different for someone who is well experienced in computer programming or creating computer-based VR, but as someone with little experience in this field apart from what we have taught ourselves in Unity, a game-building platform, 360-cinematography is simpler and more cost-effective. NB: 360 cinematography still has its limits. You must decide if this method works for your method of learning. Coding is an expensive complex and specialist route to building VR experiences, when trying to outsource this we have been quoted in the region of £50,000 for a single app, whereas 360 cinematography can range in cost, from as little as £40 for a Gear360 on Amazon to over £15,000 for an Insta360 Titan (one of, if not the, most powerful 360-degree cameras on the market). NB: This camera requires a high-spec PC to render the 360 content and high-spec HMDs to view the content at full resolution, and for a relatively unpolished product, it can be done by anyone who is willing to experiment with the camera.

Using the Insta360 Titan as an example, it works in a similar way to any other camera. You can change the exposure, white balance, and other settings to fine-tune the image/video you capture, but the standard or auto settings have sufficed for us, as long as the photographer keeps a few key principles in mind:

Distance from the camera: If you or objects get too close to the camera, they could end up behind or too close to the stitch lines discussed earlier. This distorts the image and renders the 360-degree image visibly off, which can be discomforting for the user and reduces the feeling of presence that we are trying to achieve. Playing with the settings in a professional camera can help limit this. We have found that 3D 360 imaging can help with objects too close to the camera; this takes trial and error to test and may still not fix your issue if too close to the camera.

Lighting: As with standard photography/cinematography, lighting is key. Shooting in the dark requires the lenses to remain open for longer to capture more light. If something is moving, this will blur in the image. The more natural light you can get in your scene, the better the output image. When shooting in a home environment, we tried to make sure that the curtains were all open and we were shooting on a sunny day. We also got creative with lights and lamps, trying to generate as much light in the space as possible. Again, this takes trial and error to get the best effect.

Positioning: As mentioned earlier, you will want your stitch lines on an area of non-interest, trying to keep your focus area in the center of one of the lenses. This cannot always be helped, but should be minimized where possible.

Test shoot: Whenever possible, you should always do a test shoot before filming the real thing. This gives you a chance to practice with the equipment and make sure that everything is ready and working before filming the real event. This is also an opportunity to see where your stitch lines are and how well the finished image has coped with the stitching. The test shoot is not just about taking a few practice shots but also about preparing yourself for the actual shoot, trying to identify challenges, and ensuring a successful day for all involved.

Audio: This is just as important as anything else in 360-cinematography. When filming a video with a professional-grade camera, you will need to be mindful of the cameras built in fans. The Insta360 Pro cameras have a setting to disable the camera's fans for periods of up to 15 minutes. If the fans are not turned off during audio capture, the resulting audio may be rendered unusable due to the noise interference. Using an external microphone may not be enough if the fans are still active, depending on the location of the microphone and the environment you are shooting in. This is part of why test shooting is so important, and you should check the quality of the audio in your test shoot.

Multiple takes: Always get multiple takes. When possible, stitch and review footage between takes. You may find a problem in the final product that you can put right in another take.

Transition takes: If shooting a video, and you want to phase someone into the shot, for example, to introduce students to a new environment, such as a surgical theatre, shoot an empty scene first, then have the person get into position, and film their part. This is all done in one continuous take. Later, when you stitch the footage, you can use standard video editing software like Premiere Pro to cut the empty scene and transition to the scene with the person of interest. By filming in a continuous shoot, you ensure continuity within the stitched footage. Each time the software stitches separate shoots, it will create slightly different images. So shooting an empty scene as one take and then trying to transition to that from another take, with cause a noticeable change in the image for the user, which can be very disturbing and uncomfortable for the user and is avoidable. This effect will make it appear as though the person of interest has appeared from nowhere, as a ghost becoming more solid (depending on how you transition) as time goes on. You can do the reverse at the end when they have finished talking.

Hardware: The hardware for consideration is the PC you are stitching the 360-content in. You will need a high-spec PC (depending on the 360-camera used—always check the recommended hardware for each camera) with a powerful graphics card, high capacity of RAM, and a solid-state drive for storage to stitch your content. It is better to over-spec your PC than under-spec, as an under-spec PC may not be powerful enough to produce any content for you or could burn out and break if overtasked with stitching high-resolution content.

HMD: The HMD/s that you are viewing your content will determine the resolution of the 360-content you need to produce from your original files. Where possible, we recommend shooting in the highest possible resolution in 2D and 3D. This maximizes the potential quality of what you can produce at a later date, giving you flexibility should you upgrade your headsets and offering potential solutions to stitching problems. When producing content for your headset, you should consider what resolution your HMD can display. The higher the resolution of the content you produce, the more powerful your PC needs to be and the longer it takes to produce. If your headsets can only display at HD resolution, it is a waste of time to produce 360-content at 8 K resolution, as the headset is unlikely to be able to display anything, as they do not tend to be equipped with the ability to scale the resolution down. It is best to scale the resolution down at the point of stitching or stitch at the highest quality and then scale the resolution of the 360-degree image down to your headset's capacity if you plan to get new higher-resolution headsets in the near future.

Image resolution: The resolution is the number of pixels that make up the 360-degree image in the horizontal and vertical axes. Monoscopic images are most commonly shot in a 2:1 aspect ratio and stereoscopic 1:1. Ideally, the pixel size for 360-degree images should match the display resolution of the headset to ensure the sharpest results. Where possible, we recommend shooting in the highest resolution that you can, even if this is higher than your headset can display. This allows for future upgrades of your HMDs without the need to re-shoot to take full advantage of them.

The Insta360 Titan, like other cameras, is supplied with software that can stitch the image for you. There are extensive guides available from the supplier and videos on YouTube that can teach you how to get the most out of this software. Simply following the instructions can produce some great results. Another widely used independent product is Mistika VR. This is a very powerful piece of software that lets you fine-tune your 360 content. There are guides and reviews online.

The easiest way to implement your 360 content is with a media player in an HMD. The limitation of this is the lack of interaction within the content. To build more complex applications that your viewer can interact with and engage with, you will need to use something like Unity, a game-building platform. There are packages available to help you build 360 tours or interactive content, but they are at an additional cost. Notably, 360 content can be posted on learning platforms like Moodle.

Reflections

The key lessons learned and points for reflection that we wish to impart to the readers are as follows:

1. Demystifying XR Technology
   - *Lesson*: Understanding the basics of XR, including its various forms and terminologies, is crucial. Knowing how VR compares to AR and other forms of XR helps in grasping its unique advantages and limitations.
   - *Reflection*: Consider how a clear understanding of XR fundamentals can influence the effective adoption and application of XR in your educational context.
2. Practical Guidance for Implementation of VR
   - *Lesson*: Practical steps for creating VR content are accessible even for those with limited technical expertise. This includes choosing the right equipment, understanding the importance of resolution, and knowing the key principles of 360-cinematography.
   - *Reflection*: Reflect on how you can start small VR projects in your own teaching environment and gradually build up your technical skills and resources.
3. Enhancing Learning Through Immersive Environments
   - *Lesson*: XR can create authentic learning environments that mirror real-world scenarios, enhancing students' understanding and preparing them for their future roles in healthcare. This immersive learning can significantly improve engagement and retention of knowledge.
   - *Reflection*: Think about where immersive XR environments can be integrated into your curriculum to compliment students' learning with a more engaging and realistic experience.
4. Interprofessional Collaboration
   - *Lesson*: XR can facilitate interprofessional dialogue and collaboration by allowing students from various health professions to engage in shared, complex patient safety scenarios.
   - *Reflection*: Reflect on the potential benefits of interprofessional learning in your context and how XR can be a tool to foster better teamwork and communication among different healthcare disciplines.
5. Future Trends and AI Integration
   - *Lesson*: The integration of AI with XR technologies promises to enhance personalized and adaptive learning experiences, providing intelligent feedback and dynamically adjusting to learners' needs.

- *Reflection*: Consider the future possibilities of AI-enhanced XR in education and how staying informed about these trends can prepare you for upcoming innovations in teaching.

6. Challenges and Ethical Considerations
   - *Lesson*: Implementing XR comes with challenges, including accessibility, user comfort, and ethical concerns related to data privacy. It is essential to address these challenges thoughtfully.
   - *Reflection*: Reflect on the ethical implications of using XR in education, such as data security and ensuring equitable access to technology for all students. Make sure that you understand what data is being collected from the equipment you are using, for example, is a company collecting data from your headsets about the user that you are not aware of?
7. Case Studies and Personal Experiences
   - *Lesson*: Drawing on a range of sources, including case studies and personal experiences, can provide valuable insights into the practical application and impact of XR in healthcare education.
   - *Reflection*: Reflect on how case studies and real-world examples can inform your approach to integrating XR into your educational practices.
8. Innovative Approaches to Teaching
   - *Lesson*: VR and XR technologies offer innovative approaches to traditional teaching methods, providing new ways to engage students and enhance their learning experiences.
   - *Reflection*: Think about how you can innovate your teaching methods by incorporating VR, and what specific areas of your curriculum could benefit the most from such technological advancements.

References

1. Buring SM, Bhushan A, Broeseker A, Conway S, Duncan-Hewitt W, Hansen L, Westberg S. Interprofessional education: definitions, student competencies, and guidelines for implementation. Am J Pharm Educ. 2009;73(4):59. https://doi.org/10.5688/aj730459.
2. Canadian Interprofessional Health Collaborative. A national interprofessional competency framework. The Collaborative; 2010.
3. Choi J, Thompson CE, Choi J, Waddill CB, Choi S. Effectiveness of immersive virtual reality in nursing education: systematic review. Nurse Educ. 2022;47(3):E57–61. https://doi.org/10.1097/NNE.0000000000001117.
4. Cieslowski B, Haas T, Kyeung Mi O, Chang K, Oetjen CA. The development and pilot testing of immersive virtual reality simulation training for prelicensure nursing students: a quasi-experimental study. Clin Simul Nurs. 2023;77:6–12.
5. Cook M, Lischer-Katz Z, Hall N, Hardesty J, Johnson J, McDonald R, Carlisle T. Challenges and Strategies for Educational Virtual Reality: Results of an Expert-led Forum on 3D/VR Technologies Across Academic Institutions. Information Technology and Libraries. 2019;38(4):25–48. https://doi.org/10.6017/ital.v38i4.11075.
6. Grassini S, Laumann K, Rasmussen Skogstad M. The use of virtual reality alone does not promote training performance (but sense of presence does). Front Psychol. 2020;11:1743. https://doi.org/10.3389/fpsyg.2020.01743.

7. Hamilton D, McKechnie J, Edgerton E. et al. Immersive virtual reality as a pedagogical tool in education: a systematic literature review of quantitative learning outcomes and experimental design. J. Comput. Educ. 2021;8:1–32. https://doi.org/10.1007/s40692-020-00169-2.
8. Kyaw BM, Saxena N, Posadzki P, Vseteckova J, Nikolaou CK, George PP, Divakar U, Masiello I, Kononowicz AA, Zary N, Tudor Car L. Virtual Reality for Health Professions Education: Systematic Review and Meta-Analysis by the Digital Health Education Collaboration. Journal of Medical Internet Research. 2019;21(1):e12959. https://doi.org/10.2196/12959.
9. Liaw SY, Soh SL, Tan KK, Wu LT, Yap J, Chow YL, Lau TC, Lim WS, Tan SC, Choo H, Wong LL, Lim SM, Ignacio J, Wong LF. Design and evaluation of a 3D virtual environment for collaborative learning in interprofessional team care delivery. Nurse Educ Today. 2019;81:64–71. https://doi.org/10.1016/j.nedt.2019.06.012.
10. Mistry D, Brock CA, Lindsey T. The present and future of virtual reality in medical education: a narrative review. Cureus. 2023;15(12):e51124. https://doi.org/10.7759/cureus.51124.
11. Oxford University Press. Virtual reality. In: Oxford English Dictionary. 2024. https://www.oed.com.
12. Pottle J. Virtual reality and the transformation of medical education. Future Healthcare Journal. 2019;6(3):181–185. https://doi.org/10.7861/fhj.2019-0036.
13. Radianti J, Majchrzak TA, Fromm J, Wohlgenannt I. A systematic review of immersive virtual reality applications for higher education: Design elements, lessons learned, and research agenda. Computers and Education. 2020;147, Article 103778. https://doi.org/10.1016/j.compedu.2019.103778.
14. Roche L, Kittel A, Cunningham I, Rolland C. 360° Video Integration in Teacher Education: A SWOT Analysis. Front. Educ. 2021;6:761176. https://doi.org/10.3389/feduc.2021.761176.
15. Reeves S, Fletcher S, Barr H, Birch I, Boet S, Davies N, McFadyen A, Rivera J, Kitto S. A BEME systematic review of the effects of interprofessional education: BEME Guide No. 39. Med Teach. 2016;38(7):656-68. https://doi.org/10.3109/0142159X.2016.1173663. Epub 2016 May 5.
16. Thistlethwaite J. Interprofessional education: a review of context, learning and the research agenda. Med Educ. 2012;46(1):58-70. https://doi.org/10.1111/j.1365-2923.2011.04143.x. PMID: 22150197.
17. World Health Organization (WHO). Framework for action on interprofessional education & collaborative practice. 2010. https://iris.who.int/bitstream/handle/10665/70185/WHO_HRH_HPN_10.3_eng.pdf?sequence=1.

Paul Dudley is the Head of Clinical Skills for the School of Health and Medical Sciences at City St George's University. He is currently working toward his Master's in Clinical Education from King's College London. Paul has been a technician since 2006 and has been working in Clinical Skills since 2014. Paul is leading on various projects to introduce extended reality, artificial intelligence, and other novel teaching modalities into healthcare education at City St George's University.

Monika Bolliger is a lecturer at the Center of Interprofessional Learning and Practice at the Zurich University of Applied Sciences, Institute of Public Health. She holds a Master of Nursing Science and is currently pursuing her Ph.D. at the Faculty of Medical Sciences, Private University in the Principality of Liechtenstein. With a Certificate of Advanced Studies in Virtual and Augmented Reality, she develops and integrates these technologies into interprofessional teaching and learning formats.

IPE Implementation: Organizing, Sustaining, Governance

Rebecca Maria Knecht
and Magdalena Cerbin-Koczorowska

Introduction

To develop innovation, you need creative ideas and a strategy to bring those ideas to life. Since innovation, by its nature, is something new, you will most likely start something that people do not know and face unknowns yourself. Welcome to the typical starting point for interprofessional education (IPE). This chapter aims to give insights and impulses about which areas to consider, which questions to ask, which answers to seek, and which thoughts to apply to your local and individual setting.

You might be new to IPE or an experienced IPE facilitator. In either case, if you aim to help IPE become more strongly embedded in the culture of your workplace and if you consider yourself a person who will support these changes, take the initiative, or orchestrate the efforts of different people, you are a change agent.

You might be a student who wants to be prepared to work in a diverse team. You might be a person working or teaching in the healthcare sector who wants to provide the next generation with the best tools to care for their patients. You might be

Rebecca Maria Knecht and Magdalena Cerbin-Koczorowska contributed equally to this work.

R. M. Knecht (✉)
Faculty of Medicine, The University of Bonn, Bonn, North Rhine-Westphalia, Germany
e-mail: rebecca.m.knecht@gmail.com

M. Cerbin-Koczorowska
Medical Education, Edinburgh Medical School, The University of Edinburgh, Edinburgh, Scotland, UK
e-mail: mcerbin@ed.ac.uk

A. Xyrichis et al. (eds.), *Building Bridges: A European Perspective on Interprofessional Education, Practice, Policy and Research*,
https://doi.org/10.1007/978-3-032-23222-9_12

working in an educational institution dealing with the quality and development of the study program. You might be part of your institution's leadership, dealing with the challenges of keeping the organization stable and future-oriented. Even though, as readers, you may represent different levels of institutional structure, and the local contexts in which you work may differ, each of you can still catalyze the change management process and help organize, sustain, and govern IPE. Implementing IPE only within a narrow scope of practice might prove effective in the short term, but without being integrated into the broader mechanics of your institution, sustaining IPE and making it part of the curriculum and organization is hard to achieve. Therefore, regardless of where you are now, we encourage you to identify different parts of (inter)institutional structures that affect whether the IPE can be successfully anchored into the organization's culture.

The uniqueness of each educational and local context makes it impossible to give precise recommendations about how to proceed. However, knowing the right questions to ask is far more helpful than trying to apply uniform answers.

Aiming to set up IPE as a stable feature of your institution, including different levels of change, we suggest following the organizational change implementation models (OCMs). In our experience from Poland and Germany, people invest great efforts in creating IPE offers, and many struggle to find the means to sustain them. We feel that part of this struggle is that IPE is often not recognized as needing to be embedded in the institution's mechanisms, but that IPE activities (IPEA) are set up as projects or isolated educational events. OCMs offer insights and strategies that help IPE move beyond the project stage and provide a pathway to organizing, sustaining, and governing IPE long term.

We have combined two popular models to address the need to think of processes and areas in an organization. Within the frame of these models, we present examples of questions that we learned to be helpful when implementing IPE. We supported the content of this chapter with our experiences in two different institutions, namely, Poznan University of Medical Sciences (PUMS) (Poland) and the Faculty of Medicine of the University of Bonn (Germany), to outline the practical dimension of the described topic in two different settings.

Organizational Change Models

To address the uniqueness of local settings and the complexity of both healthcare and higher education contexts in which IPE is embedded, we find the change management perspective a valuable framework for guiding the decision-making process so that the IPE implementation becomes meaningful and a time-lasting change.

The literature offers many models, some of which highlight the areas, while others focus on phases of organizational change. We combine two of those to acknowledge the value of both approaches and highlight the necessity of implying a broader institutional and long-term perspective for change implementation.

McKinsey 7-S Model

The McKinsey 7-S Framework or Model (see Fig. 1) comprises seven factors or areas of an organization that are non-hierarchical and interconnected around the focal point of shared values [1, 2]. The framework reflects the complexity of organizational functioning, as it depends on all areas and their interaction, as well as the individuality of each organization, as the areas and how they relate to one another may differ [3]. This fits the situation of IPE: different approaches may lead to different developments, depending on the unique local factors of the professions and institutions involved.

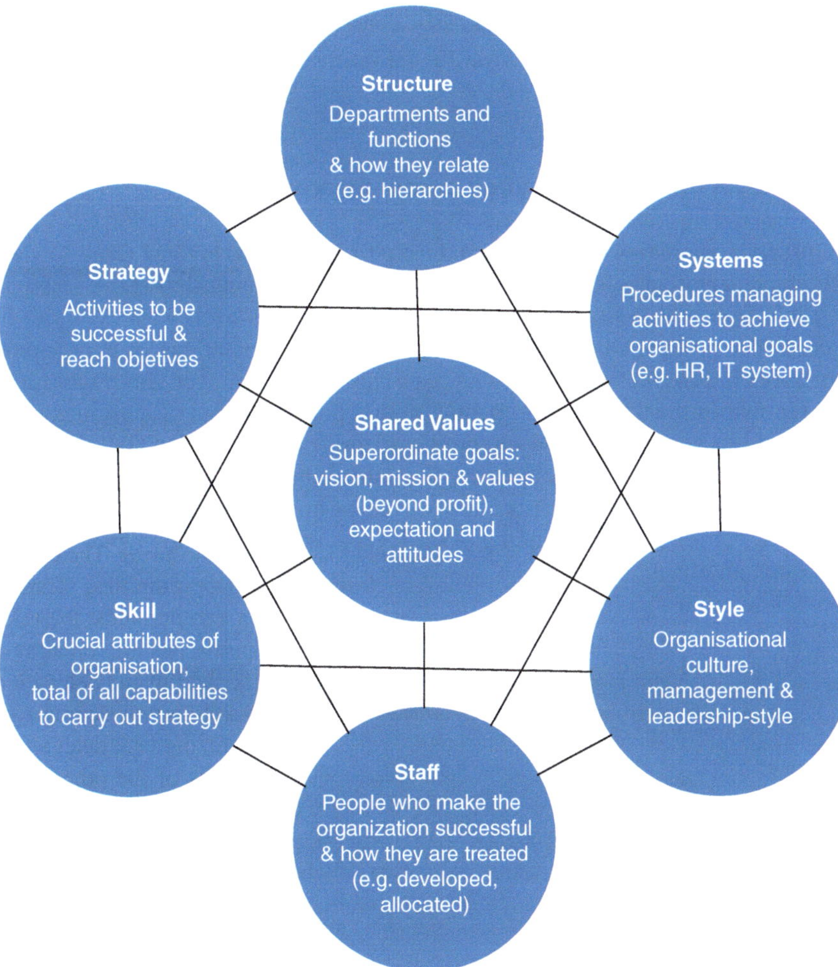

Fig. 1 Overview McKinsey 7-S Model (based on [1])

Bullock and Batten Four-Phase Model

The Bullock and Batten four-phase model (see Fig. 2) illustrates the continuity of the change process with subsequent phases that often interlink with one another [4]. The important value of this model is that it emphasizes the importance of *exploration* as a springboard for following phases, allowing for clarifying the current state, identifying needs, and leading to a more accurate diagnosis in the second phase. The *planning* phase includes generating ideas on how to achieve a previously defined goal, which, when verified, can form the action plan. Then, finally, the intervention takes place, and its evaluation is considered an integral part of the *action* undertaken. This evaluation can support both improvements and development, leading to further *integration* within the organization, visible through expanding the scope of existing activities, changing their status within the organization, or initiating further activities at different institutional levels.

Multi-Level Integrated Change Model Approach

We propose combining both OCMs and including the organizational levels to view IPE implementation as a holistic organizational change approach (Fig. 3).

Table 1 presents a short definition of the institutional levels with examples of stakeholder groups. Due to the varying nature and denotations of educational structures in different countries, this list is not exhaustive, yet you might identify the institutional level you operate on and possible types of activities most likely within your reach. You might also identify change agents and decision-makers at other levels in your setting. Establishing collaboration with others, within and outside of our institutions, was most important throughout our journeys, and getting an understanding of the levels of change and their stakeholders was quite an effort.

Exploration	Planning	Action	Integration
Need awareness	Diagnosis	Implementation	Stabilisation
Search	Design	Evaluation	Diffusion
Contracting	Decision		Renewal

Fig. 2 Overview of the Bullock and Battens Four-Phase Model [4]

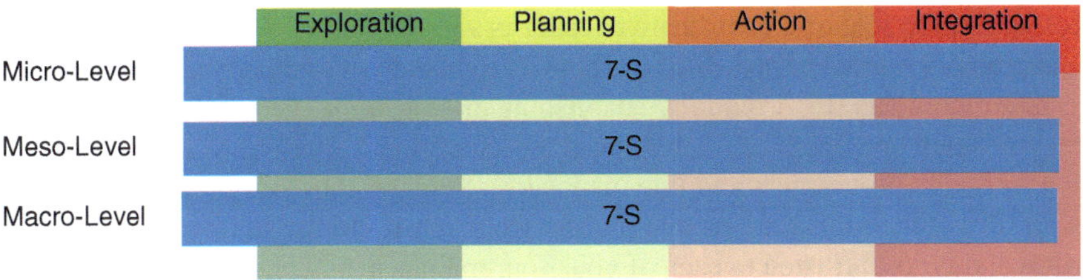

Fig. 3 Multi-level integrated change model approach

Table 1 Levels of IPE implementation and examples of their decision-makers in higher education institutions

Definitions	Examples
Macro-level—Focus on IPE governance, including strategic planning and resource management	Rectorate, University Council[a], Senate[a], Faculty Conference, Teaching and Learning Council[a], University Quality Assurance and Enhancement Committee[a]; Faculty: Deanery/office of deans, faculty councils[a]
Meso-level—Focus on sustaining IPE projects by developing the needed framework conditions	Deans, Program Curriculum Committees[a] and developers, Study Advisory Boards[a], Faculty Quality Assurance and Enhancement Committees[a], examining boards
Micro-level—Focus on organizing single IPE interventions (e.g., courses/projects)	Course Leads, Heads of the Department/Clinic, Student-Staff Liaison Board[a]

[a]Including student representatives appointed by the student government

Levels of IPE Implementation

While the levels of an institution are interdependent, it is worth recognizing the focus of each level. Therefore, we will present the relevant questions for IPE implementation as a "multi-level integrated change model approach" and examine the individual levels more closely. You can decide where you might be able to find impulses and which questions are most relevant to different stakeholders.

Organizing IPE (Micro-Level)

The micro-level refers to the area of the IPEA. It can be a learning experience or a social event established as part of a formal curriculum, an extracurricular, or a corporate activity. The main concerns at this level are how to design, organize, and establish an IPEA long term. Due to the multitude and complexity of interactions between students, different teachers and/or project workers, and potential sources of resources, the role of a coordinative leader is very important. If you operate in this area, the key questions presented in Table 2 might aid your implementation strategy.

Developing an IPEA requires establishing *Shared Values* across the broader context in which you operate. You will need the support and approval of different stakeholders (e.g., co-teachers and line managers). Some of those might not be familiar with IPE, or their motivations might differ from yours, often resulting from different roles and tasks entrusted to each of you. Your main task as a change agent would be to explore and identify similarities and synergies of those motivations to pave the way for a successful IPEA.

For example, when the first IPE course was implemented at PUMS, dated 2011/12 academic year, IPE was not recognized as a direction for strategic development. However, like many other higher education institutions in Poland, PUMS's priorities at that time were largely focused on research projects. Aligning the *Strategy* and goals for organizing IPE with these motivations allowed for building a common interest with key decision-makers, resulting in the launching of an IPEA-based Ph.D. project [5].

Making data-informed decisions about your strategy requires understanding the sheer number and origin of different stakeholders needing to be involved on various levels. A RASCI Matrix[1] can guide your exploration and planning for the *Structure* area. The role of students and staff should not be undervalued in this analysis. In PUMS, all initially launched IPEAs were available on a "first-come, first-served" basis, resulting in limited participation opportunities. High-student satisfaction scores for existing IPEAs resulted in student representatives requesting equal opportunities and access to IPEAs for all students. In 2018, while building an interprofessional training ward (IPE Ward) in pediatric cardiology at the University Hospital Bonn, ward staff not directly involved in the IPEA provided crucial feedback in all structure-related implementation phases. Another important party is the people in the IPEA and how you work together (*style*). In the IPE Ward, we emphasized the value of all perspectives and made decisions as a team. Project workers, surrounding staff, and students emerged as important stakeholders, and their strong support was an important factor in bringing IPE to the *meso-level*.

Organizing an IPEA often requires collaborating with external partners, so differences in educational and organizational *Systems* will become apparent. While building the IPE Ward in Bonn for final-year students of human medicine (HM) and

[1] The RASCI Matrix is a project management and decision-making tool used to define and clarify roles and responsibilities within a project or process. It is an extension of the RACI matrix and stands for:

- R—Responsible: The person(s) responsible for completing the task or making sure that it gets done.
- A—Accountable: The person ultimately accountable for the task's success and final approval.
- S—Supportive: The person(s) who provide resources, assistance, or expertise to help complete the task.
- C—Consulted: The person(s) who need to be consulted for input before the task is completed.
- I—Informed: The person(s) who need to be kept informed of progress or decisions but are not directly involved.

Table 2 Key questions for different stages of *organizing IPE* in relation to key areas.

	Exploration	Planning	Action	Integration
Shared value	Why do you think it is worth organizing IPEA? What are the motivations of your interprofessional partners? What are your common values and beliefs?	How can you present those values so they will be shared with key stakeholders? How can you introduce IPEA implementation in a way that can be valued by key decision-makers to gain approval?	How do you visibly incorporate the common values in your project? Have you reached shared values (e.g., regarding students' engagement)?	How will you communicate the benefits of your IPEA to other community members?
Strategy	Are other IPEAs already being implemented in your institution? Do you have to build a partnership with others outside of your institution? What resources are needed/given?	What goals do you set for this IPEA? How will your IPEA be placed in the wider curriculum? How to plan for challenges (e.g., Strengths, Weknesses, Opportunities, Threats (SWOT) analysis)?	How do you communicate IPEA'S goals and milestones? Was this IPEA successful? What changes will you consider for the future? How did different stakeholders receive the process?	What do you have to do to anchor the IPEA in the curricula? Is there a need to bring IPE to the meso-level (e.g., need for resources)?
Structure	Who are the different stakeholders? Who are the key decision-makers at this stage of implementation? Whose approval and support are needed?	How well informed and involved should the different stakeholders be (regarding different times and tasks)?	Which tasks do different stakeholders have in the action stage? Are supporting departments activated (you do not need to do everything on your own)? Who can provide meaningful feedback on different stages of the process?	Which existing programs/ initiatives can your project connect with? Who can support you in sharing positive IPEA experiences suitably with different stakeholders?

(continued)

Table 2 (continued)

	Exploration	Planning	Action	Integration
Systems	What systems/procedures exist that can facilitate or hinder the organization of IPEA (e.g., virtual learning environment)? How do the systems between educational programs/institutions differ?	Which systems will you use to organize your IPE? Can you access/use the systems, or do you need support?	Have all systems been activated? How supportive were those systems for organizing your intervention?	What kind of follow-up should be done to meet institutional requirements (quality report, student survey, etc.)?
Style	How do you consider yourself as a change agent? What strengths can you build upon?	How will you get other people on board? How will you demonstrate interprofessional leadership and teamwork (e.g., by embracing diversity)?	How do you make decisions in your interprofessional team regarding the IPEA?	How can you positively influence the continuation of received support?
Staff	Who can deliver the intervention? Will you be able to build an interprofessional teaching team? What about the administrative staff?	How will employment be arranged for the IPEA? Can you invite IPE-experienced teachers to join your initiative?	How do you acknowledge the input of different people? How did teachers experience their roles?	Can you count on the same teachers to continue to be in the project? Will it be beneficial to invite other teachers to your IPEA next time? What key decision-makers (meso-level) could support both scenarios?

(continued)

Table 2 (continued)

	Exploration	Planning	Action	Integration
Skills	What type of skills will be needed to deliver IPE? What skills will the learners need/have? Will you need further training for yourself and your team?	When and how can skill development be included in the built-up of the IPEA? How could visiting already established IPEA be arranged?	Do you have the skills to react to possible IPE-challenges? How do you reflect as a team on project processes and outcomes?	How can you promote knowledge and experience exchange with others? How can know-how be secured and transferred to the next project phase or to new staff?

nursing, the simple exploring question "When will the two learner groups be present in our area of interest?" taught us about differences in the mechanics and timelines of the clinical placement systems and delivered a lesson in problem-solving and flexibility. In nursing vocational education, the students' clinical placements are scheduled at the beginning of their program (i.e., years in advance). Final-year HM students choose if they want to have a clinical placement in pediatrics and where it should be (locally, nationally, or internationally), and the clinical departments will be informed 4 weeks before placement. These system differences posed fundamental challenges to our IPEA (i.e., presence of interprofessional learners, reliable organization, and resource management) and simultaneously stimulated its development. We devised measures, such as 1) forming an information and advertisement strategy to raise awareness and interest in participating and 2) creating a teaching design for interprofessional tandems, trios, and quartets to be flexible when dealing with varying numbers of learners. Both measures helped to manage risks and strengthen our IPEA—after a short while, we had more applications than we could accept, and if numbers fluctuated due to any reason (e.g., illness), we were confident to deal with it. It is noteworthy to say that since then, the educational systems and structures have changed, making it necessary to revisit this challenge today.

Being open to revisiting your IPEA, for example, to optimize the use of resources and address changing needs, is important. For example, the course lead of the Ph.D.-IPEA decided to close the course and transfer the developed resources to a new project designed and delivered in collaboration with medical communication and simulation experts [6] to work toward IPE diversity (*style*). Thanks to the involvement of many teachers, representing different scopes of expertise (*skills*), the new IPEA was improved by using innovative simulation methods and being open to a broader audience of learners.

Most people who invest in an IPEA hope to run their project more than once. Working toward IPE *Integration* means the changes shall become stabilized and sustainable by embedding them in the organization's mechanisms and culture, thus requiring support at other organizational levels. Different areas of your change can be considered for this purpose. You can focus on *Shared values* and *Structure* when considering which aspects of IPEA's design, delivery, and evaluation should be communicated, to whom, and how. If working in a research-focused institution, you might look at your IPEA through the lens of a research project and share the IPEA's description and its impact through publications and conference presentations [7, 8]. Focusing on *Staff*, securing future involvement, and acknowledging their input, for example, by presenting their achievements online [6, 9], are measures facilitating integration and bridging to the *meso-level*.

Sustaining IPE (Meso-Level)

Moving IPE to the *meso-level* requires broadening the focus from the IPEA itself (*micro-level*) to include necessary framework conditions, for example, curricular integration, long-term resources, and quality management (see Table 3). The lack of these can significantly affect the persistence of the IPEAs established so far and hinder further development [10]. Our experiences show that working toward this development requires particular attention to human resources, including Change Agents' broader impact.

A measure that addresses human resources and many areas of organizational change is an extensive faculty development program or system that considers training content and courses, as well as providing structures for collaboration and exchange of faculty members. It is necessary to ensure IPE quality standards, unite IPE facilitators, and benefit the staff in their (professional) development.

While leading the development of the first IPE Ward in Bonn at the micro-level, Rebecca Maria Knechts responsibilities included conducting highly individualized train-the-trainer events with a small number of participants, tailored specifically to the needs of the IPEA. These training sessions aimed to prepare trainers for their roles, facilitate the formation of interprofessional teams, and contribute to the overall design of IPEA. However, they did not contribute to the participants' official qualification or credential requirements and required significant resources. Currently, as a study developer, the focus is on advising multiple IPEA initiatives and establishing a supportive framework at the meso-level. The goal is to develop a faculty development system that integrates two interconnected approaches: 1) a platform for collaboration and 2) an interprofessional train-the-trainer concept.

When the student deanery in Bonn decided to fund IP courses, they included the creation of a network (*structure*) in their strategic funding plans. We founded the "Network of IPE Bonn," which is open to all people active and interested in IPE. Most members are IPE teachers or project workers (*staff*). The network gives them the opportunity to connect, discuss challenges and solutions, and identify common goals and interests on a broader level (*shared values*). It is a platform not only of knowledge and expertise but also of mutual support and inspiration, a community of practice. Such a dedicated structure acknowledges IPE facilitators' experiences and expertise and supports that their valuable voices can be a noticeable influence on IPE development.

Table 3 Key questions for different stages of *sustaining* IPE in relation to key areas

	Exploration	Planning	Action	Integration
Shared values	Why do you think it is worth sustaining IPE? How do different stakeholders value IPE and framework conditions (e.g., institution's strategy and faculty development)?	How can you present those values so they will be shared with different stakeholders and key decision-makers (e.g., student government)?	Have you identified additional groups of interest (e.g., patient organizations, political societies) that share and support the values of IPE?	How will you communicate the benefits of the IPE framework conditions to other community members?
Strategy	Is IPE reflected in your institution's strategy (e.g., formulated goals and action plans)? Are there regulations for using resources necessary for IPE collaboratively (different institutions/ departments)? What can you learn from previous IPEAs regarding sustainability?	Can you identify priorities regarding success factors for developing quality IPE? How does IPE impact the wider curricula?	How do you want to present the impact of the utilized resources? How did different stakeholders receive the new framework and its implementation process?	Which resources are needed and can be secured in the long term? Which resources need to be limited to secure longevity? Is there a need to bring IPE to the *macro-level* (e.g., for long-term resource management between different institutions)?
Structure	Who are the key decision-makers at this stage of implementation? Whose approval is needed to allow you to move forward?	How will different departments be involved in developing supportive framework conditions for IPE (e.g., evaluation and financial management)? Will you need more/different structures?	Was the role distribution between departments clear and efficient? Will feedback formats need to differ regarding roles/departments?	How to anchor framework factors in the different organizational structures? How to get an understanding of the macro-levels of different professions (e.g., organigrams)?

(continued)

Table 3 (continued)

	Exploration	Planning	Action	Integration
Systems	What systems and procedures (e.g., based on technologization levels or labor laws) exist that can facilitate or hinder an IPE framework?	Which systems will your IPE framework rely on? How to manage access and use of the systems for different stakeholders? How could additional procedures be created (e.g., workflows and guidelines)?	How have procedures and systems impacted the IPE framework? Did new systems meet resistance? Do you identify a need for adjustments?	What kind of follow-up should be done to meet institutional requirements? What system changes are needed for the long term? How do you transport those observations to the macro-level?
Style	What is your role, and by whom has its legitimacy been defined? Are you tasked by all involved institutions? How do you consider yourself as a change agent? What strengths can you build upon?	How will you motivate and support current leaders so they will adopt the IPE frameworks and work together? How will you promote and utilize the organizational culture for the IPE framework conditions?	How was your role received by different stakeholders (micro, meso, macro), and why? How and by whom were other leaders and supporters appreciated?	How can leadership's awareness of IPE efforts be promoted? What kind of powerful coalitions will allow you to get involved at the macro-level to integrate IPE frameworks in the organizational culture?
Staff	Is there existing space for collaboration between people involved in IPE? How are relevant staff factors (e.g., motivation, rewards, and selection) set up?	Can you promote collaboration and networking within and outside the institution? How does IPE engagement benefit staff's career goals (e.g., promotion criteria, job satisfaction) and thus support staff retention?	How is staff experience (e.g., with collaborative processes) evaluated and utilized for adjustments? How are the efforts of staff acknowledged?	How can networking and collaboration opportunities be formalized and stabilized? How can the implications of staff satisfaction in IPE be communicated to the *macro-level*? How can the *macro-level* support staff retention?

(continued)

Table 3 (continued)

	Exploration	Planning	Action	Integration
Skills	What additional skills do change agents have and need (e.g., corporate skills) to build IPE frameworks? What sort of faculty development programs (content/format) need to be available for IPE implementation?	How have you considered a needs assessment? How will identified qualification gaps be addressed? How is access to faculty development programs arranged between different institutions?	How would you evaluate skill development and its benefit for IPE?	How can institutional support ensure the ongoing skill development of staff in IPE?

For the second approach, the circumstances of people tasked with teaching (*staff*) and regulations regarding teaching qualifications (*systems and skills*) were explored, as they differ immensely among the educational systems of health professions in Germany. For example, in vocational nursing education, people teaching practical skills must complete special training (300 h) in vocational pedagogy and yearly further training (24 h) [11]. In HM, most people teaching clinical skills are practising physicians, and there is no formal obligation for further qualification in education. There are, however, some efforts in Germany to develop qualification standards and requirements for HM education [12–14]. Currently, we plan how to best comply with these requirements and design a sustainable and resource-conscious format that benefits IPE quality, as well as the IPE teachers (personally and formally, e.g., qualification portfolio).

At PUMS, the increasing number of IPE initiatives [6] highlighted the need to integrate them into the obligatory curricula to ensure recognition and sustainability. This shift necessitated a transition from Magdalena Cerbin-Koczorowskas role of IPE facilitator to that of an IPE ambassador (*style*). Key strengths that supported this transition included an M.Sc. degree in Clinical Education [15] and previous experience as Faculty Development Lead, which provided expertise in curriculum development and change management, legitimizing involvement in curriculum transformation. In collaboration with a university-wide team representing various areas of expertise, the PUMS Guidelines for designing and redesigning undergraduate curricula were developed [16], establishing an action framework for Program Curriculum Committees (*systems*). Membership in several of these committees (*structure*) provided opportunities to offer additional support and guidance for the practical implementation of these guidelines. As a result, long-term resource allocation was secured, embedding obligatory IPE courses into multiple curricula across PUMS.

Notably, the abovementioned involvement took place many years before the complete, sustainable IPE implementation at PUMS. The success of the first obligatory course, launched in 2023 and addressing approximately 600 students representing four professions yearly, was possible only thanks to the extraordinary *Staff* involvement and cooperation of many leaders of other IPEA united around *Shared values* and led by a different Change Agent [6].

Experiences from both institutions show that IPE implementation often enters a higher institutional level, accompanied by the role progression of a change agent. Therefore, we strongly encourage you to reflect on how you perceive yourself in this role, including your *Skills* and *Style*.

In conclusion, the implementation of change necessitates both the addition of new human resources and the continuous development of the existing workforce. This can be done through training, support systems, or acknowledgement, to name a few. Some approaches can be followed at the *meso-level*, while others require strategic decision-making and consistent institution-wide solutions, thus the *macro-level's* involvement.

IPE Governance (Macro-Level)

IPE governance, or macro-level, refers to steering IPE-related activities to 1) align and integrate IPE within the operational goals, 2) monitor quality systems, and 3) set directions for development. Table 4 presents examples of key questions that might benefit these purposes.

This level of decision-making (*strategy*) involves the bigger picture of healthcare education, often directly related to (federal) state laws and political developments. In the face of the healthcare workforce crisis, some countries are challenging the effectiveness and validity of the current educational approach. By developing IPE-dedicated structures and policies, they attempt to create an environment conducive to systemic changes in healthcare professions [17, 18]. Although currently, there are no nationwide agreements or regulations in Poland or Germany, IPE is gaining more supporters, and more universities are incorporating IPE into their curricula.

In Germany, in recent years, healthcare education has undergone a series of changes. In 2020, Nursing became a generalist (vocational) education with the option to study at a university. In 2023, Midwifery became an exclusively academic education (formerly vocational). Currently, HM Education is reviewing regulations on licensing physicians, causing faculties to alter their study programs. As part of these changes, the importance of interprofessional teamwork in providing holistic care and ensuring patient safety has been highlighted. However, the extent to which IPE is mentioned as an obligatory part of preparing healthcare students for interprofessional teamwork varies greatly within these regulations [19, 20].

In Poland, some governmental attempts were made to standardize IPE implementation at medical universities, but many of those institutions reacted with hesitancy and resistance. This could result not only from the fact that the proposed solution was based on proposals coming from only one of a dozen medical schools, without acknowledging the experiences of others, but also from the abruptness of the proposed changes, with a simultaneous high level of detail in the expectations set, threatening their independence in the area of curriculum design and delivery.

Table 4 Key questions for different stages of *governing* IPE in relation to key areas

	Exploration	Planning	Action	Integration
Shared values	Why is it worth integrating IPE into your institution's organizational culture? How are IPEs meaningful in your local, national, and international context? What attitudes can you identify at different levels of your institution(s)?	How can IPE support your institution's vision and mission? What actions can be taken to embed IPE values across your institution? How can you capture those shared values to promote building the community of practice for IPE?	What different perspectives of interprofessional partners did you become aware of? How effective was building the community of practice around IPE?	How will you communicate your approach to IPE to the wider community and civil society? How can you present the developments as part of the institution's image and profile?
Strategy	How do education-policy views and demands for IPE influence your strategy? Where does your institution stand in the scope of the (inter)national IPE development? What are the benefits and challenges resulting from your institution's level of IPE experience and from (not) being a pioneer in this field?	What operational goals for IPE implementation fit different areas of your IS (e.g., research, clinical work)? How will you arrange the quality assurance and enhancement (e.g., standards of excellence)? What kind of strategic partnership facilitates reaching operational goals and securing resources?	Do you have enough data to monitor progress and quality? How do different actions taken so far affect your KPIs? How can the interprofessional partnerships be maintained during the developments?	How can you support and synchronize *meso-* and *micro-levels* initiatives through strategic interventions and/or solutions? Does the current approach toward IPE allow your organization to develop in this area?

(continued)

Table 4 (continued)

	Exploration	Planning	Action	Integration
Structure	Who are IPE change agents at different levels of your organization? How are different departments currently involved in IPE? How are they collaborating with each other?	How will you allocate and communicate IPE-related authorities and responsibilities across institution(s), departments, and individuals? How can you ensure appropriate communication across different parties involved in IPE?	Were roles, responsibilities, tasks, and goals assigned and communicated clearly and appropriately? Are all areas of IPE implementation covered within the existing structure? Does the communication across different parties allow for effective delivery and management?	How can you optimize the structure to allow for IPE development and quality assurance (e.g., organigram)?
Systems	Do current systems and procedures meet the needs of IPE complexity? Which systems must be addressed and when (e.g., on boards and councils)?	How will you identify and draw standard operating procedures related to IPE? How will you gather evaluation data (e.g., financial control, enrolment) to monitor sustainability, quality, and progress?	Do any systems or procedures require updates to ensure high-quality service delivery? When dealing with interwoven systems, are workflows, offers, and demands clear?	How can you optimize systems to ease IPE delivery and quality assurance (e.g., workflows)? What systems must be involved in the next phase (e.g., boards and councils)?
Style	How have different leaders dealt with IPE implementation so far? How do you consider your role and strengths as a change agent here (e.g., transactional vs. transformational)?	What leadership skills would you need across the institution? How will you ensure current leaders will get on board and be willing to work together?	How do unwritten rules/code of conduct influence the IPE development (e.g., reciprocal exchanges)?	How do you see IPE and its organizational changes as part of your organizational culture now and in the future?

(continued)

Table 4 (continued)

	Exploration	Planning	Action	Integration
Staff	What staffing situation is needed for your IPE goals?	Do you need to hire or train key staff and support or change staffing structures?	How have appreciation and motivation mechanisms (e.g., recognition, and awards) affected staff involvement in IPE initiatives?	How can the involvement of key staff be managed long term? (e.g., career opportunities)
Skills	Which part of the skillset needed for IPE implementation does your current staff (qualifications and positions) cover?	How can the skillset be covered in-house vs. outsourcing in the short and long term?	Have you identified crucial skills that still need to be built to face new demands (e.g., for new teaching formats like eLearning)?	How do new crucial skills impact further areas, for example, structures and procedures in your institution?

This situation shows the importance of exploring prior achievements, *Strategy* and *Style*, and thus laying the foundation for *Shared Values* as a driving force for change implementation in governing IPE.

Due to the lack of national consensus, individual institutions in both countries face and master IPE implementation challenges independently, thus building a strong sense of ownership. These experiences might be applied to your institution if you plan to set a coherent policy and direction for IPE implementation (strategy), maybe even in collaboration with different institutions that may have their own varying set of external requirements, systems, and resources.

Working toward change in large institutions often depends on its alignment with their mission, vision, and strategic goals, all stated in the Institutional *Strategy* (IS). Although implementing IPE may not become a strategic goal itself, linking it with different areas of your IS is a milestone for IPE governance, as resource allocation and management will most likely reflect the directions adopted within the IS. In PUMS, "Increasing the number of IPE classes" was stated within its *Development Strategy for the years 2021–2030* [21] as an operational goal supporting the broader strategic goal of readying medical staff to serve national and world health. Although many factors described in the 7s model are not yet fully adapted to the needs of IPE, adding IPE to the PUMS's IS is believed to make securing resources for dedicated work easier in the coming years.

Notably, some of the changes and decisions made by PUMS authorities benefiting IPE governance were not initiated by IPE implementation itself. For example, due to the increasing professionalization of different areas of education at PUMS, many academics decided to give up their research careers and concentrate their efforts on innovative teaching projects. This movement forced the development of a distinct, teaching-centered career path aimed at providing educational leaders (including those involved in IPE) with suitable development and career progression opportunities, promoting *staff* satisfaction and retention enhancement.

Another important aspect of IPE governance is the presence of IPE Change Agents in decision-making *structures* (e.g., Senate or Teaching and Learning Council). Their awareness of the institution's systems and planned changes enables them to lobby (*style*) for IPE needs to be appropriately addressed.

Operating at the macro-level will require demonstrating the progress toward your operational goals, with key performance indicators (KPIs) as a measure of performance over time (*strategy*). Within the PUMS IS, we referred to the number of IPE classes, but other KPIs can suit your strategy more. For example, IPE development at PUMS can be viewed through the increase in the number of publications on IPE and related topics from 5 before the year 2010 to approximately 60 by May 2024, including 4 Ph.D. dissertations [22]. Progress in the quality of IPEA can also be monitored through changes in IPEAs' student evaluation results (*systems*); *staff* engagement can be observed by the number of teachers who completed IPE training and/or joined the network. In Bonn, the student deanery recognized the importance of such indicators, for example, arranging measures to raise the number of IPE classes by starting with a lighthouse project (IPE Ward) and then developing a funding program to raise the number from 1 to 10 within 1 year. While these indicators are considered on the *meso-level*, data-wise governance requires exploring and formalizing these aspects on the *macro-level*.

These examples illustrate how activities operate on the *micro-level*, frame a broader context on the *meso-level*, and cement decisions on the *macro-level*, highlighting the collaborative interactions of all organizational change levels, which may develop from and in several directions (top-down, bottom-up, and countercurrent).

Conclusion

We hope the content of this chapter conveyed the complexity of *"IPE implementation"* and provided you with impulses to help conduct structured actions at individual stages of your journey. Recent research [17, 23] delves deeper into multi-level organizational change and its role for IPE, confirming our belief in the need not only to perceive a broader perspective but also to recognize the specificity of a particular setting. We are looking forward to future findings and guidelines for implementing IPE.

While we acknowledge a lack of a "one-fits-all" approach to implementing IPE, we would like to direct your particular attention to three convictions we gained in our multi-national and interprofessional experience writing this chapter: First, your role as a change agent is crucial. Without their advocates, IPEAs can become fragile and easily replaceable, so devote as much attention to preparing yourself for this journey as you do to prepare IPE implementation. Second, IPE is never a one-person show, so take care to build and acknowledge your wider community, which will allow you to operate successfully and enjoyably. Finally, be patient. Implementing a lasting change is not a project for days or weeks. It requires consistency, adaptability to unforeseen circumstances, and often compromises. However, we strongly believe that by staying on course and skillfully maneuvering through the meanders of IPE complexity, together with your travel companions, you will be able to look with satisfaction at the effects of the change that you will be the authors of.

Building bridges highlights the idea that we can breach gaps and build something lasting and path-breaking in connection and collaboration with others. As two strangers from two different nations who independently strived for IPE, we have connected our experiences through this writing process and found many similarities and inspirations. We leave this experience understanding more of the IPE perspective and feeling great excitement for the future of IPE. Stay connected and build your bridges.

References

1. Waterman RH, Peters TJ, Phillips JR. Structure is not organisation. Bus Horiz. 1980;23(3):14–26. https://doi.org/10.1016/0007-6813(80)90027-0
2. Chmielewska M, Stokwiszewski J, Markowska J, Hermanowski T. Evaluating organizational performance of public hospitals using the McKinsey 7-S framework. BMC Health Serv Res. 2022;22(1):7.
3. Malan A. Applying McKinsey's 7s model within managed healthcare systems (MHS) to assess the organisation's effectiveness and ability to adapt. Rand Afrikaans University; 2003.
4. Bullock RJ, Batten D. It's just a phase we're going through: a review and synthesis of OD phase analysis. Group Organ Stud. 1985;10(4):383–412.
5. Cerbin-Koczorowska M. The development of an educational tool designed to promote pharmacist-physician cooperation and foster pharmaceutical care implementation in Poland. Poznan University of Medical Sciences; 2016.
6. PUMS. Interprofessional Education Initiatives at Poznan University of Medical Sciences. PUMS; 2024. Available from: https://ipe.ump.edu.pl/inicjatywyinterprofesjonalne.
7. Cerbin-Koczorowska M, Skowron A. Edukacja interprofesjonalna szansą na upowszechnienie współpracy pomiędzy lekarzem i farmaceutą. Farm Pol. 2017;73(6):389–96. Available from: https://ptfarm.pl/en/wydawnictwa/czasopisma/farmacja-polska/103/-/27027.
8. Cerbin-Koczorowska M, Przymuszała P, Michalak M, Skowron A. Effective interprofessional training can be implemented without high financial expenses—a pre-post study supported with cost analysis. Farmacia. 2022;70(5):976–84.
9. Medical Faculty of the University Bonn. Interprofessional Education Initiatives at the Medical Faculty of the University Bonn. Medical Faculty of the University Bonn; 2024. Available from: https://www.medfak.uni-bonn.de/de/studium-lehre/lehrqualitaet/curriculumsentwicklung/ipl.
10. Beckingsale L, Brown M, McKinlay E, OLeary M, Doolan-Noble F. Sustainable interprofessional education programmes: what influences teachers to stay involved? J Interprof Care. 2023;37(4):637–46.
11. Buzer. Educational and Examination Regulations for Care Professions—Paragraph 4. Buzer; 2020. Available from: https://www.buzer.de/PflAPrV.htm.
12. Program of Medical Didactic Bonn. 2024. Available from: https://www.medfak.uni-bonn.de/de/studium-lehre/lehrqualitaet/didaktik-und-lehre/dot.med.
13. State Academy of Medical Education North Rhine-Westphalia. [LAMA] Certificate of Medical Didactics. Medizin; 2024. Available from: https://www.medizin.hhu.de/lama.

14. Masters of Medical Education. 2024. Available from: http://www.mme-de.net/.
15. University of Edinburgh. Clinical Education Programme overview. 2024. Available from: https://www.ed.ac.uk/medicine-vet-medicine/postgraduate/clinical-education.
16. Uruska A, Cerbin-Koczorowska M, Ciastiowicz-Tomczak I, Majewska N, Marciniak R. Guidelines for developing the curriculum using the SPICES model. UMP; 2020. Available from: https://www.ump.edu.pl/media/uid/dfc510_e5-91ef-4_f-c/c2c2b7.pdf.
17. Thistlethwaite JE, Dunston R, Yassine T. The times are changing: workforce planning, new health-care models and the need for interprofessional education in Australia. J Interprof Care. 2019;33(4):361–8.
18. Yahya M, Dalal A, Eiad AA, Alfaris A, Mohammad H, Ciraj A, et al. In: Alnaami MY, editor. Novel Health Interprofessional Education and Collaborative Practice Program: strategy and implementation. Springer Singapore; 2023.
19. Educational and Examination Regulations for Care Professions—Annex 2. 2020. Available from: https://www.buzer.de/PflAPrV.htm</div>.
20. Educational and Examination Regulations for Midwives. 2020. Available from: https://www.buzer.de/HebStPrV.htm.
21. PUMS. Resolution No. 59/2021 of the Senate of the Poznan University of Medical Sciences regarding the adoption of the UMP Development Strategy for 2021–2030. 59/2021 Mar 31, 2021. https://www.ump.edu.pl/media/uid/cabe36229-_59-8e2_-2/f23e3c.pdf
22. PUMS Library Repository. PUMS employees' bibliography. 2024. Available from: http://150.254.179.40/bazy/publikacje/new/.
23. D'Amour D, Oandasan I. Interprofessionality as the field of interprofessional practice and interprofessional education: an emerging concept. J Interprof Care. 2005;19(SUPPL. 1):8–20.

Rebecca Maria Knecht (M.Sc. Psychology) pursued IPE implementation as study and program developer for IPE at the Medical Faculty of Bonn, Germany, focusing on curricula design, organizational change, and faculty development. She was the project lead of conception and coordination for the first IPE Ward in North Rhine-Westphalia at the University Hospital Bonn and leading founder of the "Network IPE Bonn". As resilience coach and counselor she also focuses on mental and emotional health, embedding them into her project work.

Magdalena Cerbin-Koczorowska (D.Sc., Ph.D., M.Sc. ClinEd, M.A. Psych, FHEA) is the Program Director for Clinical Education at the University of Edinburgh. During her career, she led Interprofessional education (IPE) implementation at Poznan University of Medical Sciences (Poland) and was appointed an expert for medical vocational programs at the Polish Ministry of National Education. Her research area focuses on different aspects of healthcare professionals' education, with a particular interest in IPE and faculty development. She is also a founder of the Teaching Excellence Academy.

Interprofessional Collaboration in Healthcare in Europe: A Case Study and Overview

Heike Wieser and Maria Mischo-Kelling

Introduction

Worldwide healthcare systems still suffer from the impact of the COVID-19 pandemic, as core health indicators such as lower life expectancy or death rates from heart attacks, stroke, or other circulatory diseases show [30]. Cardiovascular diseases are the leading cause of death worldwide, including in Europe [10], followed by cancer. These chronic conditions could be prevented by a healthier lifestyle if current knowledge is applied. One lesson learned by the COVID-19 pandemic is the need to invest in health and prevention. The demand on healthcare systems and the healthcare workforce has increased due to the increasing burden of chronic diseases and the rapid population aging. In light of the realization of the Sustainable Development Goals, healthcare systems must shift their focus from curative approaches to prevention. They should provide a comprehensive range of health services throughout the lifespan, encompassing self-care promotion, disease prevention, curative treatments, rehabilitation, and palliative care [9].

The pace of adaptation and change in current health systems will accelerate due to global challenges such as climate change and related disasters, growing violent conflicts between countries, or due to the trend toward extensive digitalization of all areas of life. All these challenges place different demands on the current and future health workforce. Against this background, there seems to be

H. Wieser (✉)
Claudiana Research, University Center for Health Professions, Bolzano, Italy
e-mail: heike.wieser@claudiana.bz.it

M. Mischo-Kelling
RWU Hochschule Ravensburg-Weingarten, University of Applied Sciences, Weingarten, Germany

A. Xyrichis et al. (eds.), *Building Bridges: A European Perspective on Interprofessional Education, Practice, Policy and Research*,
https://doi.org/10.1007/978-3-032-23222-9_13

an international consensus that interprofessional collaboration (IPC) between different healthcare professions is key to meet the challenges of current and future healthcare [11, 24].

The landmark World Health Organization (WHO) paper "Framework for Action on Interprofessional Education & Collaborative Practice" urged countries worldwide to invest in interprofessional education (IPE) to prepare future health professionals to be "collaborative-practice ready" [52].

Globally, different Interprofessional Competency Frameworks and the Lancet Report by Frenk et al. [12] have spurred initiatives in both IPE and IPC. In 2022, Julio Frenk and a group of internationally recognized experts [13] published another report, looking at what had been done in the meantime. While the group reported transformative developments in competency-based education, IPE, and the large-scale application of information technology in education, knowledge about the use of the acquired competencies in the clinical setting, as well as knowledge about the readiness of the clinical practice for IPC, seems to be rather unclear or fragmented [37]. Therefore, a key question is how the transfer of acquired competencies into clinical practice can be ensured. As IPC is necessary for coping with current and future challenges, we cannot afford to wait year after year before systematically implementing IPC [11, pp. 188–190].

While research on IPE and IPC is well supported and developed in countries such as the United States, Canada, the United Kingdom, and Australia, the focus of this chapter is on IPC in the European Region. Building on the ideas of Schot et al. [37], we wanted to explore what IPC looks like in European countries, how the acquired IP competencies are promoted and implemented by healthcare professions (HCPs) during healthcare provision in different healthcare settings in Europe. In this chapter, the two authors build on their knowledge gained by studying the perceptions and experiences of the status quo of IPC between seven HCPs in seven hospitals and 20 health districts in Northern Italy and in outpatient Diabetes Care. Second, a brief report on IPC in Italy is given. Finally, the results of an exploratory literature review on IPC in Europe are reported.

What Is Already Known in Italy?

The Northern Italian IPC Study (2014–2016)

In 2014, when the authors started their research on IPC as members of an interdisciplinary and interprofessional team, research on IPC was scarce in Italy. A mixed-method study was developed that took place in Northern Italy, in a bilingual (German and Italian) region. It was based on a cross-sectional sequential mixed-method design [6] and aimed, among other things, to provide an empirical account of the current status quo of IPC in the studied Health Trust in Northern Italy. A brief description of the study alongside selected important results regarding IPC is presented here.

Data were collected in an online survey from March to June 2014. In addition, interviews and focus-group interviews with healthcare leaders and HCPs regarding their perceptions/experiences of IPC were performed.

The sample within the Health Trust[1] consisted of the following health professions: dieticians, nurses, occupational therapists, physicians, physiotherapists, psychologists, and speech therapists. We examined how frequently the seven health professions collaborated with each other. Two scales were used for measuring: the validated multi-group measurement scale for IPC, hereafter the IPC scale, developed by Kenaszchuk et al. [20], and the adapted nurse–physician relationship scale originally described by Kramer and Schmalenberg [22, 23] in their Magnet hospitals studies, along with sociodemographic variables. The adapted nurse–physician relationship scale consists of six relationship types: (1) hostile, (2) friendly-stranger, (3) teacher–student, (4) student–teacher, (5) collaborative, and (6) collegial relationship [28, 47].

A total of 5070 HCPs in the Health Trust who met the inclusion criteria were invited. Of these, 2238 participated in the survey [28]: 1532 out of 3225 nurses (47.5%), 337 out of 1380 physicians (24.4%), 132 out of 213 physiotherapists (62.0%), 77 out of 171 psychologists (45.0%), 71 out of 111 speech therapists (64.0%), 44 out of 64 occupational therapists (68.8%), and 45 out of 62 dieticians (72.6%) [49].

To generate "a more nuanced picture of how different professional groups assess the nature of their collaborative relations with the other professions" [47, p. 267f], the frequency of contact was examined, differentiating between each individual HCP to gain more information about how a physiotherapist collaborates with a physician, nurse, and so on.

The seven HCPs indicated on a 5-point Likert scale ranging from "every day" to "never" how often they worked together [28, 49]. Not surprisingly, the professionals who collaborated most regularly, for example, on an everyday basis, were physicians and nurses. For nurses, physiotherapists were the second professional group with whom they collaborated more frequently, followed by dieticians, psychologists, speech therapists, and occupational therapists. Furthermore, the data revealed that some professional groups rarely or never worked together. The seven professional groups described their collaboration with the other professional groups generally in a positive way, but with variations between these groups. We also found evidence that the way healthcare was organized had an impact on perceptions of IPC [49].

The analysis of the relationship types between HCPs revealed that all six relationship types did exist within the Health Trust, but were experienced by the seven professions differently. The high frequency of occurrence of the positive relationship types (collaborative and collegial) reflects aspects of the results reported by Kramer and Schmalenberg [23] and Schmalenberg and Kramer [34].

---

[1] A Health Trust is a publicly funded organization responsible for managing and delivering healthcare services within a specific region or sector, often operating under a national healthcare system like the National Health Trust (NHS) in the United Kingdom.

In their studies, the collaborative and collegial (positive) relationships are mentioned more frequently than the hostile and friendly-stranger (negative) relationships. Our study reflects these results, in that our respondents reported the collaborative and collegial relationships more frequently than the other four relationship types.

A difference in perception is particularly evident when looking at physicians. Physicians assessed the different types of relationships with the other six professions more positively than the other six professions rated their relationship with physicians. This outcome reflects previous research findings [15, 29, 38]. The lack of insight by physicians into the perceptions of other professions of their relationship with medicine is a potential barrier to future attempts to improve IPC between medicine and the other HCPs, which, in turn, could also affect the quality of patient care. We noted a similar response pattern regarding the IPC scale, where physicians were more negatively rated by all the other professions of our study [49], corroborating evidence from earlier studies [32, 53].

Of particular concern is the reporting of a negative relationship with medicine by the nursing profession. The fact that all professions examined in this study reported on some level the existence of the hostile and friendly-stranger relationship raises serious questions over the quality of IPC, and concomitantly patient safety, pointing out the high demand to improve IPC in this area.

IPC in Type 2 Diabetes Care in Northern Italy (2018–2020)

In a mixed-method study on type 2 diabetes (DM2) as an epidemiologically relevant chronic disease in Northern Italy, the focus was on the awareness of HCPs to work in an aligned manner to better activate patients in outpatient and primary care settings. The aim was to explore how far and to what extent the included health professions, such as general practitioners (GPs), dieticians, and nurses, communicate and collaborate to support patients regarding changes they should integrate into their everyday lives, applying to their nutritional and physical activity habits. A particular interest was to explore the state of alignment between the HCPs mentioned above. Alignment was defined as a "service delivery in which outpatient/primary healthcare is adapted to warrant a more patient-focused care, with better distributed (human) resources and reduced rates of errors" [50, pp. 2–3].

Problem-centered interviews were conducted in 2018 with seven GPs and five of their patients, three dieticians, and three nurses working in outpatient care. The interviewees described their views on tasks and responsibilities, as well as whom they considered to be in charge. An interesting and noticeable point is that every healthcare professional reported their views and ideas in such a way that always "someone else" seemed to be in charge.

GPs described themselves as the *first contact point for diagnosis* and in charge *of* further *monitoring* (e.g., glucose levels) and as an *intermediate contact point between visits to the diabetes centers.* A common perception among

GPs—and a reality for some—was the desire for a nurse or assistant in their practice to support patient care. Currently, nurses are only involved in managing patients with complications, but they envision an expanded role as case managers, coordinating healthcare professionals, and facilitating patient care. Dietitians typically assess patients' eating and physical activity habits by default and prioritize direct communication with patients, but often do not perceive a need for collaboration with other healthcare professionals to prevent complications.

Wieser et al. [50] concluded that collaboration and communication among the various healthcare professions studied were either lacking or inadequately supported at the organizational, processual, and system levels. Similar to findings from the Northern Italian IPC study, collaboration primarily occurred when individual HCPs were personally committed to it. However, there was little emphasis on coordinating or defining the distribution of competencies among key professional groups, as this was not considered necessary. Notably, collaboration appeared to be disconnected from patient outcomes. An intriguing finding was that while healthcare professionals recognized what other professions should do or change to improve collaboration and communication, they did not apply these insights to their own practice. As a result, patients often assumed the responsibility of informing all involved healthcare professionals.

Building on the results reported above, a survey was conducted in 2019 to explore patients' perceptions of communication and interaction with HCPs. A total of 364 individuals with DM2, all members of a local patient organization, were invited to participate, with 109 responding to a paper-based survey. Here, we report findings related to the frequency of patient interactions with different healthcare professionals—diabetologists, GPs, nurses, and dietitians—in both inpatient and outpatient settings.

Assessing patients' experiences provided insights into how patient–professional relationships and related perceptions influenced their willingness to modify nutritional and physical activity habits. The analysis examined the frequency of contact, interaction, and communication with different healthcare professionals, as no previous study had explicitly applied behavior change variables to patient interactions with various healthcare providers as potential facilitators of behavior change. According to Kelly and Barker [19], these interactions could have impacted patients' stage of change and psychological processes, ultimately influencing their ability to adopt and sustain behavioral modifications.

It was striking to discover that even among patients with over 10 years of experience living with DM2, the diabetologist remained the healthcare professional they had the most frequent contact with, followed by their GP and hospital nurses. However, contact with dietitians or outpatient care nurses was rare or non-existent. Patients who demonstrated a higher readiness for behavior change—related to both dietary and physical activity habits—reported better interaction and communication with their GP and hospital nurses. Additionally, they exhibited higher self-efficacy and stability in maintaining change, along with lower levels of temptation and perceived discrepancy [51].

Selected Other Studies on IPC in Italy

In Italy, the focus of research to date has been on translating and adapting instruments of IPC. In 2021, Carradore et al. [3] used the Italian validated IPC scale [47] to assess IPC between HCPs in Reggio Emilia. In another study by Carradore et al. [4], the same IPC scale was applied to nurses working in emergency services throughout Italy. Both studies focused on the validation and re-validation of the IPC scale with different samples working in various settings. In both studies, the results of the validation of the IPC scale were confirmed, so that this scale can now be used to measure IPC in Italy. Another study by Tonarelli et al. [43] validated the Italian version of the Chiba Interprofessional Scale (CICS29). The validation of the Italian scale produced results comparable to the original Japanese scale.

Federica Dellafiore et al. [7] studied Interprofessional Team Collaboration (ITC) in Italy. They aimed to "describe the ITC domains (i.e. partnership, cooperation, coordination) and the simultaneous contribution of the major individual-level determinants (i.e. sociodemographic and individual perception of general working satisfaction) on each ITC domain" [7, p. 763]. The results showed that physicians were "less inclined to partnership and inclined to coordination" [7, p. 765].

Finally, Migotto et al. [25] explored how gender impacted physician–nurse collaboration in healthcare teams in Italy. Milani et al. [27] reported on the development of an innovative delivery model in primary care, called House of Community, aiming at strengthening comprehensive primary healthcare in which collaboration between the different healthcare providers is paramount.

In summary, our review of research on IPC in Italy reveals that this topic is emerging slowly; however, it is still under-researched, even though its relevance is recognized by HCPs and policymakers [27].

IPC in Europe: An Overview

To gain an overview of the state of IPC in Europe, we searched for scoping reviews (ScRs) in PubMed and CINAHL, the Journal of Interprofessional Care, BMC Health Service Research, and the International Journal of Integrated Care published between 2010 and 2024, which had been conducted in Europe, demonstrating research in the field of IPC. ScRs were excluded if IPC was not the focus and if the ScR only dealt with the evaluation (measurement properties) of IPC instruments.

Four ScRs conducted in Norway, Finland, Belgium, and the Netherlands were identified [21, 39, 40, 44]. Their focus was on the primary care setting. Due to the nature of ScRs, although conducted in Europe, they did not limit their search strategy to the European context. These reviews investigated the following topics:

- Facilitating factors (organizational, procedural, relational, and contextual) of multiprofessional collaboration in primary care [40];
- Professional care at home, with IPC as a subtheme of the ScR by Vaartio-Rajalin and Fagerstrom [44];

- Strategies and interventions to improve or facilitate "interprofessional collaboration and integration" (IPCI) in primary care at the micro-, meso- and macro-level to develop "an evidence-based toolkit guiding HCP in their transition toward IPCI" [39];
- Identifying and analyzing approaches of IPC in the field of palliative dementia care [21].

Across the included studies in the ScRs, only a third originated (23/62) from Europe. The practice setting in all four ScRs was located in primary care, in particular within home care, nursing homes, and care homes. Sirimsi et al. [39] identified five themes to improve or facilitate IPC in their ScR: (1) acceptance and team readiness toward collaboration, (2) acting as a team and not as an individual, (3) communication strategies and shared decision-making, (4) coordination in primary care, and (5) integration of caregivers and their skills and competences. These five themes present essential "building blocks" for interventions and strategies to improve IPC and integration in primary care. The attitudes, competencies, skills, and roles described within each theme must be developed within HCPs. According to Sirimsi et al. [39], none of the interventions and strategies can advance IPC in isolation. They are interdependent and build on each other that means that a mix of interventions/strategies could enhance IPC in primary care. Khemai et al. [21] identified three elements: "collaborative themes" such as managing pain or shared decision-making, "collaborative processes" such as communication or assessing and monitoring, and "resources in collaboration" such as material and immaterial resources (competences). Both Sirimsi [39] and Khemai et al. [21] described among their identified themes activities necessary for preparing HCPs for IPC, concrete IPC approaches such as assessments, care plans, shared decision-making, structured team meetings, or skills needed for IPC, such as communication or shared values. In the specific area of dementia care, skills needed are, for example, "pain management" and skills for managing the "care in the dying phase" of a person's life.

The four ScRs dealt with prerequisites or preparatory steps for the implementation of IPC in general or in specific areas of primary care in Europe. This could be seen as an indicator for a gradual or step-by-step introduction and implementation of IPC in this sector of healthcare in Europe. However, it still seems to be very difficult to explore how IPC is actually implemented or practiced.

Following the identification of research according to ScRs performed in Europe, the next step was to explore the state of research on IPC in Europe by means of an additional exploratory literature review. We searched in the aforementioned databases, primarily in PubMed/Medline between August 2023 and June 2024, for further studies focusing on IPC. We will now report on 16 studies that focused on IPC in Europe. The following data was extracted: European country, first author, year, study design/method, aim of the study, practice setting, and HCPs involved.

Table 1 shows the country (as site of the study), first author (all from Europe), year, aim of study, study design/methods, setting, and number of the professions involved in the included studies.

Table 1 Categorizes the 16 studies according to European region: Continental Europe, Scandinavia, and the United Kingdom

Country	First author	Year	Aim of study/project	Study design/methods	Setting	Professions involved
Continental Europe						
Netherlands	Romijn	2017	… aimed to understand how different care professionals in obstetrical teams assess their collaboration in order to gain insight into the extent to which their perceptions are aligned	Cross-sectional, quantitative study	Hospital and primary care	3 (MD, CM, RN)
	Van Dongen	2016	… is to explore influential factors of IPC regarding patient goals and the patient-centered care plan	Qualitative focus group study, four focus groups	Primary care	6 (GP, RN, PT, OT, PSY, SW)
	Van Dongen	2017	… was therefore to examine current practices in IPT meetings in primary care, as well as “how” they are conducted, as well as to explore healthcare professionals’ personal opinions regarding the current practice	A qualitative study involving both observations of team meetings and individual semi-structured interviews with participating healthcare professionals	Primary care team meetings	6 (OT, PT, RN, MD, SW, PHARM)

Country	First author	Year	Aim of study/project	Study design/methods	Setting	Professions involved
Belgium	Pype	2018	… aims to: 1. Systematically identify all complex adaptive systems (CAS) principles as expressed in healthcare providers' accounts of collaboration in a network structure 2. Describe the whole-team functioning according to the CAS principles 3. Explore factors influencing workplace learning in a distributed team as emergent behavior of a CAS	Qualitative study, interviews	Palliative home-care teams (PHCTs)	2 (MD, RN [CN, PCHC nurses])
	Karam	2022	… Overall, the study 1. assesses IPC between GPs and nurses 2. identifies target priorities for improving IPC 3. facilitates the planning and implementation of the improvement strategies proposed by participants	Participatory action research (PAR, using qualitative methods such as focus groups and a survey)	Primary care	2 (MD, RN)
	Horlait	2022	… aims to explore non-physician care professionals' perceived current and aspired roles within cancer MDTMs Additionally, it sought to identify the perceived hindering factors for these non-physician care professionals to fulfill their specific role	Exploratory qualitative design using focus groups and in-depth interviews	Medical oncology department; (multidisciplinary oncology consult [MOC])	3 (PSY, RN, SW + data managers)

(continued)

Table 1 (continued)

Country	First author	Year	Aim of study/project	Study design/methods	Setting	Professions involved
Switzerland	Schmitz	2017	… was to explore, in five different settings (…) what is described by practitioners as successful or unsuccessful IPC and, from this, to derive strategies for improving collaboration between health professionals	25 qualitative, narrative interviews	Primary care, surgical care, internal medicine, psychiatric care and palliative care	5 (MD, RN, PSY, OT, PT)
	Schmid	2021	… to explore the perspective of specific healthcare professionals and their perception of IPC in comprehensive healthcare of people with MS (PwMS)	Qualitative methodology by using focus groups (FG) in an outpatient setting A semi-structured interview guide for FG 13 participants = 3 FG's	In- and outpatient setting specialized clinics for PwMS	3 (PT, SLT, OT)
Austria	Wieczorek	2016	… investigate the ways in which different healthcare professionals struggle to work together to successfully integrate the BFHI (baby-friendly hospital initiative) into practice	Qualitative approach with semi-structured interviews 35 HCP + 1 data manager	Hospital maternity care	3 (MD, CM, RN)

Country	First author	Year	Aim of study/project	Study design/methods	Setting	Professions involved
Scandinavia						
Norway	Steihaug	2017	… aimed to explore how structural conditions facilitate or restrain collaboration in practice between GPs and other providers in the municipalities	Qualitative study a series of semi-structured interviews with health personnel in four Norwegian municipalities during spring 2011	Primary care and municipalities (structural conditions)	3 (GP, RN, PT)
	Battin	2021	… explores how professionals contribute to interprofessional collaboration in their day-to-day interactions during teamwork using a narrative lens that emphasizes therapeutic emplotment	Ethnographic research project that enabled the exploration of social processes characterizing interprofessional collaboration using observation and interviews	Biosocial pain rehabilitation ward in a hospital (social interactions during teamwork)	6 (GP, PT, OT, RN, PSY, SW)
	Johansen	2022	… to explore how rural health professionals in Northern Norway experience collaboration regarding palliative care patients, both locally and with hospital-based specialists, including perceived facilitators and barriers to optimal collaboration and the consequences of non-optimal collaboration	A qualitative focus group and interview study	Primary care and palliative care collaboration	2 (MD, RN)
	Sorenson	2020	… to explore the experience of GPs, nurses, and medical secretaries in some of these practices	Qualitative and exploratory study, drawing on interviews with six GPs, three nurses, and two medical secretaries	Primary care, five general practices	2 (GP, RN), medical secretaries

(continued)

Table 1 (continued)

Country	First author	Year	Aim of study/project	Study design/methods	Setting	Professions involved
Sweden	Mangrio	2023	… is to illuminate the experiences that health, social, and dental professionals have had during their work within grow safely	Descriptive qualitative study	Child healthcare, home-visit program (grow safely)	4 (RN, CM, SW, dental assistant)
United Kingdom						
United Kingdom	Atwal	2005	… aimed to analyze and improve multidisciplinary teamwork in discharge planning, and was supported by both the hospital management and the Local Research Ethics Committee	This study is part of an action research project, (…); observational study to record interactions of the team members using the bales' interaction process analysis (IPA)	Hospital, older people care	5 (MD, OT, PT, SW, RN)
	Hunter	2014	… to explore how the pathway was used in real-life settings and evaluate its implementation from the perspectives of all key players: midwives, doctors, mothers, and midwifery managers	Policy ethnographic approach Data were collected between October 2004 and October 2006 in two research sites Three phases; Phase 1 semi-structured interviews with experts Phase 3 + 3; semi-participant observation of midwives using the pathway in the two units, focus groups + semi-structured interviews	Hospital, maternity care unit A unit B	2 (CM, midwife managers, MD)

Continental Europe covers nine studies, as illustrated

MD medical doctor, *GP* general practitioner, *RN* registered nurse, *PT* physiotherapist, *OT* occupational therapist, *CM* certified midwife, *PSY* psychologist, *SLT* speech and language therapist, *SW* social worker, *RD* registered dietician, *PHARM* pharmacist

The studies took place between 2005 and 2023. Primary care, especially specialized care such as palliative care, seems to be a setting that interests researchers. In the hospital, maternity care [16, 48] and older people care [1] are practice settings that rely on professionals with different professional backgrounds. The number of professions involved in the studies ranged from two (e.g., nurses and GPs/physicians) to six different professions. In three of the studies, other occupations were also involved, such as medical secretaries [41], dental assistants [26], and data managers [14]. Besides HCPs, social workers are included in five studies due to the setting, such as primary care [46], or to the specific focus of the study, such as discharge planning [1]. Pharmacists are another profession included in the studies in this review [46].

Five studies were conducted within the Scandinavian *countries*, four of them in Norway [2, 17, 41, 42], and two studies [1, 16] were performed in the United Kingdom.

From a *methodological perspective*, 14 of the 16 studies pursued a qualitative approach using observation and/or interviews. Three of these studies were part of an action research project [1], or part of participatory action research (PAR), such as the study of Karam et al. [18], or part of a longitudinal qualitative design, such as an ethnographic study [2].

In discussing the results, we focus on 11 of the 16 studies found. Out of these, seven studies took place in primary care [17, 18, 31, 41, 42, 45, 46]. The other four studies addressed the hospital and primary care setting [33, 35, 36], and one explored IPC in child healthcare crossing health and social care sectors [26]. Of the five Scandinavian studies examining IPC in primary care, four were conducted in Norway [2, 17, 41, 42] and one in Sweden [26]. Two of these described concrete approaches of IPC, such as "talking together" versus "not talking together" [17] or "doing a home visit" [26]. The other two studies aimed to explore how structural conditions facilitate or restrain IPC between GPs and other HCPs [42] and focused on IPC within GP offices between GPs, nurses, and medical secretaries taking care of a specialized patient population, patients with DM2 [41]. These results from Norway indicate that the primary care sector does not yet seem to be IPC-ready and that existing different organizational logics do not fit together, for example, the logic of a GP office versus an institutional logic that frames the working conditions of other HCPs. The dominant role of the GP runs like a red thread through the Norwegian studies. Whether IPC succeeds or fails seems to depend on the attitude or motivation of the GP. Furthermore, the different financing of health services of the various HCP or legal regulations represents a major barrier to IPC. The Swedish study, in which GPs were not part of the study, demonstrated that HCPs could work well together to the benefit of the client. The results clearly indicated that IPC needs an organizational frame/structure and requires funding.

Looking at seven of nine studies [18, 31, 33, 35, 36, 45, 46] carried out in Continental Europe, four of them explored IPC in practice [18, 31, 45, 46]. Van Dongen et al. [45] explored IPC with regard to patient-centered care planning and team meetings. Karam et al. [18] conducted a PAR project, while Pype et al. [31] explored IPC from a theoretical lens such as complexity theory. Based on empirical findings regarding IPC in six Local Action Research Groups (LARGs), three in rural and three in urban areas, the study participants of each of the LARGs chose approaches for improving IPC that were suitable for their specific needs. The empirical results, summarized in a Strengths, Weaknesses, Opportunities, Threats (SWOT) analysis, highlighted strengths and weaknesses in two domains: the relational and contextual domains. Examples of the chosen approaches are: creating a shared patient's record at the patient's home, promoting task sharing and delegation to better distribute the workload, implementing a multidisciplinary screening tool for frailty screening, clarifying professional roles and formalizing task delegation, or enhancing the use of electronic communication. The results of the other three studies, concerned with the perception of HCPs of IPC, give an impression of what facilities and hinders IPC [33, 35, 36], reconstructing experienced types of collaboration ranging from coordinative to co-creative collaboration and modes of collaboration ranging from programmed, hub and network.

In summary, the studies show that supportive factors of IPC in primary care are getting to know each other personally, physical proximity, the development of a common mindset, and structured meetings. All HCPs must learn how to work together, how to learn from each other, how to actively involve the patient, and how to set goals together in order to be able to align profession-specific interventions with the common goal.

All HCPs have to abandon their old routines, have to learn new work routines, and must be able to adapt these flexibly to the given patient situation. They must learn to let go of their narrow focus on the illness and base their actions on the life of the person they are caring for and the patient's network. This can be far from easy for the HCPs involved. Psychological safety [8] is necessary so that IPC can function in highly diverse teams and so that HCPs can collaborate with each other in a trusting and respectful manner.

Supporting or hindering factors are partly similar in the different European countries, but also country-specific due to the organization of health systems in the respective countries, as well as to legal and financial conditions.

All studies exemplify that IPC, whether in the hospital [1, 16, 33, 35, 36, 48], primary care [17, 18, 31, 41, 42, 45, 46], or in specialized areas [2, 14, 26], is a complex endeavor. The type and form of IPC is not only context specific, but also person specific (the one who is cared for), as well as situation specific (e.g., crisis). In sum, IPC does not materialize automatically and by itself. Instead, it is dependent on clear organizational structures, as well as on legal and financial regulations.

Discussion

We started this chapter with selected findings from our two studies conducted in Northern Italy, describing the situation found in this field in Italy. When comparing the findings of this overview with the Northern Italian IPC study and the Diabetes Type 2 Care study, we can state that our first study with seven HCP has investigated the highest number of HCP within one study in Europe to date. Looking at the studies performed, in the European context, the number of professions included in the studies varied from two to six professional groups. While the setting of the Northern Italian IPC study [28, 47, 49] was both hospital and primary care, we noted that the studies found in our explorative literature were predominantly in primary care.

We found only a few ScRs performed in Europe by European researchers; when looking at these more closely, the ScRs performed by European researchers did not focus on the specific situation of IPC in Europe but used this form of literature review to analyze the situation of IPC worldwide. In contrast, the aim of this chapter was to obtain an initial overview of the state of research on IPC in Europe in order to be able to advance the field of research in Europe based on this empirical knowledge.

When performing research within IPC, researchers need to consider that healthcare systems around the world differ greatly. Although they seem to be close together, due to their historical and organizational development, healthcare systems in Europe are not alike and comparable. This also applies to the qualification and educational background of nurses, allied healthcare professionals, and physicians at the vocational, graduate, and post-graduate levels, although all are based on a common European legislative framework. This leads to different approaches to promote IPC in the respective European countries.

The 16 studies reported here reveal that IPC seems to offer persons in need of healthcare a lot, such as patients with varying and complex needs along their care trajectories. Maybe this is the reason why research on IPC focuses on patient groups with specific chronic diseases, such as dementia or persons in need of palliative care.

On a national, European, and international level to date, it seems difficult to state exactly what outcomes can be reached with IPC in terms of patient, professional, and/or organizational outcomes. The findings are highly variable and hardly comparable, as emphasized in an overview of reviews by Carron et al. [5]. This underlines the need for research at a European level, as well as research that focuses on how HCPs translate IPC into concrete action in their various practice settings. The study by Battin et al. [2] points in this direction, just as the systematic review by Schot et al. [37] conducted in the Netherlands, offering suggestions for future research on the basis of existing knowledge. In their review, they focused on what the various HCPs contribute to IPC. They categorized the contributions of the professions as bridging gaps, negotiating overlaps, and creating spaces. It became apparent that the contributions differed from one another. Differences also became obvious in relation to the collaborative setting, close-knit team setting, or more networked forms of collaboration, and in relation to the area, for example, hospital, mental health, primary care, and so on [37].

Summary and Prospect

The purpose of this chapter was to give an overview of what we know about IPC in Europe, starting with Italy. Our search for ScRs carried out in Europe revealed that there is no comprehensive ScR with a focus on the state of IPC in the European region. The ScRs undertaken by researchers from Europe did not focus on elucidating the situation of IPC in the European region. The findings of this work support the authors' impression that ScRs regarding the situation/state of IPC in Europe are missing. We clearly see a need for interventions (quality improvement strategies) and systematic research in the area of IPC in Europe. Mapping the knowledge in the field of IPC is as urgent as working on a common agenda for improving IPC.

To develop IPC in all healthcare settings, a Europe-wide cooperation and research agenda on IPC would be preferable. It should be complemented by corresponding national agendas. To improve the field of IPC, much work needs to be done in the educational, legal, and organizational fields to create conditions that foster and sustain IPC in each country within Europe. Regular updates of the current state of IPC in each European country are the foundation for moving ahead and for learning from each other. Furthermore, this basis is the starting point to explore what interventions or practices work in the clinical and primary care setting in which country and under which circumstances.

Reflective Questions

- Why do you think so little European-specific research has been carried out? What difference would a European research agenda make in the European/international IPC arena?
- What do you think about creating/promoting an overarching research agenda on how IPC is implemented?
- Imagine how HCPs actualize IPC in various practice settings (Hospital, primary care, long-term care): what tools/concepts facilitate them working "interprofessional"?
- From your point of view, how could collaborative work/research, which is less oriented at local or specific issues, move the whole area/field forward?
- Think about the further development/consolidation of IPC: How important is it to always rush into new areas of application? How can the purpose and benefits of IPC be brought more into the focus of research?
- What is known about the effects of IPC? How are the short-term, medium-term, and long-term effects of IPC between the professions involved? How does IPC improve the care of the people being cared for and their relatives and carers?

References

1. Atwal A, Caldwell K. Do all health and social care professionals interact equally: a study of interactions in multidisciplinary teams in the United Kingdom. Scand J Caring Sci. 2005;19(3):268–73. https://doi.org/10.1111/j.1471-6712.2005.00338.x.
2. Battin GS, Romsland GI, Christiansen B. The puzzle of therapeutic emplotment: creating a shared clinical plot through interprofessional interaction in biopsychosocial pain rehabilitation. Soc Sci Med. 2021;277:113904. https://doi.org/10.1016/j.socscimed.2021.113904.

3. Carradore M, Michelini E, Caretta I, Carpi S, Corradini L, Ganapini S, Lumetta F, Paterlini G, Pedroni E, Russo A, Sarli L, Artioli G. Interprofessional collaboration between different health care professions in Emilia Romagna. Acta Biomed. 2021;92(S2):e2021033. https://doi.org/10.23750/abm.v92iS2.11954.
4. Carradore M, Guasconi M, Giusti GD, Artioli G, Sarli L. Re-evaluation of the Interprofessional Collaboration Scale validation between nurses towards other health care professionals occupied in Italian emergency medical services. Acta Biomed. 2022;93(4):e2022287. https://doi.org/10.23750/abm.v93i4.13514.
5. Carron T, Rawlinson C, Arditi C, Cohidon C, Hong QN, Pluye P, Gilles I, Peytremann-Bridevaux I. An overview of reviews on interprofessional collaboration in primary care: effectiveness. Int J Integr Care. 2021;21(2):31. https://doi.org/10.5334/ijic.5588.
6. Cresswell JW, Piano Clark VL. Designing and conducting mixed methods research. 2nd ed. SAGE Publications; 2011.
7. Dellafiore F, Caruso R, Conte G, Grugnetti AM, Bellani S, Arrigoni C. Individual-level determinants of interprofessional team collaboration in healthcare. J Interprof Care. 2019;33(6):762–7. https://doi.org/10.1080/13561820.2019.1594732.
8. Edmondson AC. The fearless organization: creating psychological safety in the workplace for learning, innovation, and growth. John Wiley & Sons; 2018.
9. European Union (2023) State of Health in the EU Synthesis Report ISBN 978-92-68-09705-2/doi:10.2875/458883 https://health.ec.europa.eu/system/files/2023-12/state_2023_synthesis-report_en.pdf.
10. Eurostat. Major causes of death in the EU in 2022. 2022. Retrieved 4 Apr 2025 from https://ec.europa.eu/eurostat/statistics-explained/index.php?title=Causes_of_death_statistics#Major_causes_of_death_in_the_EU_in_2022.
11. Fitzgerald L, McDermott AM. Changing perspectives on change. In: Challenging perspectives on organizational change in health care, vol. 3. Routledge; 2017. p. 183–98.
12. Frenk J, Chen L, Bhutta ZA, Cohen J, Crsip N, Evans T, Fineberg H. Health professionals for a new century: transforming education to strengthen health systems in an interdependent world. Lancet. 2010;376(9756):1923–58. https://doi.org/10.1016/S0140-6736(10)61854-5.
13. Frenk J, Chen LC, Chandran L, Groff EOH, King R, Meleis A, Fineberg HV. Challenges and opportunities for educating health professionals after the COVID-19 pandemic. Lancet. 2022;400(10362):1539–56. https://doi.org/10.1016/S0140-6736(22)02092-X.
14. Horlait M, De Regge M, Baes S, Eeckloo K, Leys M. Exploring non-physician care professionals' roles in cancer multidisciplinary team meetings: a qualitative study. PLoS One. 2022;17(2):e0263611. https://doi.org/10.1371/journal.pone.0263611.
15. House S, Havens D. Nurse's and physician's perceptions of nurse-physician collaboration. A systematic review. J Nurs Adm. 2017;47(3):165–71.
16. Hunter B, Segrott J. Renegotiating inter-professional boundaries in maternity care: implementing a clinical pathway for normal labour. Sociol Health Illn. 2014;36(5):719–37. https://doi.org/10.1111/1467-9566.12096.
17. Johansen ML, Ervik B. Teamwork in primary palliative care: general practitioners' and specialised oncology nurses' complementary competencies. BMC Health Serv Res. 2018;18(1):159. https://doi.org/10.1186/s12913-018-2955-7.
18. Karam M, Macq J, Duchesnes C, Crismer A, Belche JL. Interprofessional collaboration between general practitioners and primary care nurses in Belgium: a participatory action research. J Interprof Care. 2022;36(3):380–9. https://doi.org/10.1080/13561820.2021.1929878.
19. Kelly MP, Barker M. Why is changing health-related behaviour so difficult? Public Health. 2016;136:109–16. https://doi.org/10.1016/j.puhe.2016.03.030.
20. Kenazchuk C, Reeves S, Nicholas D, Zwarenstein M. Validity and reliability of a multiple-group measurement scale for interprofessional collaboration. BMC Health Serv Res. 2010;10(83):2–15.
21. Khemai C, Leão DLL, Janssen DJA, Schols JMGA, Meijers JMM. Interprofessional collaboration in palliative dementia care. J Interprof Care. 2024;38(4):675–94. https://doi.org/10.1080/13561820.2024.2345828.

22. Kramer M, Schmalenberg C. Staff nurses identify essentials of magnetism. In: McCure ML, Hinshaw AS, editors. Magnet hospitals revisited: attraction and retention of professional nurses, vol. 25–29. American Academy of Nursing. American Nurses Publishing; 2002. p. 25–9.
23. Kramer M, Schmalenberg C. Securing “good” nurse physician relationships. Explore the link between collaboartion and quality patient care. Nurs Manag. 2003;34(7):34–8.
24. Lackie K, Najjar G, El-Awaisi A, Frost J, Green C, Langlois S, Lising D, Pfeifle AL, Ward H, Xyrichis A, Khalili H. Interprofessional education and collaborative practice research during the COVID-19 pandemic: considerations to advance the field. J Interprof Care. 2020;34(5):583–6. https://doi.org/10.1080/13561820.2020.1807481.
25. Migotto S, Garlatti Costa G, Ambrosi E, Pittino D, Bortoluzzi G, Palese A. Gender issues in physician–nurse collaboration in healthcare teams: Findings from a cross-sectional study. J Nurs Manag. 2019;27:1773–83. https://doi.org/10.1111/jonm.12872.
26. Mangrio E, Hjortsjo M. Health, social, and dental professionals’ experiences of working within an extended home-visit program in the child healthcare: a qualitative interview study in Sweden. BMC Health Serv Res. 2023;23(1):820. https://doi.org/10.1186/s12913-023-09791-z.
27. Milani C, Naldini G, Baggiani L, Nerattini M, Bonaccorsi G. How to promote changes in primary care? The Florentine experience of the House of community. Front Public Health. 2023;11:1216814. https://doi.org/10.3389/fpubh.2023.1216814.
28. Mischo-Kelling M, Wieser H, Vittadello F, Cavada L, Lochner L, Fink V, Naletto C, Kitto S, Reeves S. Application of an adapted relationship scale for assessing the occurrence of six different relationships as perceived by seven health care professions in Northern Italy. J Interprof Care. 2021;35(3):419–29.
29. Nair DM, Fitzpatrick JJ, McNulty R, Click ER, Glembocki MM. Frequency of nurse-physician collaborative behaviors in an acute care hospital. J Interprof Care. 2012;26(2):115–20. https://doi.org/10.3109/13561820.2011.637647.
30. OECD. Health at a glance 2023. OECD Indicators; 2023. https://doi.org/10.1787/7a7afb35-en.
31. Pype P, Mertens F, Helewaut F, Krystallidou D. Healthcare teams as complex adaptive systems: understanding team behaviour through team members’ perception of interpersonal interaction. BMC Health Serv Res. 2018;18(1):570. https://doi.org/10.1186/s12913-018-3392-3.
32. Reeves S, Lewin S, Espin S, Zwarenstein M. Interprofessional teamwork in health and social care. Wiley-Blackwell; 2010.
33. Romijn A, Teunissen PW, de Bruijne MC, Wagner C, de Groot CJM. Interprofessional collaboration among care professionals in obstetrical care: are perceptions aligned? BMJ Qual Saf. 2018;27(4):279–86. https://doi.org/10.1136/bmjqs-2016-006401.
34. Schmalenberg C, Kramer M. Nurse-physician relationships in hospitals: 20,000 nurses tell their story. Crit Care Nurse. 2009;29(1):74–83. https://doi.org/10.4037/ccn2009436.
35. Schmid F, Rogan S, Glässel A. A Swiss health care professionals’ perspective on the meaning of interprofessional collaboration in health Care of People with MS—a focus group study. Int J Environ Res Public Health. 2021;18(12):6537. https://www.mdpi.com/1660-4601/18/12/6537. https://mdpi-res.com/d_attachment/ijerph/ijerph-18-06537/article_deploy/ijerph-18-06537-v2.pdf?version=1623992802.
36. Schmitz C, Atzeni G, Berchtold P. Challenges in interprofessionalism in Swiss health care: the practice of successful interprofessional collaboration as experienced by professionals. Swiss Med Wkly. 2017;147:w14525. https://doi.org/10.4414/smw.2017.14525.
37. Schot E, Tummers L, Noordegraf M. Working on working together. A systematic review on how healthcare professionals contribute to interprofessional collaboration. J Interprof Care. 2019;34:332–42. https://doi.org/10.1080/13561820.2019.1636007.
38. Siedlecki SL, Hixon ED. Relationships between nurses and physicians matter. Online J Issues Nurs. 2015;20(3):6. https://doi.org/10.3912/OJIN.Vol20No3PPTO3.
39. Sirimsi MM, De Loof H, Van den Broeck K, De Vliegher K, Pype P, Remmen R, Van Bogaert P. Scoping review to identify strategies and interventions improving interprofessional collaboration and integration in primary care. BMJ Open. 2022;12(10):e062111. https://doi.org/10.1136/bmjopen-2022-062111.

40. Sorensen M, Stenberg U, Garnweidner-Holme L. A scoping review of facilitators of multi-professional collaboration in primary care. Int J Integr Care. 2018;18(3):13. https://doi.org/10.5334/ijic.3959.
41. Sorensen M, Groven KS, Gjelsvik B, Almendingen K, Garnweidner-Holme L. The roles of healthcare professionals in diabetes care: a qualitative study in Norwegian general practice. Scand J Prim Health Care. 2020;38(1):12–23. https://doi.org/10.1080/02813432.2020.1714145.
42. Steihaug S, Paulsen B, Melby L. Norwegian general practitioners' collaboration with municipal care providers—a qualitative study of structural conditions. Scand J Prim Health Care. 2017;35(4):344–51. https://doi.org/10.1080/02813432.2017.1397264.
43. Tonarelli A, Takeshi Yamamoto T, Foa C, Miraglia Raineri A, Artioli G, Baccarini E, Giampellegrini P, Masciangelo I, Moggi E, Toni D, Valcavi L, Sarli L. Italian validation of the Chiba Interprofessional Competency Scale (CICS29). Acta Biomed. 2020;91(2-S):58–66. https://doi.org/10.23750/abm.v91i2-S.9172.
44. Vaartio-Rajalin H, Fagerstrom L. Professional care at home: patient-centredness, interprofessionality and effectivity? A scoping review. Health Soc Care Community. 2019;27(4):e270–88. https://doi.org/10.1111/hsc.12731.
45. van Dongen JJ, Lenzen SA, van Bokhoven MA, Daniëls R, van der Weijden T, Beurskens A. Interprofessional collaboration regarding patients' care plans in primary care: a focus group study into influential factors. BMC Fam Pract. 2016;17:58. https://doi.org/10.1186/s12875-016-0456-5.
46. van Dongen JJ, van Bokhoven MA, Daniëls R, Lenzen SA, van der Weijden T, Beurskens A. Interprofessional primary care team meetings: a qualitative approach comparing observations with personal opinions. Fam Pract. 2017;34(1):98–106. https://doi.org/10.1093/fampra/cmw106.
47. Vittadello F, Mischo-Kelling M, Wieser H, Cavada L, Lochner L, Naletto C, Fink V, Reeves S. A multiple-group measurement scale for interprofessional collaboration: adaptation and validation into Italian and German languages. J Interprof Care. 2018;32(3):266–73. https://doi.org/10.1080/13561820.2017.1396298.
48. Wieczorek CC, Marent B, Dorner TE, Dur W. The struggle for inter-professional teamwork and collaboration in maternity care: Austrian health professionals' perspectives on the implementation of the Baby-Friendly Hospital Initiative. BMC Health Serv Res. 2016;16:91. https://doi.org/10.1186/s12913-016-1336-3.
49. Wieser H, Mischo-Kelling M, Vittadello F, Cavada L, Lochner L, Fink V, Naletto C, Reeves S. Perceptions of collaborative relationships between seven different health care professions in Northern Italy. J Interprof Care. 2019;33(2):133–42. https://doi.org/10.1080/13561820.2018.1534810.
50. Wieser H, Piccoliori G, Siller M, Comploj E, Stummer H. Living on the Own Island? Aligned collaboration between family physicians, nurses, dieticians, and patients with diabetes type 2 in an outpatient care setting in Northern Italy: findings from a qualitative study. Glob Adv Health Med. 2020a;16:1–10. https://doi.org/10.1177/2164956120946701.
51. Wieser H, Vittadello F, Comploj E, Stummer H. Do health professionals sufficiently address patients' disposition toward changing their nutritional and physical activity habits? Findings from a pilot study among people with type 2 diabetes in Northern Italy. Healthcare. 2020b;8(524):1–15. https://doi.org/10.3390/healthcare8040524.
52. World Health Organization. Framework for action on interprofessional education and collaborative practice. 2010. Retrieved from http://www.who.int/hrh/nursing_midwifery/en/.
53. Zwarenstein M, Rice K, Gotlib-Conn L, Kenaszchuk C, Reeves S. Disengaged: a qualitative study of communication and collaboration between physicians and other professions on general internal medicine. BMC Health Serv Res. 2013;13(494):2–9. http://www.biomedcentral.com/1472-6963/13/494

Heike Wieser is a researcher at the University Center for Health Professions Claudiana in Italy, where she co-leads the implementation of interprofessional education. She is a nutritional scientist with a Ph.D. in public health and brings several years of experience in health services research.

Maria Mischo-Kelling is a professor of nursing science at the University of Applied Sciences Ravensburg-Weingarten, a registered nurse, social economist, and sociologist with a doctorate in public health, who has held healthcare leadership roles in Germany and Italy. At the University Center for Health Care Professions, Claudiana, Bolzano, she undertook several research projects with researchers from different healthcare professions.

Case Studies of Interprofessional Learning in Healthcare Education in Europe

Heidi Schimatzek and Ranjev Kainth

Introduction and Purpose of the Chapter

The aim of this chapter is to provide interprofessional learning (IPL) educators with an understanding of when, where, and how IPL activities can be used, the challenges and barriers that need to be overcome when implementing them, and to present best practices from Europe.

The opportunities for students to learn and interact with other courses and professions are still limited in most educational institutions because teaching is rather concentrated in departmental spaces or educational and professional "silos" [7]. Interprofessional education (IPE) involves not only the joint attendance of courses by students but also the creation of settings in which "students from two or more professions learn about, from and with each other to enable effective collaboration and improve health outcomes" [23].

The terms IPL and IPE are often used interchangeably. While IPL focuses on the interactive learning process between students of different professions, IPE encompasses a more structured approach to teaching and learning that prepares students to work effectively together in the healthcare sector [1]. As the focus of this chapter is on specific interactive learning opportunities, the term IPL will be used.

H. Schimatzek (✉)
Health University of Applied Sciences Tyrol, Innsbruck, Austria
e-mail: heidi.schimatzek@fhg-tirol.ac.at

R. Kainth
Faculty of Life Sciences and Medicine, King's College London, London, UK
e-mail: anjev.kainth@kcl.ac.uk

A. Xyrichis et al. (eds.), *Building Bridges: A European Perspective on Interprofessional Education, Practice, Policy and Research*,
https://doi.org/10.1007/978-3-032-23222-9_14

Background

A recent systematic review by Colonnello et al. [6] addresses IPL activities among undergraduate medical students in the European Higher Education Area (EHEA), including original publications from 14 (out of 49) EHEA countries.

The IPL activities described in the included studies are heterogeneous and range from patient examples with specific clinical conditions/symptoms (e.g., wounds, ulcers, diabetes, and breast cancer) in real or simulated scenarios, to understanding the different professional roles, communication skills, and working effectively in the interprofessional team [6].

In the following section, the limitations described in the studies will be discussed, and possible solutions will be identified.

- No explicit reference was made to underlying *theories* in the development and planning of IPL activities, although there are many theories in the medical education literature that can be used to design IPL programs [6].

Hean et al. [12] assert in their review that no single theory can comprehensively explain or predict all aspects of curriculum design, advocating instead for an integrated approach. When selecting a theoretical framework, educators should first identify the specific components they aim to address—whether design, delivery, or learner experience. By making these distinctions, researchers can refine their theoretical choices to better align with their objectives. A diverse range of theories supports IPL and its evaluation, including both group- and systems-level approaches, providing the necessary depth to advance the field.

- *Student* participation in IPL activities is often voluntary, so selection bias cannot be ruled out. In most publications, students are involved in IPL activities in their final year of study, which contradicts the need for IPL at an early stage of training. In more than half of the studies, only medical and nursing students were involved, so other health professions (up to eight professions were described) are underrepresented [6].

Voluntary IPL activities can provide positive learning experiences but may lead to lower levels of student engagement. However, a mix of mandatory and optional learning activities can increase the appeal of IPL initiatives, provide flexibility in scheduling extracurricular activities, and allow interested learners to develop leadership skills [4].

Determining the optimal timing for IPL is challenging. On one hand, students need a foundational understanding of their own profession to effectively contribute to interprofessional teams. On the other hand, introducing IPL early in the curriculum is crucial to prevent the formation of professional silos, negative stereotypes, misperceptions, and hierarchical barriers. Striking a balance between these considerations is essential for maximizing the benefits of IPL [7, 21].

- Information about the IPE training and the educators' background experience with IPL activities is rarely reported; rather, the teachers are described as a team of "experts" from different professions [6].

Research suggests that educators who lack a clear understanding of IPL concepts may struggle to develop IPL activities, which can, in turn, limit their effectiveness in teaching IPE. Resources such as the Interprofessional Education Collaborative (IPEC) guidelines [14] and the WHO Framework [23] can enhance educators' preparedness, providing a strong foundation for effective IPE [3].

Within IPL settings, it is essential for trainers to mirror the heterogeneous backgrounds of trainees. Despite guidance, grasping the viewpoints of various professions can pose difficulties. Effective facilitation necessitates a common professional understanding, emphasis on collaborative results, respect for diverse professional roles, fostering teamwork, resolving conflicts, and engaging in self-assessment [22].

Moreover, it is crucial for seasoned professionals proficient in conflict resolution to oversee IPL. Learning facilitators should possess IPL experience, expertise in interactive teaching techniques and group dynamics, as well as adaptability to foster and sustain a culture of mutual respect [7].

- The *evaluation* of the activities was often carried out using locally developed questionnaires, focusing on student satisfaction with the activities and a self-assessment of the knowledge gained; often with a post-intervention survey and without a control group [6].

Methodologically, it is important to establish standardized pre- and post-intervention measures and protocols for tracking dependent variables. The inclusion of students from heterogeneous professional backgrounds and control groups is essential. Given the limited validity of current questionnaires for measuring IPL, the development of data and consensus-based instruments is warranted. Future research should compare the impact of IPL interventions involving direct participation in interprofessional collaboration with patient-centered models to improve the evidence base [6]. However, IPL activities should not only be evaluated from a positivist perspective. An interpretivist approach emphasizes the importance of learners' experiences and perspectives. Qualitative methods, such as reflection and exchange, create a deeper understanding of interprofessional collaboration. This could be reflected in changes in attitudes, perceptions, behaviors, and the potential positive impact on patients, clients, families, and communities [11].

IPL in Europe

A systematic literature search was conducted between January and March 2024 via EBSCOHost in various databases (Cinahl Ultimate, eBook Collection, Medline Ultimate, DACH Information, Education Source Ultimate) in English and German for IPL activities, preferably from Europe.

Studies were included if they had been published within the last 5 years and, in the case of original studies, if there was a European contribution to the publication. After title and abstract screening, 28 titles were included in Citavi.

The following section describes a selection of specific IPL activities that have been used in the European training of healthcare professionals; an overview of the activities is provided in Table 1.

IPL Activities Focusing on Ethical Aspects

Levett-Jones et al. [16] describe an IPL initiative at Keele University (United Kingdom) with first-year students from various healthcare disciplines (nursing, midwifery, medicine, physiotherapy, pharmacy, and biomedical science) engaged in an IPL program to foster understanding of diverse roles, teamwork, and collaboration. The initiative aimed to challenge stereotypes, nurture professional identity, empathy, teamwork, and communication skills. Students participated in plenary sessions and small interprofessional groups to discuss compassionate care, ethics, teamwork, and healthcare roles using real cases. The activity, supported by the six Cs (care, compassion, competence, communication, courage, and commitment) and ethical principles, led to increased awareness of teamwork's impact on patient outcomes. Students valued the experience, gained insights into other professions, and committed to applying their learning in future practice [16].

Machin et al. [17] highlight the growing recognition of ethics education in health and social care as essential for preparing students to navigate complex ethical challenges in their future practice. Given that ethical dilemmas often lack clear-cut solutions, collaborative reflection is crucial for helping students develop a deeper understanding of ethical, personal, and professional values. Integrating ethics into IPE reinforces its significance across all health professions. Ethics-focused IPL activities should mirror real-world practice, incorporating elements such as simulated ethics committees or ethical debates within teams. These activities provide a structured platform for students to explore diverse ethical perspectives, including critical issues like end-of-life care. Beyond enhancing ethical decision-making skills, such activities encourage students to apply core ethical principles in practical scenarios, fostering critical thinking and professional growth. Additionally, case studies and scenario-based discussions in pre-hospital care forums facilitate engagement with key themes such as teamwork, communication, professionalism, roles, ethics, and legal responsibilities, further strengthening students' readiness for ethical decision-making in clinical practice [17].

Interprofessional Case-Based Learning

A qualification program in Freiburg (South Germany) focuses on IPL among students of medicine, social work, nursing, and related fields to jointly address the needs of geriatric patients [15]. The program consists of 16 teaching units, divided

Table 1 A selection of IPL activities in Europe

References	Country	IPL activity	Number of students (in groups)	Types of professions	Year of education	Resources	Duration	Competencies
Levett-Jones et al. [16]	United Kingdom	Patient cases (neglect, safety, death)	562 (15)	Biomedical science medicine Midwifery Nursing Pharmacy Physiotherapy	First year Partly mandatory, partly support for self-directed learning	Cases from the mid Staffordshire National Health Service Foundation	Two afternoons with online discussion in between	Effective communication Teamwork Values and ethics Patient dignity Patient safety
Machin et al. [17]	United Kingdom	Pseudo-clinical ethics committees Pre-hospital care forums Capacious suicide seminars End-of-life debates	150 (7–8) 100 (10–12) 100 (10–12) 90 (45)	Biomedical science Clinical psychology Dental hygiene Medicine Nursing Pharmacy Physiotherapy Social work	Medicine (fourth year), all other final year Not shown if mandatory/ elective	Six facilitators from each department Six to eight facilitators from each dept. Six to eight facilitators from each dept. Four tutors	2-h session 3-h session 3-h session 3 h for preparation and 2 h for the debate competition	Communication Teamwork Collaborative care Critical thinking Analytical skills Decision-making Values and ethics Respective roles

(continued)

Table 1 (continued)

References	Country	IPL activity	Number of students (in groups)	Types of professions	Year of education	Resources	Duration	Competencies
Kricheldorff et al. [15]	Germany	Introductory lecture and four workshops Patient cases in gerontology/ geriatrics and presentation in the plenary session	25-30/ year (6–8)	Medicine Nursing Nursing science Pedagogy of health professions Social work	Average second and fifth years Not shown if mandatory/ elective	Facilitators from each dept. and colleagues from clinical practice	8 h 8 h	Interprofessional teambuilding
Caduff et al. [5]	Switzer-land	Case discussion following ICF (with patient participation)	Not shown	Dietician Medicine Midwifery Nursing Occupational therapy Physiotherapy	Not shown Not shown if mandatory/ elective	Real patient	Preliminary phase (self-study) IPL study day (6 h) Follow-up phase (written reflection)	Developing a common picture of the patient situation Deriving a common treatment plan Respective roles Communication

Rinnhofer et al. [19]	Austria	Inter-university IPL with interprofessional lecture and job shadowing	300/year (10)	Biomedical science Dietetics Medicine Midwifery Nursing Occupational therapy Physiotherapy Radiological technology Speech and language therapy	Third semester (health pProf. and medicine) Mandatory	Four facilitators/ group	1-day lecture 1-day job shadowing	Knowledge on interprofessionalism Problem-based learning by casework Professional profiles and work routines
Gummesson et al. [10]	Sweden	Clinical reasoning	Not shown	Nursing Physiotherapy	Beginning second year Mandatory	Clinicians providing a real-life case Facilitators from nursing and physiotherapy	Not shown	Role of professional groups and patient Clinical reasoning fosters IPC

(continued)

Table 1 (continued)

References	Country	IPL activity	Number of students (in groups)	Types of professions	Year of education	Resources	Duration	Competencies
Posenau and Handgraaf [18]	Germany	Interprofessional case conferences	200 (20)	Midwifery Nursing Occupational therapy Physiotherapy Speech therapy	Seventh semester Mandatory		180 min/case conference (10 weeks)	Person-centered healthcare Roles and responsibilities Communication
Berger et al. [2]	Germany, New Zealand	Journal Club	67 (4–5)	Dentists Laboratory technology Medicine Midwifery Nursing Orthoptics Physiotherapy Radiographer Speech and language therapy	First year Elective	Research team (four persons)	90-min formal instruction Groups work outside the lectures Presentation at the end of the semester	Interprofessional collaboration (importance, values/ethics, communication, and teamwork)

Saaranen et al. [20]	Finland	Large-group simulation	427	Medicine Midwifery Nursing Pharmacy Psychology Social work Theology Health professionals	Not shown Not shown if mandatory/elective	Simulation scenario with professional actors designed for large groups	30-min simulation scenario 40-min debriefing	New perspectives and insights Understanding of IPC Knowledge increasement

into four parts, delivered over two full days with breaks between sessions for case-based teamwork. The faculty reflects the interprofessional team model and includes perspectives from social work, geriatrics, nursing, and medical education. Clinical practitioners from the Centre for Gerontology and Geriatrics enrich the workshops. Evaluation using the Freiburg Interprofessional Learning Evaluation Questionnaire indicates successful achievement of program objectives, particularly in clarifying individual roles within the interprofessional team. The multi-professional teaching team serves as a model for effective interprofessional collaboration [15].

Caduff et al. [5] describe an interprofessional case discussion in Zurich designed to foster a shared understanding of the patient's condition. This approach encourages a comprehensive exchange of observations, information, and perspectives, ensuring a more holistic and collaborative approach to patient care. Students work together to develop a treatment plan and involve the patient in decision-making regarding their care. Patient input is crucial for optimal care, ensuring high-quality treatment tailored to the patient's preferences and goals. Utilizing the WHO-recommended International Classification of Functioning, Disability, and Health (ICF) model promotes a common language for clinical practice. The interprofessional case discussion includes a preparatory phase where students prepare themselves with assignments. On the IPL day, students develop a patient presentation that is accepted by all, draw up a treatment plan, and finally involve the patient in the decision-making process. Reflection on the learning experience takes place in the follow-up phase through written assessments [5].

Inter-University IPL

A project in Austria outlines the feasibility of an inter-university, interprofessional lecture, including planning, implementation, and evaluation [19]. The collaboration between the University of Applied Sciences for Health Professions Upper Austria (eight programs) and the Bachelor of Medicine of the Johannes Kepler University started with the planning of a lecture and an interprofessional job shadowing initiative. This involved students observing different healthcare settings under the guidance of experienced supervisors. Organizing a 1-day lecture for three groups of 100 students each required meticulous coordination. Each group was led by a team of four lecturers from both universities. The students first discussed the importance and benefits of interprofessional collaboration in a plenary session. Subsequently, in smaller groups, they explored various healthcare professions through interactive sessions. Practical tasks allowed students to apply profession-specific skills across multiple disciplines. The project culminated in group discussions on a case study, encouraging reflection, networking, and actionable insights for improving interprofessional collaboration. The successful integration of this comprehensive interprofessional lecture into the diverse educational systems of the collaborating universities required institutional commitment and effective communication between the project team and the academic programs [19].

Clinical Reasoning as a Framework for IPL

Gummesson et al. [10] describe a project in Sweden that uses clinical reasoning to enrich the understanding of different roles in interprofessional settings. The study sought to investigate how clinical teamwork could be integrated into nursing and physiotherapy theory courses through experiential learning. Authentic narratives drawn from real-life scenarios bridged theoretical concepts with practical application, fostering a contextual understanding of clinical reasoning in patient care contexts. By emphasizing the social interactions between healthcare professionals, patients, and families, the model recognized the nuanced reasoning influenced by profession and context. By engaging students in reflective discussions of the sequential narratives, the model deepened the understanding of core competencies and promoted self-assessment in interprofessional settings. This innovative approach not only addressed educational barriers but also promoted collaborative learning and interaction between different professional groups, demonstrating the potential for increased interprofessional engagement in academic coursework [10].

Interprofessional Case Conferences

Improving interprofessional healthcare interactions through effective communication based on shared visions and mutual respect is critical to fostering teamwork, treatment coordination, and ultimately more efficient care for individuals managing chronic conditions. The introduction of interprofessional case conferences, as in the example by Posenau and Handgraaf [18] from Germany, is a valuable educational tool to enhance understanding of different healthcare roles, cultivate tailored communication strategies for goal setting and decision-making, and formulate interprofessional care plans. These conferences follow a structured, task-specific format that includes discussion of organizational aspects, clarification of health contexts, definition of interprofessional care strategies, and reflection on communication dynamics. Emphasizing the need for a comprehensive approach that goes beyond mere skills orientation, such as communication techniques, underlines the complexity and importance of these interprofessional dialogues in optimizing patient care outcomes [18].

Interprofessional Journal Clubs

Preparing students for the complexities of professional practice is a significant challenge for undergraduate health professions educators. To address this, Berger et al. [2] introduced journal clubs to provide students with immersive interprofessional experiences in moderately complex settings. They implemented an approach that began with a comprehensive 90-min introduction to journal clubs at the start of the semester, equipping students with the skills to engage critically, ask questions, and gain deeper insights. Following this, students were organized into small interprofessional groups of four to five members from various healthcare settings. Each group focused on a specific English-language research article related to interprofessional collaboration and met independently throughout the semester as journal clubs to analyze their assigned articles and prepare joint presentations. Despite having limited prior experience with teamwork, the 15 interprofessional groups demonstrated notable growth and cohesion. Their willingness to navigate cognitive and collaborative challenges, step beyond their comfort zones, and actively participate in interprofessional collaboration highlights the potential for first-year students to develop essential teamwork skills early in their education [2].

Simulation-Based IPL

Simulations provide a safe environment for healthcare practice, replicating complex real-life scenarios without putting real patients at risk. Typically conducted in small groups or larger gatherings of 20–30 participants, small group interprofessional simulations may require repetition for full participation. Recent advances have led to the development of large group simulations that can accommodate hundreds of participants and follow a structured progression from orientation to debriefing. In a Finnish study focusing on sudden infant death syndrome in a large group simulation, participants found the scenario realistic, engaging, and beneficial for gaining insight into interprofessional collaboration, highlighting the success of large group simulations in bridging education and professional practice [20].

A Contemporary Case Study from the United Kingdom

A Threaded IPE Offering at King's College London

King's College London is arguably one of the largest universities in Europe by student number and is responsible for the delivery of education to several different health profession student groups. A unique aspect of the student experience at King's is the opportunity to be involved in IPE with peers at similar stages from different programs. The IPE offering at King's includes 16 different health professions programs, from four different health faculties. Students are invited to attend IPE Workshops at different points in their program. By the end of their program, students would have had the opportunity to attend several different IPE Workshops. The overall aim is to equip students with the skills to work and learn collaboratively alongside different health professionals upon graduation.

IPE Workshops at King's College London

The number of IPE Workshops offered has varied over the years, with new workshops continually being considered and existing workshops reviewed. At the time of writing (2024), there are eight different IPE Workshops that students can attend

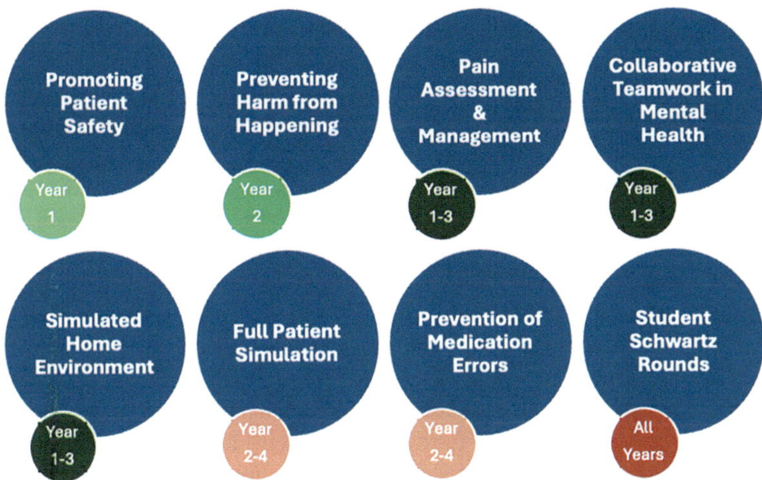

Fig. 1 IPE Workshops at King's College London (2024)

based on their year of study (see Fig. 1). The workshops are designed considering both the student groups and the intended learning outcomes. Not every workshop will necessarily include all professions; this is to ensure that students who do attend are able to contribute meaningfully to the workshop and the contents are relevant to their program.

Workshops vary in length from 1 to 9 h of didactic content with additional group-work time. For example, the Student Schwartz Round Workshop is maintained for 1 h following guidelines by the Point of Care Foundation.[1] Student group sizes also vary: there may be small groups (6–10 students) in Full Patient Simulation compared to larger facilitated groups, such as in the Pain Assessment and Management Workshop, with over 20 students. Each workshop is run several times throughout the year to accommodate for the large student numbers (>1500): either multiple workshops run in parallel on the same day, by multiple facilitators, or the workshop is spread over several workshop dates.

The educational methods are also matched to optimizing achievement of the learning outcome. For example, the Simulated Home Environment Workshop uses computer-based simulation; the Full Patient Simulation Workshop includes high-fidelity mannequins within King's three simulation centers with facilitated structured debriefing; the Pain Assessment and Management Workshop utilizes case-based discussion and whole-group discussions; and, the Collaborative Teamwork in Mental Health Workshop includes Patient Educators with lived experience. Detailed aspects of the workshop are continually evaluated and appraised, and thus, all aspects of the workshop are subject to modification.

[1] https://www.pointofcarefoundation.org.uk/our-programmes/schwartz-rounds/.

An Example Workshop in Detail: Promoting Patient Safety

The Promoting Patient Safety Workshop is open to all first-year students, some of whom will attend the workshop in the first few weeks of commencing their program. The workshop consists of three sessions, each 3 h long, delivered over 3 consecutive weeks. Sessions two and three build on the contents from the previous week. The sessions cover areas such as professionalism, role identity, teams, teamworking, and communication. A core aspect of the workshop is to foster a sense of psychological safety amongst the students and convey the value of IPE for their own learning, as well as for patient-centered care. The module includes different educational modalities, including the use of abstract tasks, small-group discussions, video analysis activities, and short didactic content. Pre-recorded material, presentations, and worksheets are used to help facilitate content delivery. There is also time at the end of the workshop for students to reflect upon their first IPL experience. Each of the three sessions also includes time for faculty reflections—a key component of the workshop lifecycle.

The IPE Workshop Lifecycle: A Continuous Process of Design, Delivery, and Improvement

The delivery of the workshop is a small part of the entire workshop lifecycle. Each workshop has a named lead or co-leads who are responsible for various stages of the workshop lifecycle. The lifecycle of an IPE workshop involves several key stages to ensure its continuous improvement and effectiveness (see Fig. 2). It begins with the design and refinement of the workshop content, followed by the preparation of a faculty pack and the development of training material. Training material may include faculty presentations, lesson plans, and pre-recorded videos by the lead(s) providing details of the workshop. This approach helps to standardize the delivery of core components. Workshop facilitators will then attend training led by the workshop lead(s). This session is recorded for future playback and is an opportunity for facilitators to ask various questions regarding the lesson plan, planned activities, and logistical issues.

The workshop is then delivered to students, after which feedback is collected from both students and faculty. Faculty feedback may be collected in multiple ways: (a) verbal feedback immediately after a workshop session; (b) written feedback in the form of a faculty evaluation survey; and (c) as part of a formal end-of-year workshop review meeting. The review meeting is a planned activity that includes core members of the IPE Steering Group—a senior group of IPE leads across Faculties—with the aim of analyzing feedback and overall effectiveness. Based on this analysis, modifications are made to the workshop content and structure. Modifications may also be made based on other considerations, such as student groups and numbers, other logistical issues, and the need to change or incorporate new learning outcomes. National and local research, frameworks, guidelines, policies, and reports may also drive change. If significant changes are required, there

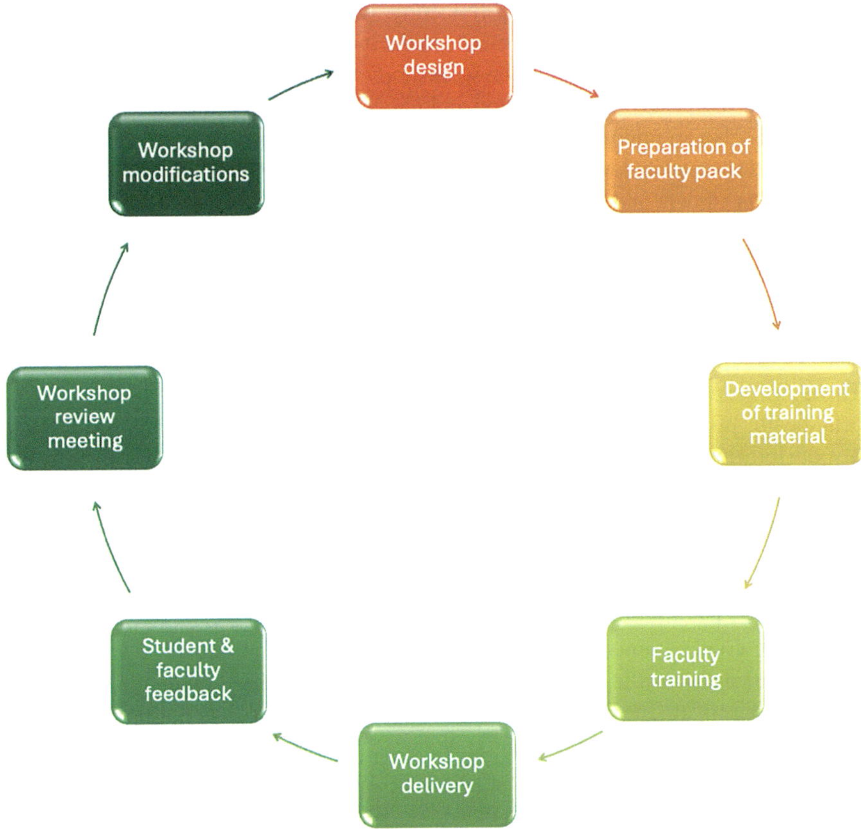

Fig. 2 The IPE Workshop Lifecycle at King's

may be benefits from the formation of a working group. The workshop is modified in preparation for delivery in the next academic year. This iterative process ensures that the workshop evolves and improves year on year.

Organization and Delivery of IPE at King's

The success of the program is driven by the strong administrative support and buy-in from senior-level decision makers at King's. Administration support is essential for aspects such as liaising with program leads to identify suitable workshop dates; facilitating room bookings; assigning students to session dates; assigning students to smaller sub-groups in the sessions; creating a faculty pool from which facilitators can be recruited; facilitating faculty and student evaluation; and helping support workshop review meetings.

Although each workshop has a designated lead, these individuals do not operate or lead workshops independently. There is a collective steering group composed of all workshop and IPE leads from each faculty, senior leaders, and research leads. Members of the steering group contribute to the individual workshop review meetings and may help support changes to the workshops. The steering group also meets four times a year to discuss each workshop and identify challenges or potential upcoming issues. It is also an opportunity to discuss potential new workshops. Finally, there is an IPE end of year review meeting that is often longer and looks at cross-workshop themes from student and faculty evaluation, reflects on success, provides an opportunity to look at recent IPE literature, and strategizes IPE delivery for the future.

Discussion and Conclusion

Through IPL activities such as case-based discussions, simulations, and team projects, health profession students across Europe gain valuable insight into the roles, responsibilities, and perspectives of other healthcare professionals [7]. The learning objectives for IPE activities in Europe are often, but not exclusively, derived from existing frameworks, such as IPEC [14]. When designing interprofessional activities, the core competencies of (a) values and ethics, (b) roles and responsibilities, (c) communication, and (d) teams and teamwork can be helpful to consider as learning outcomes [22].

Finding good patient cases is not that easy. One source of authentic and credible patient narratives is the DIPEx project (https://dipexinternational.org/), which is embedded into an international network of 14 countries, including the Czech Republic, Germany, the Netherlands, Norway, Slovakia, Spain, Switzerland, and the United Kingdom. The website covers more than 180 different diseases or health topics, which have been systematically collected, evaluated, and presented following an established method [9].

When implementing IPL, early planning, promoting student responsibility, considering cultural differences between departments, and explicitly considering teamwork are beneficial [8]. Case studies are good for promoting interprofessional interaction, preparing students to think critically, making the case for interprofessional collaboration, seeing problems through another's eyes, and sharing perspectives through constructive feedback [13].

If, as at King's College London, IPL opportunities are a focus in health professions education, it requires a variety of well-designed programmed sessions offered throughout the undergraduate curriculum. Administrative support, site identification, and facilitators training are all important, as is the evaluation of the activities to inform possible modifications to the workshops.

Reflective Questions for the Reader

The examples shared in this chapter aim to inspire educators to replicate, modify, and integrate these innovative and practical IPL activities within their unique educational settings. Although organizing interprofessional courses requires the combined efforts of organizations, teams, and individuals and is challenging, especially when several institutions work together, it is worth the effort.

- What are some of the fundamental interprofessional skills and attributes we want to equip European health profession students upon graduation?
- Which theories and teaching methods are best suited to underpinning IPE in Europe?
- When during education are IPL activities useful, and which student groups should participate?
- How can the effectiveness of IPL activities be measured to determine the benefit for students and ultimately for healthcare?
- How can decision-makers be convinced that the effort (personnel, administration, time for the entire workshop lifecycle, rooms, etc.) is worthwhile?
- What are some of the challenges of initiating and maintaining an IPL offering?
- What does a successful interprofessional faculty development program look like in your European context?
- How can educators gain competencies to develop IPL activities?

References

1. Barr H. Interprofessional education: today, yesterday and tomorrow: a review. London: Higher Education Academy, Health Sciences and Practice Network; 2005. (Occasional Paper no 1).
2. Berger S, Whelan B, Mahler C, Szecsenyi J, Krug K. Encountering complexity in collaborative learning activities: an exploratory case study with undergraduate health professionals. J Interprof Care. 2019;33(5):490–6. https://doi.org/10.1080/13561820.2018.1562423.
3. Berghout T. How are nurse educators prepared to teach interprofessional practice? Nurse Educ Today. 2021;98:104745. https://doi.org/10.1016/j.nedt.2021.104745.
4. Bogossian F, New K, George K, Barr N, Dodd N, Hamilton AL, et al. The implementation of interprofessional education: a scoping review. Adv Health Sci Educ Theory Pract. 2023;28(1):243–77. https://doi.org/10.1007/s10459-022-10128-4.
5. Caduff U, Bärlocher A, Staudacher D. Interprofessionalität lernen und leben. PADUA. 2021;16(4):223–7. https://doi.org/10.1024/1861-6186/a000632.
6. Colonnello V, Kinoshita Y, Yoshida N, Bustos Villalobos I. Undergraduate interprofessional education in the European higher education area: a systematic review. IME. 2023;2(2):100–12. https://doi.org/10.3390/ime2020010.
7. Da Rodrigues Silva Noll Gonçalves J, Noll Gonçalves R, Da Rosa SV, Schaia Rocha Orsi J, Santos de Paula KM, Moysés SJ, Werneck RI. Potentialities and limitations of interprofessional education during graduation: a systematic review and thematic synthesis of qualitative studies. BMC Med Educ. 2023;23(1):236. https://doi.org/10.1186/s12909-023-04211-6.
8. Evans CH, Cashman SB, Page DA, Garr DR. Model approaches for advancing interprofessional prevention education. Am J Prev Med. 2011;40(2):245–60. https://doi.org/10.1016/j.amepre.2010.10.014.
9. Glässel A, Zumstein P, Scherer T, Feusi E, Biller Andorno N. Case vignettes for simulated patients based on real patient experiences in the context of OSCE examinations: workshop experiences from interprofessional education. GMS J Med Educ. 2021;38(5):Doc91. https://doi.org/10.3205/zma001487.
10. Gummesson C, Sundén A, Fex A. Clinical reasoning as a conceptual framework for interprofessional learning: a literature review and a case study. Phys Ther Rev. 2018;23(1):29–34. https://doi.org/10.1080/10833196.2018.1450327.

11. Guraya SY, Barr H. The effectiveness of interprofessional education in healthcare: a systematic review and meta-analysis. Kaohsiung J Med Sci. 2018;34(3):160–5. https://doi.org/10.1016/j.kjms.2017.12.009.
12. Hean S, Green C, Anderson E, Morris D, John C, Pitt R, O'Halloran C. The contribution of theory to the design, delivery, and evaluation of interprofessional curricula: BEME guide no. 49. Med Teach. 2018;40(6):542–58. https://doi.org/10.1080/0142159X.2018.1432851.
13. Henry B, Garner C, Guernon A. Teaching and learning about interprofessional collaboration through student-designed case study and analysis. Int J Teach Learn High Educ. 2018;30(3):560–70. https://eric.ed.gov/?id=EJ1199345
14. Interprofessional Education Collaborative. IPEC core competencies for interprofessional collaborative practice. Version 3. Washington, DC: Interprofessional Education Collaborative; 2023. Online verfügbar unter https://www.ipecollaborative.org/ipec-core-competencies. Zuletzt aktualisiert am 27.03.2024, zuletzt geprüft am 27.03.2024.
15. Kricheldorff C, Heimbach B, Himmelsbach I, Schumann H. Interprofessionelle Teambildung—ein hochschulübergreifendes Qualifizierungsprogramm. Z Gerontol Geriatr. 2022;55(3):197–203. https://doi.org/10.1007/s00391-022-02021-x.
16. Levett-Jones T, Burdett T, Chow YL, Jönsson L, Lasater K, Mathews LR, et al. Case studies of interprofessional education initiatives from five countries. J Nurs Scholarsh. 2018;50(3):324–32. https://doi.org/10.1111/jnu.12384.
17. Machin LL, Bellis KM, Dixon C, Morgan H, Pye J, Spencer P, Williams RA. Interprofessional education and practice guide: designing ethics-orientated interprofessional education for health and social care students. J Interprof Care. 2019;33(6):608–18. https://doi.org/10.1080/13561820.2018.1538113.
18. Posenau A, Handgraaf M. Framework for interprofessional case conferences - empirically sound and competence-oriented communication concept for interprofessional teaching. GMS J Med Educ. 2021;38(3):Doc65. https://doi.org/10.3205/zma001461.
19. Rinnhofer C, Steininger-Kaar K, Igelsböck E, Hochstöger D, Öhlinger S. Joint learning for improvement - interprofessional competence development within the framework of a co-operative project between the University of Applied Sciences for Health Professions Upper Austria and the Medical Faculty of Johannes Kepler University Linz. GMS J Med Educ. 2022;39(2):Doc18. https://doi.org/10.3205/zma001539.
20. Saaranen T, Silén-Lipponen M, Palkolahti M, Mönkkönen K, Tiihonen M, Sormunen M. Interprofessional learning in social and health care-learning experiences from large-group simulation in Finland. Nurs Open. 2020;7(6):1978–87. https://doi.org/10.1002/nop2.589.
21. Shakhovskoy R, Dodd N, Masters N, New K, Hamilton A, Nash G, et al. Recommendations for the design of interprofessional education: findings from a narrative scoping review. FoHPE. 2022;23(4):82–117. https://doi.org/10.11157/fohpe.v23i4.608.
22. van Diggele C, Roberts C, Burgess A, Mellis C. Interprofessional education: tips for design and implementation. BMC Med Educ. 2020;20(Suppl 2):455. https://doi.org/10.1186/s12909-020-02286-z.
23. WHO. Framework for action on interprofessional education & collaborative practice. World Health Organization; 2010. https://www.who.int/publications/i/item/framework-for-action-on-interprofessional-education-collaborative-practice. Zuletzt geprüft am 28.03.2024.

Heidi Schimatzek is the head of the Bachelor's and Master's programs in Biomedical Sciences at the Health University of Applied Sciences Tyrol, Innsbruck. In 2009, she developed and implemented an interprofessional Master's program in Health Professions Education. As the person responsible for interprofessional modules, she is committed to networking with teachers and students at the Health University. Heidi is involved in the D-A-CH Association for Medical Education—Section Austria and is on the extended board of the Society of Interprofessional Health Care, IP-Health.

Ranjev Kainth is a general pediatrician in London with a special interest in clinical education. He is an Interprofessional Fellow at King's College London, where he also leads the Simulation in Clinical Education module as part of the postgraduate program in clinical education. Ranjev's research interests include interaction analysis, clinical education, and simulation-based education, focusing particularly on simulation debriefing.

Think Big, Start Small: Interprofessional Learning in a Workplace-Based Context

Catrine Buck Jensen, Tove Törnqvist, Anika Mitzkat, Marion Huber, and Rene Ballnus

Abbreviations

IPE	Interprofessional education
IPL	Interprofessional learning
IPTW	Interprofessional training ward

C. Buck Jensen
Department of Health and Care Sciences, UiT The Arctic University of Norway, Tromsø, Norway
e-mail: catrine.b.jensen@uit.no

T. Törnqvist
Department of Health, Medicine and Caring Sciences, Linköping University, Linköping, Sweden
e-mail: tove.tornqvist@liu.se

A. Mitzkat
Department of General Practice and Health Services Research, University Hospital Heidelberg, Heidelberg, Germany
e-mail: Anika.Mitzkat@med.uni-heidelberg.de

M. Huber
Institute of Public Health, Zurich University of Applied Sciences – ZHAW, School of Health Sciences, Winterthur, Switzerland
e-mail: marion.huber@zhaw.ch

R. Ballnus (✉)
Unit of Teaching and Learning, Karolinska Institutet, Solna, Sweden
e-mail: rene.ballnus@ki.se

A. Xyrichis et al. (eds.), *Building Bridges: A European Perspective on Interprofessional Education, Practice, Policy and Research*,
https://doi.org/10.1007/978-3-032-23222-9_15

Introduction

So far in this book, we have learnt about the importance of interprofessional collaboration, what it is, and how it can be executed in different situations. With this chapter, we aim to continue to unravel the complexity of interprofessional collaboration by focusing on interprofessional learning in workplace-based contexts.

The foundation of this chapter is based on the claim that "learning occurs best in context" ([5], p. 36). This statement is in line with learning theories that focus on contextual and experiential learning [57]. Knowledge is hereby situated within a context, and learning is a response to and constructed within this context. Learning that comes from interacting with patients or clients in a real practical context is fundamental to the education of healthcare professionals; there is simply no alternative [39]. Workplace-based contexts provide students with authentic learning experiences and the experience of responsibility for real persons in need of care, where they encounter various people either for healthcare prevention, actively receiving care and treatment, or following up previous treatments [20].

What Is the Purpose of This Chapter?

The goal of this chapter is to motivate and guide educators across various settings to initiate and enhance interprofessional learning activities within their workplace environments. We aim to empower those involved in interprofessional education and practice to embrace ambitious ideas while recognizing the value of starting with manageable initiatives—think big but start small. This chapter will explore a range of interprofessional learning activities, highlighting their complexity, the level of student responsibility in patient care, and the extent to which they are structured or occur spontaneously.

We will present and discuss several examples of interprofessional activities. Some are well-established and thoroughly evaluated within the field, and these will be discussed in greater detail. Others may be newer or less recognized, and while we will not delve as deeply into these, it is important to note that their value is not diminished. The selection and depth of discussion are influenced by the available literature and our own experiences with conducting interprofessional workplace-based learning, which we are eager to share.

Understanding Workplace-Based Interprofessional Learning

In Europe, various linguistic conventions have evolved to describe clinical interprofessional education and learning. This chapter employs the term "workplace-based learning", which aptly consolidates these diverse methodologies. It encompasses all educational activities within the daily work setting, characterized by three core elements: practical/clinical work, learning processes, and the environment [39]. The Josiah M. Jr. Foundation [28] defines learning environments as "…social interactions, organizational cultures and structures, and physical and virtual spaces that surround and shape participants' experiences, perceptions, and learning" (p. 36). Given current challenges like labor shortages, it is crucial that the learning environment also fosters educational opportunities, optimizing both climate and workload. Ma et al. [33] note, "the pressure to perform impairs learning opportunities, leading to cognitive overload" (p. 8). Poor communication and collaboration among professionals can result in adverse patient outcomes and increased clinical errors (e.g., [21, 27]). Thus, workplace-based interprofessional learning is advocated as a strategy for students and professionals to acquire teamwork skills and understand colleagues' roles [29]. Activities vary in complexity and resource requirements. This chapter outlines these activities across a complexity spectrum, emphasizing real-life scenario handling. Learning extends beyond students to include professional teams and patients, fostering interprofessional skills development and aligning with lifelong learning concepts.

Historical Perspectives and Early Initiatives

Historically, interprofessional collaboration has been recognized as crucial for advancing healthcare over several decades, with significant discussions on preparing and supporting healthcare professionals to develop interprofessional competencies [2, 15, 55, 56]. Over the past 30 years, there has been a global rise in interprofessional education initiatives [14], with workplace-based interprofessional learning being a key component.

The first European initiatives in this domain emerged in the mid-1990s in Linköping, Sweden, where the world's first interprofessional training ward (IPTW) was established through a partnership between Linköping University and Linköping University Hospital. This initiative expanded the university's IPE curriculum from theoretical to more practical-oriented studies.

Subsequently, a political decision in Stockholm led to the creation of IPTWs in four hospitals as a 3-year project, which, after a positive evaluation, became an implemented practice. Initially, IPTWs were set up in orthopedic wards for practical reasons and because orthopedic patients benefited from the competencies of the involved professional study programs. Later, IPTWs expanded to other disciplines such as geriatric and stroke units.

In these settings, undergraduates typically engage in learning activities in their senior years, ideally after theoretical and, in some cases, interprofessional simulation-based activities. Recent literature indicates emerging new models for organizing interprofessional workplace-based training [3, 34, 54], emphasizing the need for students to practice, not just learn about, interprofessional collaboration in practical settings.

Foundations for Interprofessional Learning in a Workplace-Based Context

Interprofessional learning in a workplace-based context features three key elements: (1) patient encounters, (2) facilitator support, and (3) reflection on actions.

Role of Patients

In workplace-basede settings, students interact with individuals receiving care or treatment, including clients and service users. The term "patients" is used broadly here. Recently, the Interprofessional Education Collaborative (IPEC) core competencies [22] have recognized patients as equal team members. Historically, the role of patients in interprofessional learning has been underemphasized, but there is a growing call for their active involvement, recognizing their experiences as valuable learning resources [23, 25, 46, 51].

Role of Facilitators

Facilitators are crucial in supporting interprofessional learning. They are often referred to by various terms, such as mentors, clinical supervisors, or placement teachers. Their role extends beyond profession-specific learning, sometimes challenging them to focus on broader educational aspects such as communication, roles, ethics, and teamwork [10, 12, 22]. There is potential for enhancing patient-centeredness in facilitation [24, 25], and efforts are underway to develop frameworks for training and assessing facilitator competencies [43].

Role of Reflection

Critical reflection is a major domain of interprofessional learning as defined by the World Health Organization [55]. It involves examining and exploring issues triggered by experiences, leading to new perspectives [6]. Reflection can occur individually or collaboratively and is supported by frameworks like Gibbs' reflective cycle [17]. Effective reflection requires shared experiences among students to trigger meaningful dialogue and learning [58].

Cultivating Foundational Skills

In the following, we focus on current workplace-based interprofessional activities along a complexity continuum that serve the purpose of cultivating foundational skills. We start with structured and very complex interprofessional learning activities, which may also require a high level of resources. Moreover, a variety of less complex activities are highlighted to inspire small-scale activities. See a visualization of the variety of activities in Fig. 1.

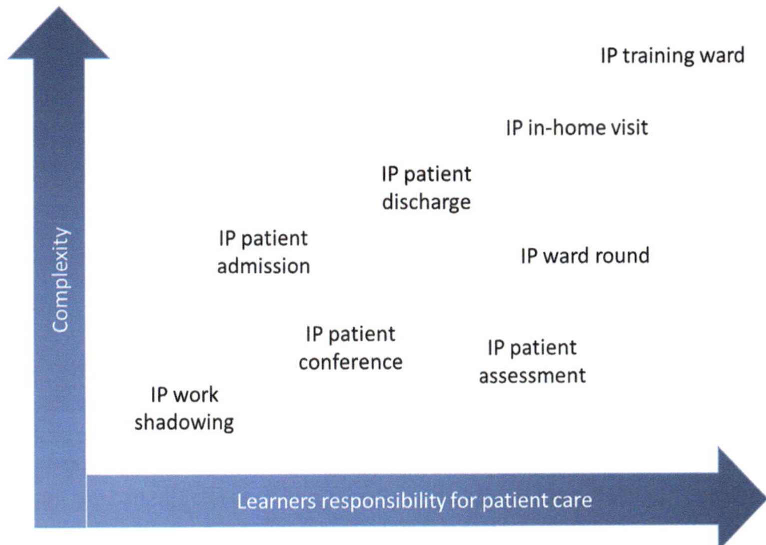

Fig. 1 Visualization of interprofessional workplace-based learning activities based on our experiences and presented in the text (own presentation)

Structured Initiatives

By structured activities, we mean learning activities that are organized, for instance, by a higher education institution, often in close collaboration with the organization where the activity takes place. These activities are included in a curriculum as elective or compulsory learning activities and serve to support students in developing a deep understanding of interprofessional collaboration and holistic person-centered care.

Interprofessional Training Wards

An IPTW is a clinical ward where students from multiple healthcare professions (e.g., medical, nursing, physiotherapy, occupational therapy, and pharmacy) collaboratively manage patient care [42]. Across Europe, IPTWs are implemented with varying designs, but generally, they involve students working as interprofessional teams for 2–4 weeks in a hospital ward or primary care facility dedicated to student learning. Supported by a facilitator, these teams are responsible for the comprehensive care of four to six patients, managing these patients from admission to discharge [48, 53].

In Sweden, IPTWs include a range of student professions and are a mandatory part of the curriculum. The first IPTWs in Germany were established in 2017 in cities such as Heidelberg [36]), Mannheim [35], and Freiburg [4] and have since expanded to other locations. The first IPTW in Zurich, Switzerland, "ZIPAS", was introduced in 2019 [52].

Studies have highlighted IPTWs as safe learning environments that foster interprofessional collaboration [18, 19]. Recent findings suggest that IPTWs enhance short-term collaborative competencies, though long-term impacts are less understood [37, 38, 42].

Key success factors for IPTWs include a joint office for all involved professions, facilitating knowledge exchange and integrating interprofessional patient conferences into daily routines [49, 52]. Interprofessional ward rounds, where professions take turns leading, promote a holistic approach to patient care.

Despite positive outcomes, careful planning is essential for IPTWs to effectively convey the complexities of interprofessional collaboration. Recent studies emphasize the importance of arrangement and conscious decision-making in organizing interprofessional learning activities. For instance, Törnqvist et al. [47–49] and Jensen et al. [23, 24] point to the arrangement and how it can support students to share knowledge, negotiate tasks and competencies, as well as include patients or clients in their interprofessional collaboration. These studies bring attention to the importance of becoming aware of how educators do things, matter for students' learning, and how conscious decisions are important when arranging interprofessional learning activities.

In-Home Visits

In-home visits involve interprofessional student teams visiting a person's home with specific learning objectives tailored to the nature of the interprofessional activity. These visits can target individuals already receiving services like home care or aim to assess and recommend preventive or health-promotion measures for demographics such as elderly individuals living independently [16] or families with complex needs [32].

The structure of in-home visits typically encompasses several phases: a preparatory phase, the visit itself, and a debriefing phase. For example, in Norway, Jentoft [26] details how students review the person's discharge summaries and discuss key issues as a team before the visit. Similarly, Toth-Pal et al. [50] describe a process where students familiarize themselves with a brief patient summary and delineate team responsibilities ahead of the visit. The visit may be conducted as an informal conversation or a more structured interview with prepared questions.

In Switzerland, a specialized version of in-home visits focuses on providing low-threshold support to single-parent families. Here, interprofessional teams consisting of two students each work closely with a single-parent family. This initiative also follows a three-phase approach: defining the family's needs and available resources, providing support over approximately 6 months, and concluding with a final reflection meeting. Throughout this period, students receive monthly online coaching from facilitators.

In-home visits can vary in duration. Longer visits emphasize relationship building and are also structured in three phases: identifying support needs and building trust, implementing practical support, and concluding with a reflective or debriefing session led by a supervisor or facilitator. According to Larsen et al. [31], trust and security are crucial for effective interprofessional collaboration from the perspectives of patients and service recipients.

Other Structured Learning Activities

Further, we present a variety of structured learning activities, some of which are well implemented, while others are pilot projects that have not yet been fully implemented.

The Centre for Interdisciplinary Workplace Learning (TVEPS) in Bergen, Norway, annually brings together senior year students from 17 professions and disciplines to engage with individuals with diverse needs across various settings. In the healthcare setting, students are mainly located in primary care, such as nursing homes. The arrangement also includes in-home visits, interaction with inmates in correctional services, or service users of Healthy Life Centers, which address lifestyle-related issues. The interprofessional student teams interview the patients/service users they encounter and develop care plans with suggestions to improve their health conditions and quality of life, which they share with the staff in the workplace in a dialogue meeting [1]. This model has proven to be a sustainable approach to interprofessional learning since its inception in 2012.

In Stockholm, Sweden, an innovative approach for interprofessional learning has been piloted in a prehospital setting. Here, undergraduate medical and nursing students joined the ambulance service for one day. The findings from a follow-up-study on the initiative showed how students had learning outcomes throughout the chain of care. From the moment, they received information about the patient to the arrival at the place where the person was located and the measures being implemented at the location and in the ambulance on the way to the emergency care unit [8]. Conte et al. [8] emphasize how interprofessional training in the ambulance service is an unfamiliar environment, with no hierarchical structures or stereotypes that often exist in other parts of healthcare. This serves students with good opportunities for interprofessional learning.

In Switzerland, students from five healthcare professions (midwifery, nursing, physiotherapy, health prevention, and occupational therapy) are brought together to solve joint tasks in pairs during their placements. Learners choose an interprofessional activity or process that they subsequently analyze. This could include a joint diagnostic process or a joint treatment. In addition to the profession-specific significance, the aim is to identify the interprofessional core aspects of the activity. Each student writes their own reflection report, and their partner provides feedback. Once the report and the feedback have been completed, students register for an educator-led World Café where experience-sharing and reflection are central.

In Northern Norway, a pragmatic interprofessional learning activity is integrated into an ordinary clinical placement in a community health center by having students from different study programs whose placements overlap working collaboratively for 2–4 days (see context description in, for instance, [23, 24, 47–49]). Organization varies between the different placement periods; however, common to them all is a shared responsibility for daily care and follow-up of two to four patients.

The final example we present is a pilot recently conducted in the United Kingdom, where interprofessional student teams undertook 6-week cycles in care homes, encountering a small number of residents working on the residents' personal goals. In this project, like the Norwegian initiative TVEPS, students from disciplines outside health care also joined the placement (e.g., sports rehabilitation students). The students' presence varied; some were on-site full-time, while other students were present part-time. The interprofessional student teams met weekly following the principles of action learning when reflecting on their encounters. [45].

Seizing Everyday Opportunities

Interprofessional learning activities do not have to include extensive organization and access to resources to be realized. It is unnecessary to turn a ward upside-down or to restructure a whole department for interprofessional students. Facilitators who have knowledge and experience in interprofessional education will be able to identify many daily situations where students have interprofessional learning opportunities. In the following, we will exemplify different interprofessional learning activities that can be feasible on the go.

Interprofessional Patient Conferences

Interprofessional patient conferences are essential in both specialized and primary care settings, known variably as interprofessional case conferences [41] or interprofessional ward rounds [38]. According to O'Brien et al. [41], these conferences are "interactive, facilitated, case-based group discussions with specific educational goals, involving members from at least two health professions working collaboratively to enhance patient care" (p. 1214).

Interprofessional patient conferences must set explicit goals for both students and patients and be structured to ensure these objectives are met. Students may facilitate interprofessional communication, or a facilitator might assist, emphasizing the unique and overlapping competencies of the different professions attending.

Key considerations include coordinating participants (patients, students, and facilitators), accessing resources (e.g., electronic patient records), and ensuring that the physical space supports team interaction [41].

Patient conferences can be integrated into daily routines, focusing on patients involved in the students' regular care, although involvement of all students in direct care is not mandatory. Regular discussions can be scheduled if all students are involved in care. If only one student is actively involved, they should brief the team on the patient's status. Ideally, the patient participates, sharing their history and needs, which then informs the care plan and goal setting during the conference.

Interprofessional Ward Rounds

If more than one profession works with a patient/client, an interprofessional ward round can be planned without major difficulties. Goals for the ward round and roles (e.g., who will lead the conversation with the patient), as well as the questions for the visit, must be clarified in advance. Subsequently, a conversation and, if need be, an examination takes place with the patient. The aim for the ward round could, for instance, be to articulate a common goal for the next 7 days. If there are existing ward round guidelines in the institution, it is worth basing an interprofessional ward round on these.

A pivotal aspect of interprofessional clinical learning is recognizing that a ward round need not always be led by a physician, although this remains the common practice. Implementing a rotational leadership model can be highly beneficial, where each professional takes a turn at leading the round. Different professions prioritize different types of information: nurses might focus on self-care or care needs, occupational therapists on elements crucial for daily activities, physiotherapists on structural and functional issues, and medical professionals on clinical aspects. Embracing these diverse perspectives in conducting ward rounds can foster a more holistic view of patient care, aligning with the goals of an interprofessional approach.

Interprofessional Assessments, Examinations, Treatment, and Care

Interprofessional assessments, examinations, treatment, and care can be seamlessly integrated into daily routines, like interprofessional ward rounds. These activities might involve students collaborating on diagnostic tests or patient care.

A crucial step is the comparison and preparation of diagnostic instruments and objectives. It is important for all involved to understand the specific "tests" being used, addressing questions like "How do you measure this or that?" in the assessment process.

From the patient's perspective, it often appears that tests are duplicated across professions due to different diagnostic goals. For instance, the Romberg test, used to identify specific neurological impairments [13], serves multiple purposes: doctors use it for diagnosis, physiotherapists assess balance for functional interventions, and occupational therapists might use it to practice daily activities with the patient. The key is not who performs the test but ensuring the results are communicated across all relevant professions, ideally with all present during the test.

In cases of high patient complexity, dual treatment or care, such as assisting with morning routines or mobilization, is common. These activities can be managed by interprofessional students under the guidance of a facilitator. It's essential to discuss common goals and clarify roles and responsibilities beforehand, as multiple professions might perform the same tasks. For example, mobilizing a patient with severe tetraparesis from bed to wheelchair involves nurses, occupational therapists, and physiotherapists. The focus should be on preventing complications and stabilizing circulation, with clear communication about who leads and who handles specific tasks.

Interprofessional Admissions, Discharge, and Handovers

Integrating joint patient admissions, particularly for elective admissions, offers a practical approach to interprofessional learning. This setting is ideal for nursing and medical students to collaborate on planning and conducting the admission process. The activity typically involves a comprehensive conversation with the patient about their medical and health history, followed by the development of an interprofessional care and treatment plan. Prior to admission, it is crucial to clarify roles, such as who will lead the session and which examinations are needed, along with who will perform them. This planning stage emphasizes the importance of negotiation, a key component of this learning activity. Through negotiation, participants not only enhance their communicative skills but also gain insights into the dynamics of power and hierarchy within clinical settings, which are often perceived as fluid and varying [40]. Following the initial admission, a follow-up period is necessary to finalize the interprofessional care and treatment plan, ensuring that roles and responsibilities are clearly defined and documented.

Discharge planning inherently involves multiple professions, making it an organic interprofessional learning activity. To enhance this aspect further, it is beneficial to allow students ample preparation time. Ideally, discharge planning should commence at the time of admission, particularly given the trend toward shorter hospital stays.

A crucial element of effective discharge management is the transfer of comprehensive patient information (handovers) to subsequent service providers. Handovers are defined as "The exchange between health professionals of information about a patient accompanying either a transfer of control over, or of responsibility for, the patient" ([7], p. 494). These are situations that occur every day within healthcare and serve as a natural opportunity for training in interprofessional communication.

Students can utilize standardized communication tools such as (I)SBAR [11], which was specifically designed to accommodate varying communication styles [44]. Tools like ISBAR may ensure clear and consistent communication during transitions like discharge or handovers. Additionally, visualizing the care trajectory can aid in making interprofessional discharge planning a practical learning opportunity. This approach encourages students to consider the needs of all service providers involved, focusing on the specific information each requires.

Incorporating training on standardized handover protocols can significantly enhance interprofessional communication and can be seamlessly integrated into both clinical and outpatient settings. This not only improves the discharge process but also enriches the educational experience for students, preparing them for real-world interprofessional collaboration.

Work Shadowing

The primary goal of work shadowing is to foster an understanding of another profession and familiarize participants with its core tasks.

Work shadowing is an accessible interprofessional learning activity that can vary in duration, from brief periods focusing on specific tasks to full-day or multiple-day experiences. This practice allows students to gain insights into the roles of other professionals, as highlighted by Kusnoor and Stelljes [30], and can be implemented as a short-term intervention.

Reflective questions such as "What can I learn from this profession?" or "What do I know about the core task of the other profession?" can facilitate brief yet meaningful discussions. To further enhance and solidify this understanding, organizing several short workshops during workplace-based training can be effective. These workshops can be planned or initiated spontaneously, providing flexible and practical learning opportunities that deepen interprofessional knowledge and collaboration.

Challenges with Workplace-Based Interprofessional Learning

Given the diverse forms and conditions of workplace-based learning, questions arise regarding how these can be effectively integrated into the curricula of various health professions. This integration must consider the comparability of skill acquisition, the assessment of learning outcomes, and the organization of practical training in health profession education. One potential solution is to involve all relevant professional groups in the planning stages of interprofessional learning interventions. Additionally, piloting interventions within the elective or compulsory elective segments of curricula before incorporating them into mandatory components can be beneficial once positive outcomes are observed.

The organizational effort required for interprofessional workplace-based learning activities can be substantial. For instance, establishing an IPTW demands significant institutional resources, including human, financial, and spatial allocations. Moreover, it is crucial that such initiatives receive strong support from institutional management.

Effective interprofessional workplace-based learning also requires competent facilitators and supervisors. These individuals ensure a safe learning environment, safeguarding both patient safety and providing space for students to develop self-directed learning strategies and personal responsibility. Concurrent with the implementation of workplace-based interprofessional learning, there should be opportunities for faculty development in interprofessional teaching.

While promoting individual competencies and interprofessional teamwork is vital, these alone may not suffice to enhance interprofessional collaborative practice in the long term. Addressing this issue may require broader interventions aimed at changing the overall culture of collaboration.

Final Words on Bridging Theory and Practice

The literature repeatedly emphasizes that interprofessional workplace-based learning should not be a one-off intervention. Implementing workplace-based learning activities raises a classic dilemma: which should come first, akin to the chicken or the egg? If a workplace already practices interprofessional collaboration, integrating students can naturally enhance their learning. Conversely, in environments lacking such practices, introducing interprofessional student activities can illuminate potential benefits and challenges, potentially fostering a collaborative culture among health professionals involved in training.

Starting with small-scale activities, such as a reflective phone call with another professional (ideally a health professions student), can be effective. These activities can then be expanded to include work shadowing or interprofessional ward rounds, eventually scaling up to more comprehensive initiatives like IPTWs.

Research highlights a gap between interprofessional clinical student training and post-graduate clinical reality, with a notable but temporary boost in interprofessional competencies post-training. This suggests that entrenched uni-professional structures often prevent the sustained application of interprofessional skills. Transitioning to an interprofessional care culture requires interventions in both education and healthcare delivery. For instance, interprofessional structures like IPTWs should be integrated into standard care, including interprofessional ward rounds and handovers. New staff from all healthcare professions could benefit from interprofessional induction concepts, and specific training courses could promote teamwork and communication.

We would like to conclude this chapter with some recommendations based on our knowledge and experience when you aim to arrange interprofessional workplace-based activities:

- Start with manageable interactions, such as phone calls or handovers, and consider everyday opportunities like patient conferences and bedside teaching.
- Scale initiatives to include activities like work shadowing or interprofessional ward rounds, which can lay the groundwork for more complex endeavors such as IPTWs and in-home visits.
- Ensure coordination, access to resources, and adequate physical space to support successful interprofessional activities. Regular discussions, patient involvement, and clear communication of roles enhance both learning and patient care.
- Address challenges, including skill acquisition comparability, learning success assessment, and resource allocation.
- Promote faculty development and a cultural shift toward collaborative practice for sustainable interprofessional learning and practice.
- Provide students with diverse experiences involving different peers, patients, and health issues throughout their training.
- Recognize the disparity between interprofessional learning and clinical realities post-graduation, using these activities to better prepare students for professional challenges.
- Use reflective questions to identify and enhance interprofessional learning opportunities, aiming to align interprofessional collaborative practice with students' workplace-based learning processes.

Reflective Questions for the Reader

As you conclude this chapter, consider your specific context and what interprofessional learning opportunities might be feasible and beneficial. Reflect on the importance and advantages of interprofessional learning in a workplace-based setting.

- Why is it crucial for your environment?
- What initiatives could serve as a common ground for multiple professions?
- Are there any easily implementable activities, or "low-hanging fruits", that could kickstart interprofessional interactions?
- What resources are available, including location, finances, personnel, and time?
- How can these resources support your interprofessional learning goals?
- Consider the role of patients or clients in these learning experiences. How can their involvement enrich the learning process?
- What kind of facilitation is needed for effective learning, and who should provide it?
- Who are the stakeholders necessary for successful implementation? What strategies can you employ to ensure their active participation?
- Do the people involved need to be trained for the intervention? How could you do that?

By addressing these questions, you can lay a strong foundation for fostering interprofessional collaboration and learning in your workplace.

References

1. Baerheim A, Raaheim A. Pedagogical aspects of interprofessional workplace learning: a case study. J Interprof Care. 2020;34(1):59–65. https://doi.org/10.1080/13561820.2019.1621805.
2. Barr H. Working together to learn together: learning together to work together. J Interprof Care. 2000;14(2):177–9. https://doi.org/10.1080/jic.14.2.177.179.
3. Bivall A-C, Lindh Falk A, Gustavsson M. Students' interprofessional workplace learning in clinical placement. Prof Prof. 2021;11(3):e4140. https://doi.org/10.7577/pp.4140.
4. Bode SFN, Friedrich S, Straub C. 'We just did it as a team': learning and working on a paediatric interprofessional training ward improves interprofessional competencies in the short- and in the long-term. Med Teach. 2022:1–8. https://doi.org/10.1080/0142159x.2022.2128998.
5. Boud D, Cohen R, Walker D, editors. Using experience for learning. The Society for Research into Higher Education & Open University Press; 1993.
6. Boyd E, Fales A. Reflective learning: key to learning from experience. J Humanist Psychol. 1983;23(2):99–117. https://doi.org/10.1177/0022167883232011.
7. Cohen MD, Hilligoss PB. The published literature on handoffs in hospitals: deficiencies identified in an extensive review. BMJ Qual Saf. 2010;2010(19):493–7. https://doi.org/10.1136/qshc.2009.033480.
8. Conte H, Wihlborg J, Lindström V. Developing new possibilities for interprofessional learning- students' experience of learning together in the ambulance service. BMC Med Educ. 2022;22(1):192. https://doi.org/10.1186/s12909-022-03251-8.

9. Dahlberg J, et al. The Linköping journey. Sustainability and interprofessional collaboration. Ensuring leadership resilience in collaborative health care. In: Forman D, Jones M, Thistlethwaite J, editors.. Springer; 2020.
10. Davys A, Fouché C, Beddoe L. Mapping effective interprofessional supervision practice. Clin Superv. 2021;40(2):179–99. https://doi.org/10.1080/07325223.2021.1929639.
11. Denham CR. SBAR for patients. J Patient Saf. 2008;4(1):38–48. http://www.jstor.org/stable/26637647
12. Ericson A, Masiello I, Bolinder G. Interprofessional clinical training for undergraduate students in an emergency department setting. J Interprof Care. 2012;26(4):319–25. https://doi.org/10.3109/13561820.2012.676109.
13. Forbes J, Munakomi S, Cronovich H. Romberg test [Updated 2023 Aug 13]. In: StatPearls [Internet]. Treasure Island: StatPearls Publishing; 2024. Available from: https://www.ncbi.nlm.nih.gov/books/NBK563187/.
14. Fox L, Onders R, Hermansen-Kobulnicky CJ, Nguyen TN, Myran L, Linn B, Hornecker J. Teaching interprofessional teamwork skills to health professional students: a scoping review. J Interprof Care. 2018;32(2):127–35. https://doi.org/10.1080/13561820.2017.1399868.
15. Frenk J, et al. Health professionals for a new century: transforming education to strengthen health systems in an interdependent world. Lancet. 2010;376(9756):1923–58. https://doi.org/10.1016/S0140-6736(10)61854-5.
16. Friden C, Olsson C. Interprofessionellt samarbete i primärvården. Fysioterapi. 2018;3:36–41.
17. Gibbs G. Learning by doing: a guide to teaching and learning methods. Oxford: Oxford Further Education Unit; 1988.
18. Hallin K, Kiessling A. A safe place with space for learning: experiences from an interprofessional training ward. J Interprof Care. 2016;30(2):141–8. https://doi.org/10.3109/13561820.2015.1113164.
19. Hallin K, Gordon M, Sköldenberg O, Henriksson P, Kiessling A. Readmission and mortality in patients treated by interprofessional student teams at a training ward compared with patients receiving usual care: a retrospective cohort study. BMJ Open. 2018;8(10):e022251. https://doi.org/10.1136/bmjopen-2018-022251.
20. Huber M, Spiegel-Steinmann B, Schwärzler P, Kerry-Krause M, Dratva J. Kompetenzen zur Interprofessionellen Zusammenarbeit und geeignete Unterrichtsformate, Schlussbericht der Studie M3, ZHAW. 2019. https://www.bag.admin.ch/dam/bag/de/dokumente/berufe-gesundheitswesen/Interprofessionalitaet/Forschungsberichte1/studie-m3-kompetenzen-ipz-zhaw-schlussbericht.pdf.download.pdf/Studie%20M3_Kompetenzen%20zur%20IPZ%20%20%20Unterrichtsformate_ZHAW_Schlussbericht.pdf. Zugegriffen am 20.12.2020.
21. Institute of Medicine. To err is human: building a safer health system. Washington, DC: The National Academies Press; 2000. https://doi.org/10.17226/9728.
22. Interprofessional Education Collaborative. IPEC Core competencies for Interprofessional collaborative practice: version 3. Washington, DC: Interprofessional Education Collaborative; 2023.
23. Jensen CB, Norbye B, Abrandt Dahlgren M, Iversen A. Getting real in interprofessional clinical placements: patient-centeredness in student teams' collaborative learning. Adv Health Sci Educ. 2022;28(3):687–703. https://doi.org/10.1007/s10459-022-10182-y.
24. Jensen CB, Norbye B, Abrandt Dahlgren M, Törnqvist T, Iversen A. Students in interprofessional clinical placements: how supervision facilitates patient-centeredness in collaborative learning. Clin Superv. 2023;42(2):352–74. https://doi.org/10.1080/07325223.2023.2223204.
25. Jensen CB, Iversen A, Dahlgren MA, Norbye B. "Everyone who wants to can practice on me"–a qualitative study of patients' view on health profession students' learning in an interprofessional clinical placement. BMC Med Educ. 2024;24(1):255. https://doi.org/10.1186/s12909-024-05194-8.
26. Jentoft R. Boundary-crossings among health students in interprofessional geropsychiatric outpatient practice: collaboration with elderly people living at home. J Interprof Care. 2021;35(3):409–18. https://doi.org/10.1080/13561820.2020.1733501.

27. Joint Commission. The joint commission announces the 2008 National Patient Safety Goals and requirements. Jt Comm Perspect. 2007;27(7):1:9–22.
28. Josiah M Jr, Foundation. Improving environments for learning in the health professions. In: Recommendations from the Macy foundation conference. New York: Josiah Macy Jr. Foundation; 2018. Retrieved from: https://macyfoundation.org/assets/reports/publications/macy_monograph_2018_webfile.pdf.
29. Kent F, Francis-Cracknell A, McDonald R, et al. How do interprofessional student teams interact in a primary care clinic? A qualitative analysis using activity theory. Adv in Health Sci Educ. 2016;21:749–60. https://doi.org/10.1007/s10459-015-9663-4.
30. Kusnoor AV, Stelljes LA. Interprofessional learning through shadowing: insights and lessons learned. Med Teach. 2016;38(12):1278–84. https://doi.org/10.1080/0142159X.2016.1230186.
31. Larsen A, Broberger E, Petersson P. Complex caring needs without simple solutions: the experience of interprofessional collaboration among staff caring for older persons with multimorbidity at home care settings. Scand J Caring Sci. 2017;31(2):342–350.
32. Lima AWSD, Alves FAP, Linhares FMP, Costa MVD, Coriolano-Marinus MWDL, Lima LSD. Perception and manifestation of collaborative competencies among undergraduate health students. Rev Lat Am Enfermagem. 2020;28:e3240. https://doi.org/10.1590/1518-8345.3227.3240.
33. Ma K, Houben M, Telgen S, Cohen MX, Paffen CL. The pressure to perform impairs learning opportunities, leading to cognitive overload. J Cogn Neurosci. 2021;33(10):2063–76. https://doi.org/10.1162/jocn_a_01676.
34. McKinlay E, White K, Garrett S, Gladman T, Pullon S. Work-place cancer and palliative care interprofessional education: experiences of students and staff. J Interprof Care. 2023;37(1):29–38. https://doi.org/10.1080/13561820.2021.1981259.
35. Mette M, Baur C, Hinrichs J, Oestreicher-Krebs E, Narciß E. Implementing MIA – Mannheim's interprofessional training ward: first evaluation results. GMS J Med Educ. 2019;36(4):Doc35. https://doi.org/10.3205/zma001243.
36. Mihaljevic AL, Schmidt J, Mitzkat A, Probst P, Kenngott T, Mink J, Fink CA, Ballhausen A, Chen J, Cetin A, Murrmann L, Muller G, Mahler C, Gotsch B, Trierweiler-Hauke B. Heidelberger Interprofessionelle Ausbildungsstation (HIPSTA): a practice- and theory-guided approach to development and implementation of Germany's first interprofessional training ward. GMS J Med Educ. 2018;35(3):Doc33. https://doi.org/10.3205/zma001179.
37. Mink J, Mitzkat A, Krug K, Mihaljevic A, Trierweiler-Hauke B, Götsch B, Wensing M, Mahler C. Impact of an interprofessional training ward on interprofessional competencies—a quantitative longitudinal study. J Interprof Care. 2021;35(5):751–9. https://doi.org/10.1080/13561820.2020.1802240.
38. Mitzkat A, Mink J, Arnold C, Mahler C, Mihaljevic AL, Möltner A, Trierweiler-Hauke B, Ullrich C, Wensing M, Kiesewetter J. Development of individual competencies and team performance in interprofessional ward rounds: results of a study with multimodal observations at the Heidelberg Interprofessional training ward. Front Med. 2023;10:1241557. https://doi.org/10.3389/fmed.2023.1241557.
39. Nordquist J, Hall J, Caverzagie K, Snell L, Chan MK, Thoma B, et al. The clinical learning environment. Med Teach. 2019;41(4):366–72. https://doi.org/10.1080/0142159X.2019.1566601.
40. Nugus P, Greenfield D, Travaglia J, Westbrook J, Braithwaite J. How and where clinicians exercise power: interprofessional relations in health care. Soc Sci Med. 2010;71(5):898–909. https://doi.org/10.1016/j.socscimed.2010.05.029.
41. O'Brien BC, Patel SR, Pearson M, Eastburn AP, Earnest GE, Strewler A, Gager K, Manuel JK, Dulay M, Bachhuber MR, Shunk R. Twelve tips for delivering successful interprofessional case conferences. Med Teach. 2017;39(12):1214–20. https://doi.org/10.1080/0142159X.2017.1344353.
42. Oosterom N, Floren LC, ten Cate O, Westerveld HE. A review of interprofessional training wards: enhancing student learning and patient outcomes. Med Teach. 2019;41(5):547–54. https://doi.org/10.1080/0142159X.2018.1503410.

43. Paignon A, Schwärzler P, Kerry M, Stamm D, Bianchi M, Xyrichis A, Gilbert J, Cornwall J, Jill Thistlethwaite I-I, Huber M. Interprofessional educators' competencies, assessment, and training—IPEcat: protocol of a global consensus study. J Interprof Care. 2022;36(5):765–9. https://doi.org/10.1080/13561820.2021.2001445.
44. Ruhomauly Z, Betts K, Jayne-Coupe K, Karanfilian L, Szekely M, Relwani A, et al. Improving the quality of handover: implementing SBAR. Future Healthc J. 2019;6(Suppl 2):54.
45. Stephens M, Kelly S, Chadwick A, Clark A, Walker SH, Chesterton L. Investigating the long-term impact of Interprofessional Education (IPE) initiatives in care home settings. University of Salford; 2024.
46. Thistlethwaite J, Towle A, Canfield C, Lauscher D. When I say… the patient voice. Med Educ. 2023;57(10):898–9. https://doi.org/10.1111/medu.15121.
47. Törnqvist T, Tingström P, Falk AL, Abrandt Dahlgren M. Students' Interprofessional collaboration in clinical practice: ways of organizing the patient encounter. Prof Prof. 2022;12(1) https://doi.org/10.7577/pp.4289.
48. Törnqvist T, Lindh Falk A, Tingström P. Sharing knowledge: final-year healthcare students working together at an interprofessional training ward. J Interprof Educ Pract. 2023a;33:100670. https://doi.org/10.1016/j.xjep.2023.100670.
49. Törnqvist T, Lindh Falk A, Jensen CB, Iversen A, Tingström P. Are the stars aligned? Healthcare students' conditions for negotiating tasks and competencies during interprofessional clinical placement. BMC Med Educ. 2023b;23(1):648. https://doi.org/10.1186/s12909-023-04636-z.
50. Toth-Pal E, Fridén C, Asenjo ST, Olsson CB. Home visits as an interprofessional learning activity for students in primary healthcare. Prim Health Care Res Dev. 2020;21:e59. https://doi.org/10.1017/S1463423620000572.
51. Towle A, Farrell C, Gaines ME, Godolphin W, John G, Kline C, Lown B, Morris P, Symons J, Thistlethwaite J. The patient's voice in health and social care professional education: the Vancouver statement. Int J Health Gov. 2016;21(1):18–25. https://doi.org/10.1108/IJHG-01-2016-0003.
52. Ulrich G, Flury C, Beerli S, Vega V, Wick A, Huber M. Erfolgsfaktoren der Zürcher inter-professionellen Ausbildungsstation (ZIPAS). Eine Synopse aus Erfahrungen, Evaluationsberichten und Lessons-Learned-Sitzungen. Zürich: ZIPAS Verbund; 2023.
53. Wahlström O, Sandén I, Hammar M. Multiprofessional education in the medical curriculum. Med Educ. 1997;31:425–9.
54. Walker L, et al. Mapping the interprofessional education landscape for students on rural clinical placements: an integrative literature review. Rural Remote Health. 2018;18(2):1–18.
55. World Health Organization [WHO]. Framework for action on interprofessional education & collaborative practice. Geneva: WHO; 2010.
56. World Health Organization (WHO). Learning together to work together for health, WHO technical report series. Geneva: WHO; 1988.
57. Worrell JA, Profetto-McGrath J. Critical thinking as an outcome of context-based learning among post RN students: a literature review. Nurse Educ Today. 2007;27(5):420–6.
58. Zarezadeh Y, Pearson P, Dickinson C. A model for using reflection to enhance interprofessional education. Int J Educ. 2009;1(1):e12.

Catrine Buck Jensen is a registered nurse (RN) and an associate professor at UiT The Arctic University of Norway. She currently holds her main position in the Bachelor's program in nursing at UiT and a part-time position as a home care nurse in Tromsø Municipality. Catrine's research interests concerns interprofessional education and supervision, the patient perspective in IPECP, and active patient involvement in health professions education. Since 2022, Catrine has been the chair of the Norwegian Network for Interprofessional Education and Collaborative Practice and are a current board member of the Nordic Interprofessional Network (NIPNET).

Tove Törnqvist is a registered occupational therapist and an assistant professor at the Department of Health, Medicine and Caring Sciences, Linköping University, Sweden. Tove's research interests are focused on interprofessional collaboration and learning with emphasis on students' learning. She is also engaged in education and pedagogical development within the bachelor's program in occupational therapy, the master's program in medical sciences, as well as specific interprofessional learning activities such as interprofessional simulations at Linköping University.

Anika Mitzkat is a health and nursing scientist and works in the field of nursing science and interprofessional healthcare in the Department of General Practice and Health Services Research at Heidelberg University Hospital. Anika is a lecturer in the Bachelor program "Interprofessional Healthcare" and is involved in interprofessional curriculum development and faculty development as part of the "Interprofessional Qualification Programme Steering Group" of the Heidelberg Medical Faculty. Her research focuses on the learning processes that take place in interprofessional education and fostering strategies.

Marion Huber is a qualified physiotherapist, psychologist, and neuroscientist. She leads the Interprofessional Learning and Practice Unit of the Institute of Public Health at the Department of Health Sciences at the Zurich University of Applied Sciences. Her research focuses on competence development for interprofessional collaboration, but also on competence development of teachers who design interprofessional learning settings, both classroom-based and in clinical settings. Methodologically, the focus is on mixed-method designs.

Rene Ballnus is an RN, a pedagogical developer, and an area manager at the Unit for Teaching and Learning at Karolinska Institutet, focusing on faculty development for workplace based learning for healthcare students in Stockholm county. Rene was the previous director and founder of the Center for Clinical Interprofessional Learning and Collaboration. Rene has extensive experience as a lead of one of the clinical interprofessional training wards in Stockholm. He is a current board in the Nordic Interprofessional Network (NIPNET) and the Swedish equivalent (Svipnet).

Toward a European Vision for Interprofessional Science: Reflections, Realizations, and Future Directions

Andreas Xyrichis, Cornelia Mahler, Maria Kvarnström, and Marion Huber

Introduction

As we conclude this comprehensive exploration of interprofessional education and collaborative practice (IPECP) across Europe, we find ourselves at a pivotal moment in the field's evolution. The preceding chapters have illuminated both the remarkable diversity and underlying unity that characterize European approaches to IPECP, while simultaneously revealing the persistent challenges that require coordinated attention. This concluding chapter synthesizes the key insights emerging from our collective endeavor, examines the extent to which we have achieved our stated aims, and charts a course for the future development of interprofessional science in Europe.

The journey documented in this volume reflects more than an academic exercise; it represents a collaborative attempt to map the terrain of IPECP across a continent characterized by linguistic diversity, varied healthcare systems, and distinct professional traditions. Through the voices of contributors spanning multiple countries and professional backgrounds, we have endeavored to create a shared understanding of where European IPECP stands today and where it might develop tomorrow.

Synthesis of Key Messages: A Tapestry of European IPECP

The chapters in this book collectively paint a rich tapestry of IPECP implementation across Europe, revealing both convergent themes and contextual variations that characterize the field. From the foundational frameworks explored in chapter "Exploring European IPECP Frameworks: A Comprehensive Overview and Analysis" to the workplace learning initiatives detailed in chapter "Think Big, Start Small: Inter professional Learning in a Workplace-Based Context", several overarching messages emerge that warrant particular attention.

A. Xyrichis et al. (eds.), *Building Bridges: A European Perspective on Interprofessional Education, Practice, Policy and Research*,
https://doi.org/10.1007/978-3-032-23222-9

Perhaps most prominently, the imperative for theoretical grounding appears consistently across chapters. Whether examining curriculum development models in the Nordic countries, simulation-based approaches in central European contexts, or technology-enhanced learning through Extended Reality, contributors consistently emphasize that sustainable IPECP requires robust theoretical foundations. This aligns with the call for interprofessional science articulated in our introductory chapter, suggesting that the field has indeed recognized the necessity of moving beyond atheoretical implementations toward evidence-informed practice.

The centrality of patient and student voices emerges as another critical theme threading through multiple chapters. The explicit focus on patient narratives in chapter "Focus on Patient Voices: Benefits for Learners and Experienced Health Professionals in Everyday Practice in Interprofessional Healthcare Settings" and student perspectives in Chapter "Student Voices" reflects a broader recognition that IPECP cannot be developed in isolation from those it aims to serve and educate. This emphasis on co-creation and participatory approaches represents a maturation of the field, moving away from expert-driven models toward more inclusive, democratic approaches to interprofessional learning.

The role of technology as both enabler and challenger of IPECP implementation features prominently across several chapters. From simulation-based education to Extended Reality applications, contributors demonstrate how technological innovations can transcend geographical and institutional boundaries while creating new opportunities for interprofessional learning. However, the chapters also reveal the digital divide that exists across European countries and institutions, highlighting equity considerations that require attention as the field advances.

Sustainability emerges as perhaps the most pressing concern identified across chapters. Whether discussing curriculum integration, organizational change, or policy implementation, contributors consistently emphasize the challenges of moving beyond pilot projects toward systematic, institutionally embedded IPECP. This concern resonates strongly with the gaps identified in our introductory analysis and suggests that the field requires more sophisticated approaches to change management and institutional transformation.

Mapping the European Landscape: Progress and Persistent Gaps

Our exploration across these chapters provides valuable insights into the current state of IPECP across Europe, while simultaneously revealing the complexity of achieving comprehensive continental coverage. The countries represented in this volume—spanning Northern, Southern, Western, and Eastern Europe—offer important perspectives on IPECP implementation within diverse healthcare and educational contexts.

However, our mapping exercise also illuminates significant blank spots in our understanding of European IPECP. Several countries, particularly in Eastern and Southeastern Europe, remain underrepresented in our analysis, limiting our ability to claim truly comprehensive coverage of the European landscape. Countries such as Albania, Belarus, Bosnia and Herzegovina, North Macedonia, Moldova, and several others represent important gaps in our understanding, each potentially offering unique insights shaped by their distinct healthcare systems, educational traditions, and socio-political contexts.

Beyond geographical gaps, our exploration reveals profession-specific limitations in current IPECP discourse. While nursing, medicine, and allied health professions feature prominently across chapters, professions such as social work and emerging healthcare roles receive less systematic attention. This professional bias may reflect historical patterns in IPECP development but potentially limits the field's ability to address the full spectrum of collaborative practice required in contemporary healthcare.

The linguistic diversity of Europe presents both an opportunity and a challenge that requires more systematic attention. While this volume operates primarily in English, the reality of European IPECP implementation occurs across dozens of languages, each carrying cultural and professional nuances that may not translate directly. The development of multilingual resources, terminology frameworks, and translation protocols emerges as a critical infrastructure requirement for advancing European IPECP.

Collaborative Endeavors: Lessons From the Writing Process

The process of creating this volume has itself provided valuable insights into the challenges and opportunities of European IPECP collaboration. Establishing writing rapport across linguistic, cultural, and professional boundaries required sustained effort and patience, reflecting in microcosm the challenges faced by interprofessional teams in practice settings.

The negotiation of common language and terminology proved particularly illuminating. Contributors from different countries and professional backgrounds often used familiar terms—collaboration, teamwork, and interprofessionalism—with subtly different meanings, requiring explicit discussion and clarification. This experience reinforces the need for more systematic attention to definitional clarity and cross-cultural communication in IPECP development.

Perhaps most significantly, the collaborative writing process revealed the importance of creating safe spaces for intellectual vulnerability and learning. Contributors needed time and encouragement to share practices, challenges, and uncertainties that might be perceived as weaknesses within their national or institutional contexts. This finding has important implications for how European IPECP networks might be developed and sustained, suggesting that relationship-building and trust development represent essential preconditions for meaningful collaboration.

Patient and Student Agency: Toward Democratic IPECP

The emphasis on patient and student voices throughout this volume reflects a broader recognition that IPECP cannot be developed without meaningful participation from the very individuals it aims to reach. However, our exploration also reveals that such participation remains inconsistent and often tokenistic across European implementations.

Moving forward, the field requires more sophisticated approaches to involving patients and students as genuine partners in IPECP design, implementation, and evaluation. This involves moving beyond consultation models toward genuine co-design approaches that recognize patients and students as experts in their own experiences and needs. Such approaches will require new methodologies, funding mechanisms, and institutional commitments that support sustained partnership rather than episodic involvement.

The cultural and linguistic diversity of European healthcare contexts adds complexity to patient and student involvement initiatives. Approaches developed in one cultural context may not translate directly to others, requiring careful attention to local adaptation while maintaining core principles of participation and empowerment. This suggests the need for European-level guidance that can support contextual adaptation while ensuring meaningful involvement across diverse settings.

Diversity, Culture, and Inclusion: The European Imperative

The diversity that characterizes Europe—linguistic, cultural, religious, socio-economic—represents both a strength and a challenge for IPECP development. Our chapters reveal that successful IPECP implementation requires careful attention to cultural sensitivity and inclusive practice, yet systematic approaches to addressing diversity remain underdeveloped across many European contexts.

The increasing mobility of healthcare professionals across European borders, documented in our introductory chapter, creates new imperatives for developing culturally responsive IPECP approaches. Healthcare teams increasingly comprise professionals trained in different countries, speaking different languages, and bringing diverse cultural perspectives to collaborative practice. This reality requires IPECP curricula and professional development programs that explicitly address cultural competence and cross-cultural communication.

Furthermore, the patient populations served by European healthcare systems reflect increasing diversity, requiring interprofessional teams capable of providing culturally responsive care. This adds another layer of complexity to IPECP development, as programs must prepare professionals not only to collaborate effectively with each other but also to work together in serving diverse communities with varying health beliefs, communication styles, and care preferences.

European Policy Landscape: Opportunities and Imperatives

The policy analysis presented in our introductory chapter and reinforced throughout subsequent chapters reveals both significant opportunities and persistent barriers within the European regulatory landscape. The alignment between workforce development imperatives, quality improvement goals, and interprofessional competency requirements creates a policy window that could support substantial advancement in European IPECP.

However, realizing this potential requires more coordinated action at the European level. Current policy frameworks, while supportive of general principles of collaboration and quality improvement, lack the specificity and coordination mechanisms necessary to drive systematic IPECP implementation across member states. The development of European standards for interprofessional competencies, quality indicators for collaborative practice, and funding mechanisms for cross-border IPECP initiatives emerges as a critical priority.

The task shifting agenda, as outlined in our introductory analysis, provides a particularly compelling policy lever for advancing IPECP. As European healthcare systems grapple with workforce shortages, demographic transitions, and sustainability pressures, the rational redistribution of tasks across professional boundaries becomes both necessary and inevitable. This creates opportunities for positioning IPECP as essential infrastructure for safe, effective task shifting rather than an optional enhancement.

The Future of European IPECP: Strategic Directions

Looking forward, several strategic directions emerge from our collective analysis that could significantly advance European IPECP over the coming decade. These directions reflect both the insights generated through our collaborative exploration and the broader trajectories visible within European healthcare and education systems.

The development of European infrastructure for IPECP emerges as perhaps the most critical priority. This infrastructure would encompass several interconnected components: a European body for scholarly IPECP coordination, shared standards and quality indicators, multilingual resource repositories, research collaboration mechanisms, and funding programs specifically designed to support cross-border IPECP initiatives. Such infrastructure would provide the foundation for moving beyond fragmented national efforts toward coordinated European advancement.

The integration of digital technologies presents both opportunities and challenges that require strategic attention. As healthcare delivery increasingly incorporates digital health solutions, artificial intelligence, and remote care modalities, interprofessional teams must develop new forms of collaborative competence. This creates opportunities for developing innovative IPECP approaches while also requiring attention to digital equity and access across European contexts.

The evolution toward personalized and precision medicine, combined with increasing emphasis on prevention and health promotion, will require new forms of interprofessional collaboration that extend beyond traditional healthcare boundaries. This suggests the need for IPECP approaches that encompass social care, public health, community development, and other sectors involved in supporting health and wellbeing.

Network Building and Sustainable Collaboration

The European networks identified in our introductory chapter, such as CAIPE and Nordic Interprofessional Network (NIPNET), provide important foundations for coordinated action, yet their current reach and capacity remain limited relative to the scope of challenges identified throughout this volume. Strengthening and expanding these networks emerges as a critical priority, requiring sustained investment and strategic development.

Effective network building requires more than periodic conferences and information sharing. The insights from our collaborative writing process suggest that meaningful collaboration requires sustained relationship development, trust building, and shared commitment to common goals. This points toward the need for more intensive collaboration models that enable deep professional relationships and genuine intellectual partnership across European borders.

The development of early career researcher networks emerges as particularly important for sustaining long-term European IPECP advancement. Creating opportunities for doctoral students and early career academics to develop international collaborations, engage in cross-border research projects, receive training and supervision from IPECP experts, and build a shared understanding of European IPECP challenges could provide the foundation for more sustained collaboration over time.

Research Priorities and Evidence Development

Throughout this volume, contributors consistently identify the need for more robust research evidence to support IPECP implementation and effectiveness. However, the fragmented nature of current research efforts across European countries limits the cumulative impact of individual studies and inhibits the development of a comprehensive understanding.

The development of coordinated European research agendas emerges as a critical priority, requiring attention to both methodological innovation and collaborative infrastructure. This includes developing shared outcome measures that can support comparative analysis across different European contexts, methodological approaches that can capture the complexity of interprofessional interventions while maintaining rigor, and ethical frameworks that can guide research involving multiple countries and cultural contexts.

Longitudinal studies tracking the development of interprofessional competencies and collaborative practice over time represent a particular priority, as current evidence remains heavily skewed toward short-term outcomes and immediate impacts. Understanding how interprofessional competencies develop and are sustained throughout healthcare careers requires sustained research investment and cross-border collaboration.

Funding Mechanisms and Sustainability

The sustainability challenges identified across multiple chapters reflect, in part, the absence of dedicated funding mechanisms for IPECP development at the European level. While current funding opportunities through programs such as Erasmus+ and Horizon Europe provide important support, they do not feature IPECP as a clear priority. The broad remit of these programs, while beneficial in many ways, may inadvertently discourage targeted IPECP engagement and systematic advancement. Funding streams that explicitly spotlight the advancement of IPECP across Europe are still missing.

The development of dedicated European funding streams for IPECP research, implementation, and evaluation emerges as a critical infrastructure requirement. Such funding could support multi-country research collaborations, cross-border educational program development, and systematic evaluation of different implementation approaches across European contexts.

However, sustainable funding requires more than new programs; it requires demonstrating value and impact in terms that resonate with policymakers and institutional leaders. This suggests the need for more sophisticated approaches to measuring and communicating the benefits of IPECP investment, including economic evaluation methodologies that can capture the complex impacts of collaborative practice on health outcomes, system efficiency, and professional satisfaction.

Reflecting on Our Achievements

As we conclude this volume, it is appropriate to reflect on the extent to which we have achieved the aims articulated in our introduction. Our goal of providing comprehensive insight into the state, challenges, and future of IPECP in Europe has been partially realized, with important contributions from multiple countries and professional perspectives that illuminate both successes and ongoing challenges.

The establishment of conceptual linkages between education, practice, research, and policy has progressed through our collective exploration, though significant work remains to translate these linkages into practical coordination mechanisms. The concept of interprofessional science has provided a useful organizing framework, yet its operationalization across diverse European contexts requires continued development.

Perhaps most significantly, this collaborative endeavor has demonstrated both the potential and the challenges of European IPECP collaboration. The richness of perspectives, diversity of approaches, and shared commitment to advancing the field are evident across our contributors and provide genuine cause for optimism about the future of European IPECP.

What Comes Next: A Call to Action

This volume concludes not with answers but with an enhanced understanding of the questions that require collective attention. The path forward for European IPECP demands sustained commitment, collaborative investment, and strategic coordination that extends far beyond the pages of this book.

We call upon European institutions, funding bodies, professional organizations, and individual practitioners to recognize IPECP not as an optional enhancement but as essential infrastructure for twenty-first-century healthcare. This recognition must translate into sustained investment in infrastructure development, research collaboration, and systematic implementation support.

The development of a European Charter for Interprofessional Science could provide a unifying framework for coordinated action, establishing shared principles while respecting contextual diversity. Such a charter could guide funding decisions, research priorities, and policy development while providing a foundation for sustained collaboration across European borders.

Educational institutions across Europe must move beyond peripheral IPE implementations toward systematic integration of interprofessional competencies within core curricula. This requires institutional commitment, investment in faculty development, and quality assurance mechanisms that ensure meaningful rather than tokenistic implementation.

Conclusion: Toward Interprofessional Transformation

The vision of European IPECP advancement articulated throughout this volume is ambitious yet achievable. It requires recognition that the complexity of contemporary healthcare challenges demands collaborative responses that transcend traditional professional, institutional, and national boundaries. It demands investment in infrastructure, relationships, and shared understanding that can support sustained collaboration across diverse contexts.

Most importantly, it requires commitment to the fundamental premise that patients and communities deserve healthcare teams capable of working together effectively to provide safe, high-quality, person-centered care. This commitment must animate our collective efforts to overcome the barriers, bridge the gaps, and build the collaborative relationships necessary for European IPECP advancement.

As we conclude this exploration, we invite readers to consider not only what they have learned but what they will do differently as a result. The future of European

IPECP depends not on policy declarations or funding announcements but on the countless individual and collective decisions made by practitioners, educators, researchers, and policy makers across the continent.

The journey toward truly collaborative, interprofessional healthcare is far from complete, but the foundations established through this collaborative endeavor provide genuine reason for optimism. By working together across professions, across borders, and across sectors, we can realize the vision of European healthcare characterized by seamless collaboration, shared commitment to excellence, and unwavering focus on the needs of those we serve.

The future of European IPECP is not predetermined; it will be shaped by our collective choices, commitments, and actions. This volume represents one contribution to that future; the chapters that follow will be written by all of us, together.

Reflective Questions

- How is the interprofessional education or practice in your own context currently grounded, and what specific theoretical framework could be adopted or strengthened to ensure its sustainability and rigor?
- In your setting, how could you transition from a consultative model to a truly collaborative partnership with these key stakeholders in the design and evaluation of IPECP initiatives?
- What three specific organizational or policy changes are necessary within your institution or region to ensure IPECP is systematically integrated and sustained over the long term?
- What is one personal, one institutional, and one policy-related action you are committed to taking in the next 6 months to advance the vision of interprofessional transformation in European healthcare?

Andreas Xyrichis is a reader in interprofessional science at the Florence Nightingale Faculty of Nursing, Midwifery and Palliative Care, King's College London. An intensive care nurse by background, he researches interprofessional practice-based interventions for quality, safety, and equity, working with collaborators across and beyond Europe. Andreas is a Trustee of the UK Centre for the Advancement of Interprofessional Education (CAIPE), co-founder of the European Academy for Interprofessional Science, and Editor-in-Chief of the Journal of Interprofessional Care, the leading international journal in interprofessional science.

Cornelia Mahler is the director of the Department of Nursing Science at the Medical Faculty, Eberhard Karls University, Tuebingen, Germany, and dean of studies of the bachelor's nursing program. In 2011, she developed and implemented a bachelor's degree in Interprofessional Health Care at the Medical Faculty, University of Heidelberg, Germany, and led the development of interprofessional education (IPE) and research there. She co-led and co-founded the interprofessional working group within the German Association for Medical Education and has extensive experience in the translation and validation of instruments for research and evaluation in IPE and collaborative practice. She is a nurse by background, the co-founder of the European Academy for Interprofessional Science, and serves as an associate editor for the Journal of Interprofessional Care.

Maria Kvarnström is an Associate Professor in Medical Education at the Department of Health, Medicine and Caring Sciences at Linköping University, which has the longest European tradition of IPE at a faculty of medicine. She is a member of the strategic area for interprofessional learning and collaboration at the medical faculty at Linköping University, a member of the board of the Nordic Interprofessional network, and the co-founder of the Swedish network for IPE. She is a biomedical laboratory scientist by profession, an associate editor for the Journal of Interprofessional Care, and a co-founder of the European Academy for Interprofessional Science.

Marion Huber is the Head of the Center of Interprofessional Learning and Practice at the Zurich University of Applied Sciences, Department of Health Sciences, and leads the research group of interprofessionalism. She is a qualified physiotherapist, psychologist, and neuroscientist, and she is responsible for the evaluation of the Zurich interprofessional clinical training wards. She is a co-founder of the European Academy for Interprofessional Science, the Chair of Interprofessional. Global (IP.G)—the Global Confederation for Interprofessional Education and Collaborative Practice—and the Chair of the International Society of Interprofessional Health Care (IP-Health).

GPSR Compliance

The European Union's (EU) General Product Safety Regulation (GPSR) is a set of rules that requires consumer products to be safe and our obligations to ensure this.

If you have any concerns about our products, you can contact us on ProductSafety@springernature.com

In case Publisher is established outside the EU, the EU authorized representative is:

Springer Nature Customer Service Center GmbH
Europaplatz 3
69115 Heidelberg, Germany

Batch number: 10365480

Printed by Printforce, the Netherlands